I0038347

UNDERSTANDING THE LIVED EXPERIENCE OF THE STROKE PATIENT

This book offers a comprehensive exploration of the lived experiences of stroke patients, interwoven with healthcare professional expertise to provide evidence-based guidance for nurses and other healthcare professionals. It aims to enhance clinical practice and promote patient-centred care by bridging theory with real-world application.

Edited by a team that integrates academic, professional and personal experience of stroke, the book ensures that the patient perspective remains central throughout. This approach enables healthcare professionals, students and those living with the consequences of stroke to develop a deeper understanding of stroke's clinical, emotional and social impact, reinforcing the significance of compassionate and informed care in improving patient outcomes. This textbook offers a comprehensive exploration of stroke care, with contextual chapters that examine the nature of strokes, psychological and cognitive challenges and safe environments. Subsequent sections focus on specific Activities of Daily Living (ADLs), such as eating and drinking, sleeping and communication which provide targeted insights into everyday functional recovery.

To enhance learning transfer to clinical practice, the chapters incorporate reflective activities and questions, along with key knowledge summaries. Designed for nurses and allied health professionals, this resource serves as an essential learning tool for those new to stroke care while offering valuable insights for stroke survivors and experienced practitioners seeking to refine their approach to care delivery.

Catherine Forward is a Registered Adult Nurse and Specialist Community Public Health Nurse who has worked in nursing education for over a decade. She has a master's in medical law and ethics and is a Senior Fellow of the Higher Education

Academy. Catherine has also supported a family member who had a stroke as a young adult.

Ruth Trout, with over 30 years of experience in the neurosciences specialty, Ruth has worked across neuroscience wards, intensive care and as an Advanced Nurse Practitioner. Ruth holds a BSc in Critical and Specialist Care (Neurosciences), an MSc in Advanced Practice, and a Postgraduate Certificate in Education. She has been a member of the Executive Board of the British Association of Neuroscience Nurses and remains an active contributor to both the European Association of Neuroscience Nurses and the World Federation of Neuroscience Nurses. Since 2010, Ruth has led the Stroke Care and Management module at Buckinghamshire New University, educating healthcare professionals from across the UK. Her professional expertise is complemented by her personal experience as the main carer for her grandmother, Molly, who experienced a mild ischaemic stroke in 2011, deepening her insight into patient and family perspectives in stroke care.

Jo Vincent is a retired SEND teacher who worked in further education having studied BA (Hons) in Childhood Studies with a Certificate in Education with qualified teacher status (QTS). Jo has undertaken EbE work since 2022 and talks to a variety of students and healthcare professionals regarding her experiences as a stroke patient to inform and improve quality of care.

UNDERSTANDING THE LIVED EXPERIENCE OF THE STROKE PATIENT

A Guide for Health Professionals

Edited by Catherine Forward, Ruth Trout and Jo Vincent

Routledge
Taylor & Francis Group

LONDON AND NEW YORK

Designed cover image: Getty images

First published 2026
by Routledge
4 Park Square, Milton Park, Abingdon, Oxon OX14 4RN

and by Routledge
605 Third Avenue, New York, NY 10158

Routledge is an imprint of the Taylor & Francis Group, an informa business

© 2026 selection and editorial matter, Catherine Forward, Ruth Trout and Jo Vincent; individual chapters, the contributors

The right of Catherine Forward, Ruth Trout and Jo Vincent to be identified as the authors of the editorial material, and of the authors for their individual chapters, has been asserted in accordance with sections 77 and 78 of the Copyright, Designs and Patents Act 1988.

All rights reserved. No part of this book may be reprinted or reproduced or utilised in any form or by any electronic, mechanical, or other means, now known or hereafter invented, including photocopying and recording, or in any information storage or retrieval system, without permission in writing from the publishers.

For Product Safety Concerns and Information please contact our EU representative GPSR@taylorandfrancis.com. Taylor & Francis Verlag GmbH, Kaufingerstraße 24, 80331 München, Germany.

Trademark notice: Product or corporate names may be trademarks or registered trademarks, and are used only for identification and explanation without intent to infringe.

British Library Cataloguing-in-Publication Data
A catalogue record for this book is available from the British Library

ISBN: 9781032546971 (hbk)
ISBN: 9781032546964 (pbk)
ISBN: 9781003426196 (ebk)

DOI: 10.4324/9781003426196

Typeset in Times New Roman
by Newgen Publishing UK

CONTENTS

CONTRIBUTORS

Fiona Chalk has been a Registered Nurse since 1995 and worked within acute medicine including acute stroke care in senior nurse roles. She has worked at Buckinghamshire New University since 2016 as a Senior Lecturer and leads Continuing Professional Development Education for a range of healthcare professionals.

Sarah Davies is a Registered Learning Disability Nurse who has worked within community, residential and clinical settings including stroke care. Sarah now works for Birmingham City University as a Lecturer on the Nursing Associate Degree programme. She is passionate about improving health outcomes and quality of care within nursing.

Konstantinos Eleftheriadis is a Stroke and Medical Team Lead Dietitian, Enteral Feeding Lead and Parenteral Nutrition Team member at Royal Free Hospital NHS Trusts, North Middlesex University Hospital Health Unit. With a strong clinical background across several areas of dietetics, they specialise in nutritional management of stroke and medical patients. Their research focuses on enteral feeding and quality of life in stroke patients, malnutrition risk and dysphagia in hospital settings.

Catherine Hamilton is a registered Child and Adult Nurse Educator with over 30 years' experience which traverses the lifespan from neonatal to older persons. More recently, Catherine has focussed on the delivery of tailored and effective palliative care in the acute service setting. Catherine is passionate about person-centred services and nurse education which ensures learners are empowered to deliver best practice within safe and supportive environments.

Claire Hartley is an HCPC registered Speech and Language Therapist (SLT), Senior Lecturer and Course Lead. She runs the Birmingham City University SLT Clinic for people with acquired communication needs. Claire also supports people living with communication disability to become EbyEs involved in health professional education.

Rachel Hayden qualified as a physiotherapist in 2002 and works for Buckinghamshire Healthcare NHS Trust. She began specialising in stroke and neurology in 2004. Rachel completed an MSc in Neurorehabilitation in 2011 and has recently undertaken additional master's level study. Rachel is passionate about providing person-centred care and has a particular interest in spasticity management.

Gill Hoad is an HCPC qualified physiotherapist and currently works as a Joint Team Lead for Acute Stroke at Wycombe Hospital and as an Associate Lecturer at Buckinghamshire New University. She is a passionate advocate for stroke survivors and their families, and her focus is on promoting self-management skills early in their stroke recovery to provide them with the tools required to regain their independence in the future.

Jennifer Huffadine is an Occupational Therapist and Associate Lecturer with over 20 years' experience working in the NHS. She has specialised in stroke rehabilitation and community services. Her MSc focused on patient experience and Jennifer has established collaboration groups to enable patients, carers and staff to work together to improve services.

Hilalnur Küçükakgün is a Research Assistant at Canakkale Onsekiz Mart University Faculty of Health Sciences. She completed her PhD in 2023 at Istanbul University-Cerrahpasa, focussing on the impact of a nurse-led rehabilitation coordination programme on psychosocial issues and quality of life in stroke patients. Her research area is neurology, particularly stroke.

Catherine Lamb is an Advanced Clinical Practitioner specialising in neurovascular conditions at Oxford University Hospital. She leads a nurse-led service that supports patients from admission to discharge. This role requires specialised skills in neuro assessment, complex case management, history taking, investigation, ordering and interpretation, and medication prescribing. Additionally, she facilitates a support group for patients and their families after discharge.

Claire Lynch is a Senior Lecturer and Nursing Deputy Course Leader at Birmingham City University and has a long clinical career in Neuroscience Nursing. Previously, Claire has been on the committee of the British Association of Neuroscience

Nurses and supported a number of national and international conferences in the specialty. She also regularly contributes to research within Neurosciences and Nurse Education and is passionate about supporting the development of this field of nursing.

Hannah Mosley is a Registered Nurse with a background in Neuro Critical Care, currently working as a Senior Lecturer in Adult Nursing at Birmingham City University. She teaches across the undergraduate programme and supports a variety of teaching in postgraduate modules including the Adult Critical Care Course. Hannah is passionate about nurse education, ensuring students are supported and empowered to deliver safe, high-quality, person-centred care.

Annette Palmer is a Registered Adult Nurse and Specialist Practitioner in District Nursing, a Senior Lecturer and Module Lead. She has extensive clinical experience, delivering complex nursing care at home, empowering individuals to maintain independence. Holding a BSc(Hons), MSc and Postgraduate Certificate in Education, Annette is also a Fellow of Advance HE, with specialist interests in Community Nursing and Wound Care.

Lyndsey Shawe is an HCPC registered and chartered Physiotherapist and Associate Lecturer. She has over 15 years of clinical experience in the NHS and private sectors. She has specialised in stroke and neurological conditions in clinical practice in her MSc and within her lecturing work.

Sarah Thirtle holds a specialist qualification in District Nursing, a BSc in Community Healthcare Nursing, a Post Graduate Certificate in Professional Studies in Education, an MA in Education and an Advance HE Fellowship. As a Senior Lecturer, Sarah leads the SPQ District Nursing and MSc Community Healthcare Practice programmes at Buckinghamshire New University, shaping the future of community nurse education and leadership.

Zeliha Tulek is a faculty member at Istanbul University-Cerrahpaşa Florence Nightingale Faculty of Nursing. She has specialised in neurology, particularly stroke and multiple sclerosis, since 1999, when she contributed to a project aimed at improving nursing care in one of Turkey's first stroke units. She earned her PhD in 2006 and is actively involved in professional organisations, including the European Neuroscience Nurses Association.

Julia Williams has a clinical, educational and research profile which spans over 35 years. Her main areas of interest lie within colorectal nursing, sexuality and body image. Having worked as a specialist and lead nurse for many years, she now contributes to research with a focus on understanding the patient's experience within this specialist field.

PREFACE

To facilitate learning and engagement, a series of icons have been incorporated throughout each chapter. These are intended to assist readers in locating key information efficiently and to draw attention to opportunities for active participation and deeper reflection. The icons denote the following:

	Insights from individuals with lived experience of stroke (patients and carers) who share personal perspectives on their stroke journey and the care they received.
	Reflection prompts: Structured opportunities for readers to critically reflect on their own experiences, professional practice, and the implications for future learning.
	Learning Activities: tasks designed to consolidate understanding, encourage critical thinking, and promote the application of knowledge to clinical practice.
	Practical Tips: Evidence-informed suggestions and strategies that may be implemented in clinical settings or shared with professional colleagues, patients, and carers.
	Web-Based Resources: Curated online materials recommended by contributors to support continued professional development and to provide valuable information for patients and their families.
	Family and Carer Involvement: Guidance and strategies to encourage the engagement of family members and carers in supporting stroke survivors throughout their recovery journey.

ACKNOWLEDGEMENTS

Thank you to all of the Experts by Experience who have shared their own stories of stroke as patients or family/carers for this project.

Damian Farrell
Olive Harris
Les Hemus
Jacqueline Isaac
Malcolm Joesbury
Gill Joesbury
Karen Mollison
Alan Orchard
PJ (Philip) Jlu-Johnson
Louise Rivers
Phil Rivett
Michelle Smith
Jeremy Sowter
Jan Tanner
Steph Vincent
Jo Vincent
Kelly Williams
Nerys Wilson
Oxford Stroke Patient Group
South Birmingham (BCU) Conversation Group and Family Group

ABBREVIATIONS

ACP	Advance care planning
ACT	Acceptance and Commitment Therapy
AOS	Apraxia of Speech
BBB	Blood-brain barrier
CBT	Cognitive Behavioural Therapy
CCD	Cognitive-Communication Disorder
CPP	Cerebral Perfusion Pressure
CSF	Cerebrospinal Fluid
EbyE	Expert by Experience
FOF	Fear of falling
ICP	Intracranial pressure
ISWP	Intercollegiate Stroke Working Party
MBCT	Mindfulness-based Cognitive Therapy
MBSR	Mindfulness-based Stress Reduction
NHS	National Health Service
NICE	National Institute for Health and Care Excellence
OSA	Obstructive Sleep Apnoea
PHE	Public Health England
QoL	Quality of Life
RCP	Royal College Physicians
SAH	Subarachnoid Haemorrhage
SLT	Speech and Language Therapist
TIA	Transient Ischaemic Attack
WHO	World Health Organization
WSO	World Stroke Organization

INTRODUCTION

Catherine Forward

Fatigue is not tired; it is a completely different animal. Having a good night's sleep will help if you are tired but there is nothing that helps stroke fatigue in terms of making you feel better, like you've recharged the batteries. I can sleep for hours, and it doesn't help.

(Jo, 47, embolic stroke, 20 years post stroke)

The purpose of this textbook is to bring together the voices of stroke patients and a variety of healthcare professionals to collaborate and share their knowledge and experience. The focus is upon the lived experience and how to best support those affected by stroke. The honest and authentic experiences shared within the chapters by a number of individuals will be accompanied by current evidence-based expertise and practical information written by healthcare professionals and academics. This book will benefit the healthcare professional and student alike. Their roles are crucial in the rehabilitation of stroke patients. A further aim is also to provide a useful guide for those who have experienced stroke themselves and their families.

The idea for this collaboration came from editor Jo's very personal experiences of the life-changing impact of stroke 20 years ago, and the roller coaster ride of managing the challenges and limitations it imposes upon everyday life. As an Expert by Experience (EbyE) who shares her story with healthcare professionals and nursing, medical and allied healthcare professional students, Jo has talked openly about the multiple ways she has had to adapt her life. Her disability, as a result of endocarditis an embolic stroke, is often invisible to those who do not know her. To remain an independent adult, she has had to make alterations to all aspects of her life, but the ongoing impact and challenges of stroke remain.

DOI: 10.4324/9781003426196-1

The role of the EbyE has gained momentum in recent years. Described by the Care Quality Commission (2025) as someone who has 'personal, lived experience of using health, mental health and/or social care services, or of caring for someone who uses those services', the impact of the role is highly valued and is transforming how we improve quality and prepare and deliver education and care related to many different areas of health. Examples can be found within the NHS, social care, charity sector and higher education, to name but a few. EbyE programmes and the opportunity to be involved and share experiences provide validation that this input is valued and listened to. The involvement of the EbyE is leading to genuine change and improvement. From campaigning and policy work to developing new services, EbyEs should be at the heart of what we do within healthcare services and this book will provide inspiration and suggestions for how EbyEs can be best used.

The inclusion of the voice of the EbyE is vital for the education of future generations of healthcare professionals. This textbook aims to illustrate that the EbyE is as valued as the clinical expert, not a passive recipient of care; and that listening to the needs and experiences of our patients is key to quality care improvement. Sharing open and honest stories of real people with an active learning approach helps make the learning real and we hope that educators and lecturers will be inspired to structure some of their teaching around our chapters and to co-produce their teaching materials with EbyEs. Collaboration between academics and EbyEs during curriculum design supports the creation of an environment that is conducive to students learning to work collaboratively within a service-user-led culture (Atwal *et al.*, 2018). The EbyE also offers a unique perspective on other activities within education such as student recruitment and assessment. If undertaken with supporting policy in an authentic, non-tokenistic, way, the EbyE brings considerable value and impact.

As well as sharing narratives about their physical and mental health, the voice of the EbyE brings to life the challenges faced navigating the care system. Areas such as discrimination and inequality in provision, as well as areas of good practice, which have made all the difference to the care received, are discussed with meaning and context. Stroke research tends to focus on the acute phase and there are fewer education resources that focus on the long-term effects of stroke, unmet needs and family/carer support. For their involvement, we are grateful to our EbyEs and thank them for their contributions.

Each chapter will include key learning objectives, a brief overview of the pathophysiology related to the theme and the impact of pathology on the individual. There will be activities to undertake should the reader wish to, or these can be adapted by the educator for their classroom. Each area will also consider the psychological and emotional aspects of the lived experience for the stroke patient and provide suggestions and insight with regards to self-management strategies.

It is hoped that this book will provide a unique resource for healthcare professionals and students, stroke survivors and their families alike. Throughout the text, the lived experience and strategies for making that life better are discussed.

This is achieved by focussing on the key element which should always be at the heart of care delivery – the individual.

References

Atwal, A., *et al.* (2018) Service users and academics teaching together in nurse education. *Nursing Times* [ROM] 114(6), pp. 47–51. Available at: https://cdn.ps.emap.com/wp-content/uploads/sites/3/2018/05/180516-Service-users-and-academics-teaching-together-in-nurse-education.pdf (accessed 24 September 2022).

Care Quality Commission (2025) Experts by experience. Available at: Experts by Experience - Care Quality Commission.

1

WHAT IS STROKE?

Ruth Trout, Claire Lynch and Catherine Lamb

Learning objectives

- To review the anatomy and physiology related to stroke.
- To gain an understanding of the different types of strokes.
- To increase awareness of the risk factors relating to stroke.

Background

Globally, there are over 12.2 million new strokes each year, and it is ranked as the second leading cause of death and disability by the World Health Organization (WHO, 2020). Stroke has historically affected older people; however, cases within younger age groups (20–64 years) are rising. One in four people over the age of 25 can expect to have a stroke in their lifetime (World Stroke Organization (WSO), 2022). Public Health England (PHE) figures show that whilst many strokes do occur in the over 60s, over a third of first-time strokes occurred in middle-aged adults, an increase compared to a decade ago (PHE, 2018).

The consequences of stroke can be wide-ranging-physically, psychologically and socially impacting the individual and their families. It is therefore vital that healthcare professionals and the general population understand the risk factors for stroke and its altered physiology.

This chapter aims to provide an overview of the anatomy and physiology related to stroke but should be reviewed in conjunction with topic-specific neuroanatomy texts to support further physiological understanding.

DOI: 10.4324/9781003426196-2

Anatomy and physiology related to stroke

Cells of the central nervous system

The functional cell of the central nervous system (CNS) is the neurone (see Figure 1.1). Electrical activity, called an action potential, allows transmission of signals throughout the nervous system.

A stimulus, such as activation of a sensory receptor or neurotransmitter being released, causes the neurone to be excited at the dendrite. This causes sodium (Na^+) and potassium (K^+), powered by adenosine triphosphate (ATP), to enter and leave the cell, creating an action potential. When the axon terminal is reached, calcium (Ca^+) causes the release of a neurotransmitter, completing the neurones' action – either eliciting an action potential in a neighbouring neurone, processing sensory information or innervating a muscle or a gland (see Table 1.1). Neurones have receptors for many different neurotransmitters but will only release one neurotransmitter (Hickey, 2020a). There are more than 100 known neurotransmitters, and Table 1.1 represents some of the most common.

- Neurones are supported by glial cells (Greek for glue).
- Astrocytes store and release glucose and create the blood–brain barrier (BBB), ensuring that there is tight control of the molecules entering and leaving the brain.
- Oligodendrocytes create myelin sheath – the lipid that surrounds a neurone, ensuring smooth conduction of the action potential along a neurone (Clancy, 2017).
- Microglia are significant in the immune system function of the brain recognising antigens (molecules that initiate an immune response) and initiating phagocytosis (destruction of cells or antigens).

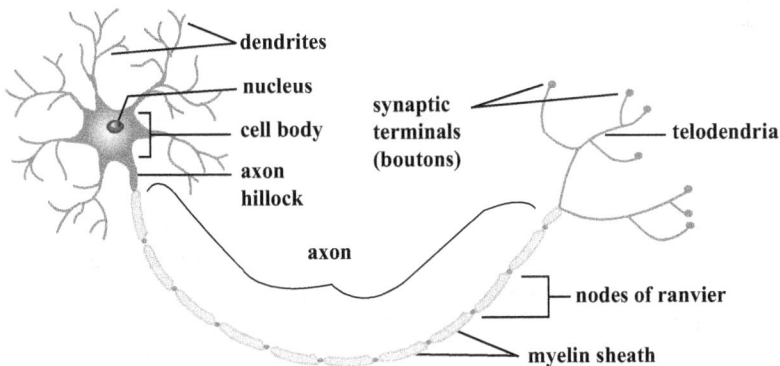

FIGURE 1.1   A neurone.
Source: Sturgeon (2018, p. 205).

TABLE 1.1 Names and functions of neurotransmitters

Substance	Homeostatic actions
Neurotransmitters	
Acetylcholine (Ach)	Released by some neuromuscular and neuroglandular synapses and at neuronal synapses in the central nervous system
	Acts mainly as an excitatory neurotransmitter but also has inhibitory functions
Serotonin (5-HT)	Concentrated in certain neurons in the brainstem
	Acts as an excitatory neurotransmitter
	May induce sleep
	Also involved in sensory perception, temperature regulation and control of mood
Noradrenaline (NA)	Released at some neuromuscular and neuroglandular synapses
	Also found in neural synapses of the brainstem: mainly excitatory
	May be involved in arousal, dreaming and regulation of mood
Gamma-aminobutyric acid (GABA)	Concentrated in the thalamus, hypothalamus and occipital lobes of cerebrum: mainly inhibitory
Dopamine (DA)	Inhibitory in substantia nigra of midbrain
	Involved in emotional responses and subconscious movement of skeletal muscles
Neuropeptides[a]	
Substance P	Excitatory in pain pathways within central nervous system
Enkephalins	Inhibitory in pain pathways within the thalamus and spinal cord
Endorphins	Inhibitory (see Enkephalins), especially within the midbrain
	May have a role in memory and learning
Dynorphin	Inhibitory (see Enkephalins): 50 times more powerful than beta-endorphin

Source: Clancy (2017, p. 192).

Note

[a] Neuropeptides are neurotransmitters, but some are also neuromodulators that are produced elsewhere but will interact with the synapse where they are also found.

All cells of the CNS require ATP, the product of cellular respiration (see Table 1.2). As there are millions of action potentials taking place at any one time, this creates a high demand for both oxygen and glucose by the CNS.

When cell oxygen levels are reduced, anaerobic respiration occurs, leading to reduced ATP production and lactic acid as a waste product. In stroke, this impacts neuronal function and is an important pathophysiological element of stroke considered throughout this chapter.

TABLE 1.2 Description of aerobic and anaerobic respiration

Aerobic respiration	Anaerobic respiration
O_2 + Glucose = ATP (energy) + CO_2 + H_2O	(reduced) O_2 + Glucose = (reduced) ATP + Lactic Acid

Types of strokes and their pathophysiology

- Do you fully understand the differences between each type of stroke?
- What else would you like to know?
- What further knowledge do you need about interventions and management?
- Other than this book, what resources are available to you to develop your knowledge?
- What national guidelines are available for reference?

A stroke is defined as a rapidly developing clinical syndrome of presumed vascular origin that results in signs of focal or global disturbance of cerebral function. This disturbance either leads to death or persists for 24 hours or longer. A transient ischaemic attack (TIA), often considered a precursor to stroke, is defined as a temporary episode of neurological dysfunction lasting less than 24 hours (WHO, 1978).

There are two main types of stroke: ischaemic and haemorrhagic. To understand the causes, types, and symptoms of stroke, it is first necessary to understand cerebral circulation. The brain has both arterial and venous circulatory systems. Although strokes resulting from venous system damage are rare, considering both systems is essential for a comprehensive understanding of cerebrovascular pathology.

Cerebral circulation

The CNS has a high metabolic demand and as a result receives between 15% and 20% of total cardiac output (Hickey, 2020a). Due to this high demand, any disruption to the perfusion (oxygen delivery) of the brain has the potential to impact neuronal function. The BBB (see Figure 1.2) and the Circle of Willis (see Figure 1.3) are designed to reduce the risk of low perfusion.

As shown in Figure 1.3, the physiological positioning of the arteries within the Circle of Willis creates 'vascular territories'. The anterior circulation provides blood to the front and top of the brain, whereas the posterior arteries supply the back and underneath of the brain. Each vascular territory perfuses a subsection of the brain with individualised functions. Therefore, the specific vascular territory affected by a stroke results in specific symptoms, which an experienced healthcare professional can evaluate to identify the vascular territory affected.

Cerebral venous flow is unlike elsewhere in the body as it does not follow arterial flow. Cerebral veins drain into venous sinuses (see Figure 1.4). The largest,

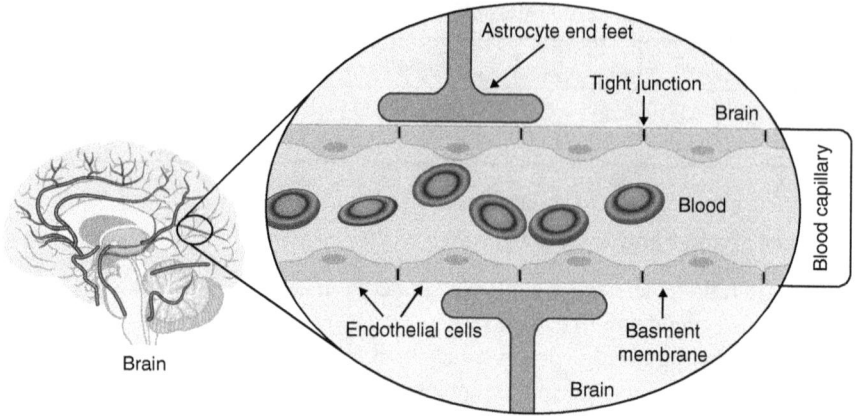

FIGURE 1.2   Cells surrounding the blood vessels of the brain, which form the BBB.

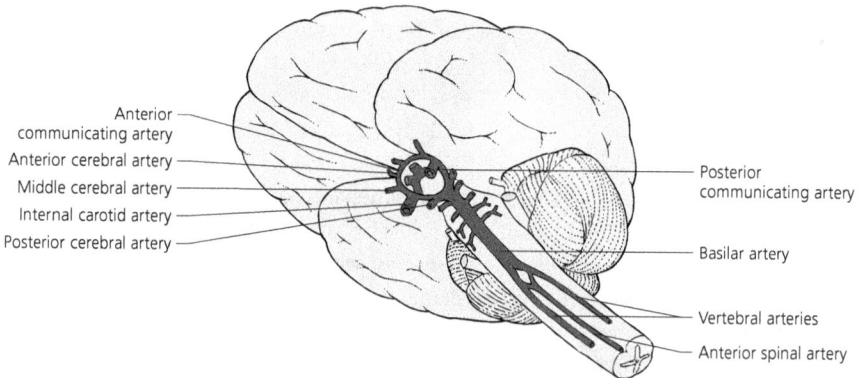

FIGURE 1.3   The Circle of Willis creates collateral circulation to prevent reduced perfusion if damaged.

Source: Clancy (2017, p. 182).

the dural venous sinuses, lie along the midline of the brain (over and in between the two hemispheres) and drain the CNS, face and scalp into the internal jugular vein.

Cerebral autoregulation, a specialised neurovascular function, allows for the maintenance of cerebral blood flow, despite changes to the systemic blood pressure. Through a complex series of metabolic processes, cerebral blood vessels can undergo vasodilation in response to hypertension, thereby reducing the risk of rupture in smaller vessels. Vasoconstriction can occur to support adequate cerebral perfusion during hypotension. This allows for a consistent cerebral blood flow, regardless of systemic changes in blood pressure.

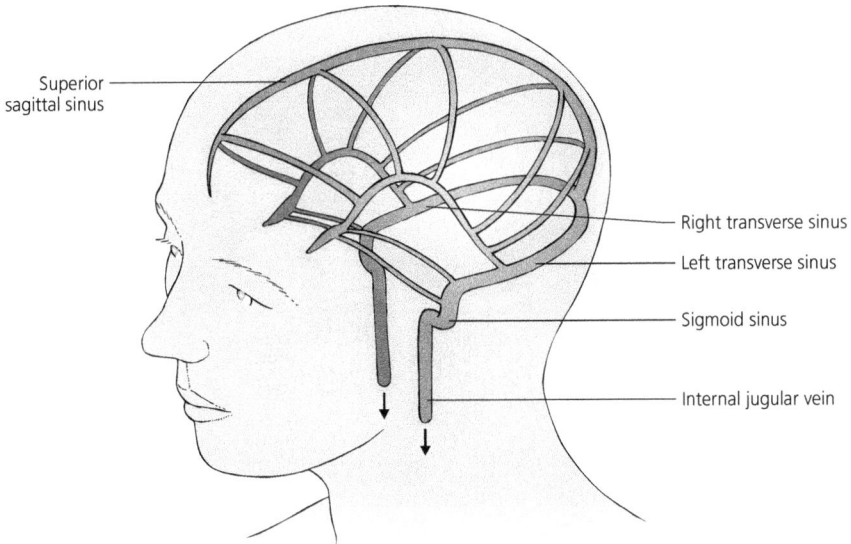

FIGURE 1.4 The venous supply of the brain.
Source: Clancy (2017, p. 182).

Some of the cerebral vasculature, along with cerebrospinal fluid (CSF), is contained within membranous coverings of the brain, the meninges (see Figure 1.5).

CSF provides protection and buoyancy to the brain within the skull. By removing cellular waste products, it supports the metabolic stability of the CNS, ensuring effective neuronal function. Around 500 ml of CSF is produced every day, with 150 ml circulating within the adult cranial vault at any one time (Hickey, 2020a). Ependymal cells within the ventricles make CSF, with microvilli helping to circulate it around the brain (see Figure 1.6).

Arachnoid villi in the arachnoid space drain CSF into the venous system. These channels are small, meaning the presence of blood or swollen cerebral tissue following stroke has the potential to block or disrupt this flow, leading to hydrocephalus.

Cerebral blood flow is directly proportional to the perfusion pressure of the cerebral tissue – known as cerebral perfusion pressure (CPP). It is also inversely proportional to the total resistance of the system (the brain) known as intracranial pressure (ICP) (Hickey, 2020a) (see Table 1.3). Raises in ICP occur because the skull is a rigid box, containing a fixed volume of approximately 150 ml blood, 150 ml CSF and 1500 ml of brain tissue (Hickey, 2020a). The brain can compensate for small increases in any of these volumes, up to around 150 ml, by increasing CSF flow to the spinal cord and through cerebral autoregulation; however, after this ICP will rise.

Dura mater — Outer layer / Inner layer — Skin

Skull bone

Superior sagittal sinus (venous blood)

Arachnoid villus

Arachnoid mater

Brain tissue

Cerebral artery or vein

Pia mater

Falx cerebri (an extension of dura mater that helps support brain tissue)

Subarachnoid space (filled with CSF)

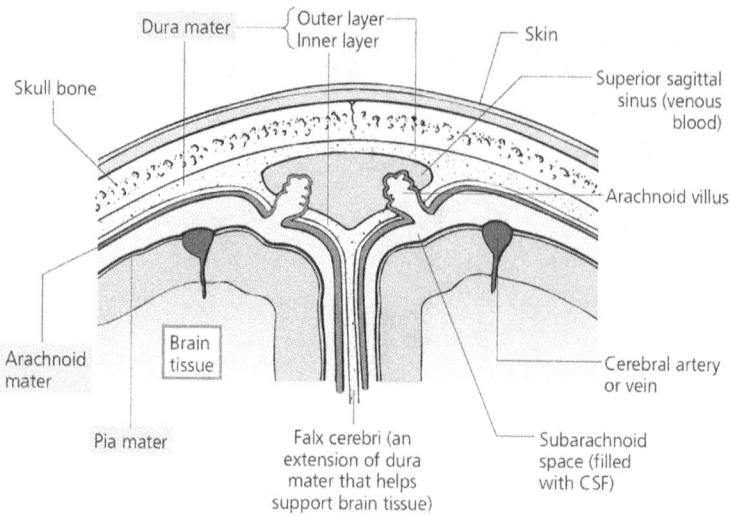

Note: Arachnoid and pia mater are connected by a network of bridging strands (called trabeculae) that help to maintain the patency of the subarachnoid space

FIGURE 1.5   The meninges.

Source: Clancy (2017, p. 179).

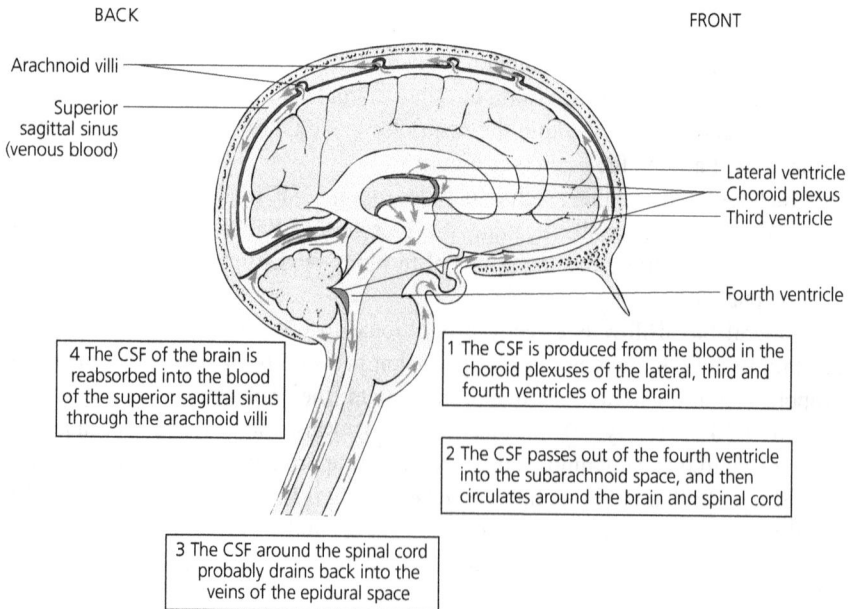

BACK

FRONT

Arachnoid villi

Superior sagittal sinus (venous blood)

Lateral ventricle
Choroid plexus
Third ventricle

Fourth ventricle

4 The CSF of the brain is reabsorbed into the blood of the superior sagittal sinus through the arachnoid villi

1 The CSF is produced from the blood in the choroid plexuses of the lateral, third and fourth ventricles of the brain

2 The CSF passes out of the fourth ventricle into the subarachnoid space, and then circulates around the brain and spinal cord

3 The CSF around the spinal cord probably drains back into the veins of the epidural space

FIGURE 1.6   CSF flow throughout the brain and spinal cord.

Source: Clancy (2017, p. 181).

TABLE 1.3 Definition and relationship of ICP, CPP and MAP in relation to cerebral blood flow

Cerebral perfusion pressure (CPP)	The net pressure that allows oxygen delivery from the blood to brain tissue
Intracranial pressure (ICP)	The pressure within the cranial vault
Mean arterial pressure (MAP)	The average pressure in the arteries through one cardiac cycle
CPP = MAP – ICP	

As discussed previously, a stroke is a change in focal or global neuronal function from a presumed vascular cause. Any damage to the vasculature or CSF systems described can reduce the neuronal function and oxygen supply reducing ATP. Anaerobic respiration further reduces ATP and causes the build-up of by-products leading to ischaemia, and cell death. This further exacerbates ICP and reduces CPP causing further cerebral damage.

Types of strokes

Ischaemic infarction

This is the most common type of stroke. It is sudden in onset and accounts for approximately 85% of all strokes (National Institute for Health and Care Excellence (NICE), 2023a). It is caused by a blockage within a cerebral artery which deprives the brain of glucose and oxygen. It presents with non-epileptic neurological deficit, due to a well-defined volume of infarcted brain tissue within a discrete vascular territory. The signs and symptoms evident can be used to localise the affected artery. The infarction may be due to one of several physiological processes including thrombosis, embolism or decreased systemic perfusion of blood.

When the pathophysiology is due to *thrombosis,* blood flow is obstructed by a localised occlusive process secondary to thickening of the artery wall and a build-up of atherosclerosis (fatty plaques) of the blood vessels that supply the brain. Blood vessels become narrower, less flexible and more brittle. Platelets adhere to the atherosclerosis, allowing further build-up of clotting components such as fibrin and thrombin. These form blood clots which further block the lumen of the artery, resulting in a stroke (Hickey and Livesay, 2020). See Figure 1.7.

An *embolism* is a piece of material that causes a blockage within a blood vessel. It may be formed of a blood clot (thrombus), fat, air or a foreign body. The embolism arises somewhere distant to the brain, which in stroke, is most frequently the heart. Malfunctioning heart valves, recent myocardial infarction and atrial fibrillation (AF) can cause clots to form within the cardiac chambers (cardio-embolism).

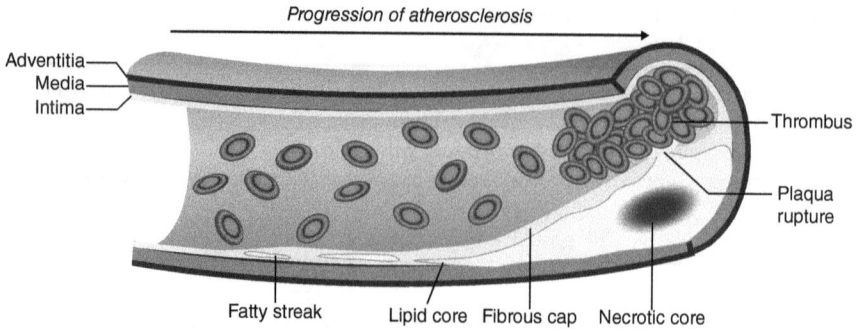

FIGURE 1.7   Image of blood vessels with atherosclerosis.
Source: www.news-medical.net/suppliers/Tocris-Bioscience.aspx

Further subtypes of ischaemic stroke are identified by the Trial of Org 10172 (Danaparoid) in Acute Stroke Treatment (TOAST) classification (Adams *et al.*, 1993). These include:

- Large artery atherosclerosis – defined as >50% stenosis of major cerebral artery
- Small artery atherosclerosis or occlusion – often called lacunar stroke
- Cardioembolic stroke
- Stroke of other determined causes
- Cryptogenic stroke – in which no cause can be determined (Adams *et al.*, 1993).

Regardless of the cause, occlusion of the blood vessels causes the territory of the brain they supply to become ischaemic and it dies quite quickly. This is known as the 'core ischaemic zone'. There is little that healthcare professionals can do to restore that area of cell death. However, surrounding the core ischaemic zone is the 'ischaemic penumbra' which is receiving a limited blood supply and therefore limited oxygen and glucose. This tissue is potentially salvageable if blood flow can be restored. Therefore, medical management is aimed at preventing the ischaemic penumbra from progressing to infarction. See Figure 1.8 for an image of the core ischaemic zone and ischaemic penumbra.

Haemorrhagic stroke

Although less common, around 11% of strokes are haemorrhagic (Intercollegiate Stroke Working Party ISWP, 2023). Haemorrhagic stroke has significantly worse mortality and morbidity rates than ischaemic stroke. The risk of rapid deterioration means patients should be admitted directly to a Hyperacute Stroke Unit for specialist assessment, monitoring and interventions (ISWP, 2023).

In haemorrhagic stroke, cerebral blood vessels burst or leak blood into the cerebral tissues. This may also be referred to as intracerebral haemorrhage or

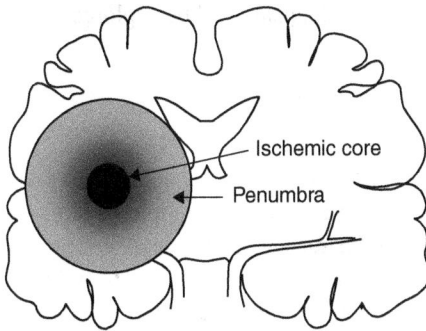

FIGURE 1.8   Ischaemic core and penumbra after stroke.
Source: Coultrap *et al.* (2011).

intraparenchymal haemorrhage. Common sites of intracerebral haemorrhage include the basal ganglia, thalamus, cerebellum, brainstem and within the lobes of the brain. Haemorrhagic stroke is usually due to *hypertension. Cerebral amyloid angiopathy* – a condition characterised by deposits of amyloid-β peptides in the smaller blood vessels is a less frequent cause.

Subarachnoid haemorrhage (SAH), a subtype of stroke, is caused by bleeding between the brain and surrounding membrane on the surface of the brain (see Figure 1.5). SAH is the cause of approximately 6%–8% of all stroke subtypes, affecting approximately 10 per 100,000 people each year (Castanares-Zapatero and Hantson, 2011). Ruptured cerebral aneurysms are the cause for approximately 85% of SAHs.

Cerebral aneurysms are acquired lesions related to haemodynamic stress on arterial walls. They generally arise where arteries branch, usually within the Circle of Willis (Luoma *et al.*, 2013). These aneurysms are specific to intracranial arteries, as the vessel walls lack an external elastic lamina and contain a thin adventitia (Becske, 2018). Other causes, including arteriovenous malformations (AVMs), account for 5% of SAHs. AVMs occur through an entanglement of vessels where arteries and veins connect without the presence of the normal capillary bed, meaning veins receive blood at higher pressure, leaving them susceptible to rupture (Hickey and Livesay, 2020). Non-aneurysmal perimesecephalic SAHs account for 10% of the incidence. This is a condition defined by a particular blood distribution in combination with normal angiographic studies (van Gijn *et al.*, 2007).

The rupturing of vessels in a haemorrhagic stroke disrupts the BBB (Figure 1.3), allowing the presence of molecules that are not normally able to enter the brain. Arterial bleeds may also increase ICP significantly, leading to a reduction in CPP and metabolic activity (the production of ATP). Both mechanisms lead to oedema (swelling of cerebral tissue), further impacting perfusion and ICP. Blood blocking CSF pathways and associated hydrocephalus can further increase ICP. Interventions to prevent and reduce the impact of these mechanisms will be explored later on in this chapter.

Transient ischaemic attack (TIA)

Colloquially referred to as a 'mini stroke', a TIA is caused by a temporary disruption in the blood supply to part of the brain, causing symptoms like a stroke. Although it is caused by ischaemia, it demonstrates no evidence of acute infarction on radiological investigation. The effects may last a few minutes to a few hours, and according to the definition of TIA, should fully resolve within 24 hours and so do not cause the amount of damage to neuronal tissue as described above (NICE, 2023a).

Cerebral venous thrombosis (CVT)

A CVT is due to a prothrombotic state (propensity to venous thrombosis) from either local infection, dehydration or malignancies (Grear and Bushnell, 2013).

Pregnancy-related strokes

These occur in approximately 30 per 100,000 pregnancies and carry a relatively high mortality rate (Miller and Leffert, 2020). Complex pregnancy-related physiological processes occur, increasing the risk of stroke. These include hypervolaemia, increased circulatory demands, decreased blood pressure and venous stasis, which combined create a hypercoagulable state (Cauldwell *et al.*, 2018). Prothrombotic changes are highest in the third trimester, which is the most common time for strokes to occur (Singhal *et al.*, 2013). The most common causes include arterial occlusions, cardiac embolism, and intra- or extracranial atherothrombosis (Grear and Bushnell, 2013). See Figure 1.9 for some mechanisms of pregnancy-related stroke.

Other causes, such as AVMs, cause 5%–12% of all maternal deaths and 17% of foetal mortality. Bleeding from an AVM during pregnancy is rare and so is generally undiagnosed until the onset of stroke (Coppage *et al.*, 2004). If it does occur, it is more prevalent after the second trimester when blood volume and cardiac output are at their greatest (Tonetti *et al.*, 2014).

Signs and symptoms of stroke and diagnosis

The signs and symptoms of stroke are dependent on the type of stroke, as well as the location of the stroke within the CNS. Whilst vascular territories provide some defined functional zones (see Figure 1.10a), functional pathways, such as movement, may involve multiple areas of the brain and therefore multiple pathophysiologies following stroke. As a result, the following discussion is

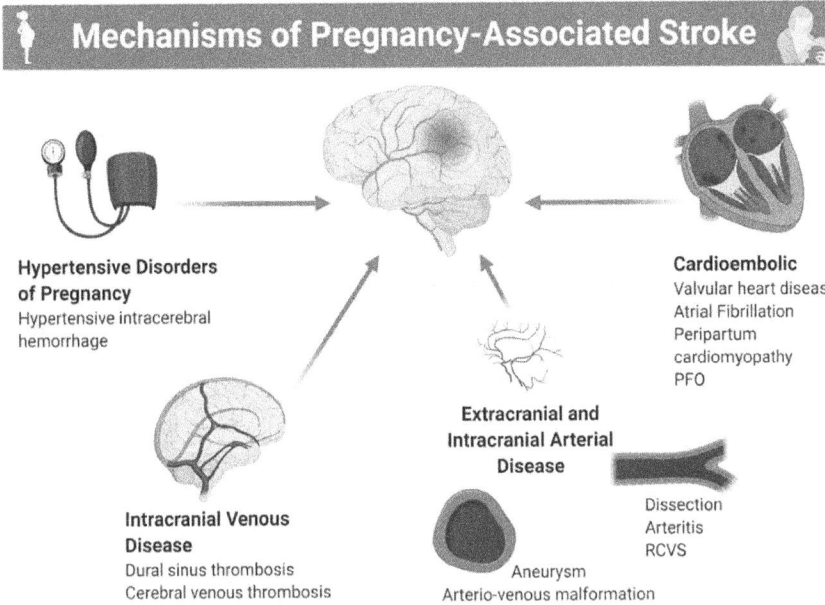

FIGURE 1.9 Mechanisms of pregnancy-related stroke.
Source: Elgendy *et al.* (2021).

not designed to be exhaustive, or to oversimplify these complexities, but to support healthcare professionals' basic understanding of the pathophysiology of stroke.

Functional areas of the brain

The brain is divided into two hemispheres, which are not identical in their function, with the dominant hemisphere generally being where important centres, such as speech, are located. The left hemisphere sends information to and receives information from the right side of the body, with the right hemisphere doing the same for the left. Therefore, someone with a stroke affecting the left hemisphere may experience motor and sensory issues on the right side of the body. The cerebral cortex (surface of the brain) can be divided into four lobes containing specific functional areas (Figure 1.10a, Table 1.4).

Stroke pathology typically combines diffuse and focal brain damage and can be associated with cognitive and emotional changes, which can be difficult to treat (Hickey, 2020b). A stroke affecting the anterior arterial circulation may damage the frontal lobe, leading to changes in a person's cognition (the ability to think or process and respond to information). Cognitive changes such as impaired memory, executive function and reduced attention are common and can make it difficult

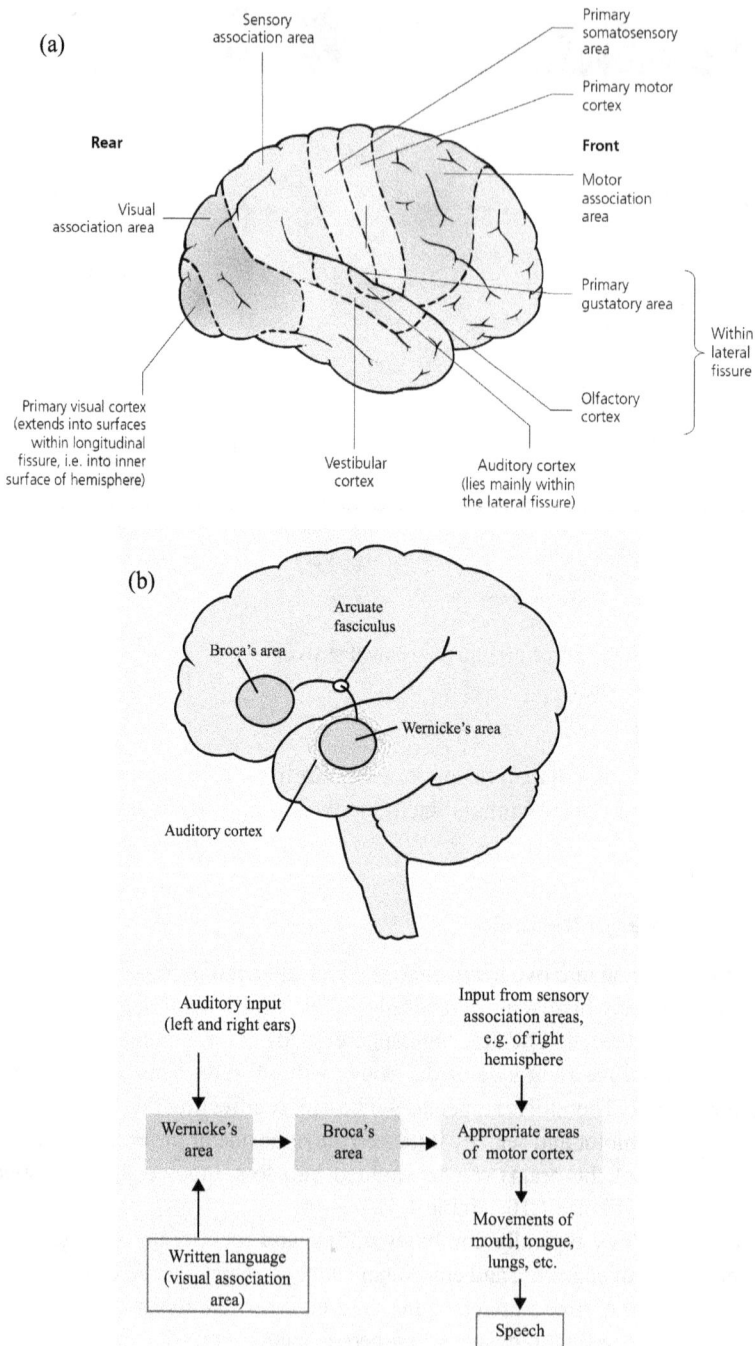

(a)

Sensory association area

Primary somatosensory area

Primary motor cortex

Rear

Front

Visual association area

Motor association area

Primary gustatory area

Within lateral fissure

Primary visual cortex (extends into surfaces within longitudinal fissure, i.e. into inner surface of hemisphere)

Olfactory cortex

Vestibular cortex

Auditory cortex (lies mainly within the lateral fissure)

(b)

Arcuate fasciculus

Broca's area

Wernicke's area

Auditory cortex

Auditory input (left and right ears)

Input from sensory association areas, e.g. of right hemisphere

Wernicke's area → Broca's area → Appropriate areas of motor cortex

Written language (visual association area)

Movements of mouth, tongue, lungs, etc.

Speech

FIGURE 1.10 (a) The functional areas of the cortex. (b) Broca's and Wernicke's area and the pathway required for speech.

Source: Sturgeon (2018, p. 221).

TABLE 1.4 Lobe functions of the cortex

Frontal lobe	• Inhibition of emotions • Executive functioning (behavioural, cognitive and motivational function) (Bennett, 2020). • Personality • Voluntary motor control • Motor control of speech (Broca's area – see Figure 1.10b)
Parietal lobe	• Somatosensory function – processing all sensations except smell and hearing • Proprioception – information that allows the brain to know where the body is in relation to its environment
Temporal lobe	• Hearing • Auditory processing of speech – Wernicke's area (see Figure 1.10b) • Limbic system • Hippocampus – long-term memory processing and retrieval • Amygdala – controls anger, fear, reproduction, thirst hunger (often referred to as 'basic instincts' (Hickey, 2020a)
Occipital lobe	• Vision – signals received from the eye • Visual association – understanding the images we see

for patients to accept and understand the changes that have occurred (Persson *et al.*, 2017).

Al-Khindi *et al.* (2010) found that stroke survivors commonly experienced deficits in memory and executive function affecting their day-to-day abilities and quality of life (QoL), with many of these deficits being further compounded by depression, anxiety, fatigue and sleep disturbances.

The motor and somatosensory areas are divided further by the area of muscle that they innervate (motor) or where they receive information from (sensory). These divisions are represented on the motor and sensory homunculus, with the body parts distorted to demonstrate how much of the cerebral cortex is devoted to that function/sensation. Healthcare professionals can use the homunculus to pinpoint the area of damage by identifying deficits following a stroke (see Figure 1.11) and to understand why not all motor or sensory function to a limb or side of the body may be lost. Damage to the parietal lobe can occur due to damage to the anterior or middle circulation and can often result in patients lacking awareness of a limb, commonly referred to as 'neglect' of that limb.

The connection between Broca's area in the frontal lobe and Wernicke's areas enables us to perform activities such as answering questions, following commands, and identifying objects we see (see Figure 1.10b). Damage to these areas can cause aphasia defined as full or partial loss of language.

Damage can precipitate ongoing challenges, including anxiety and fatigue (ISWP, 2023). The literature suggests that anxiety prevention measures may

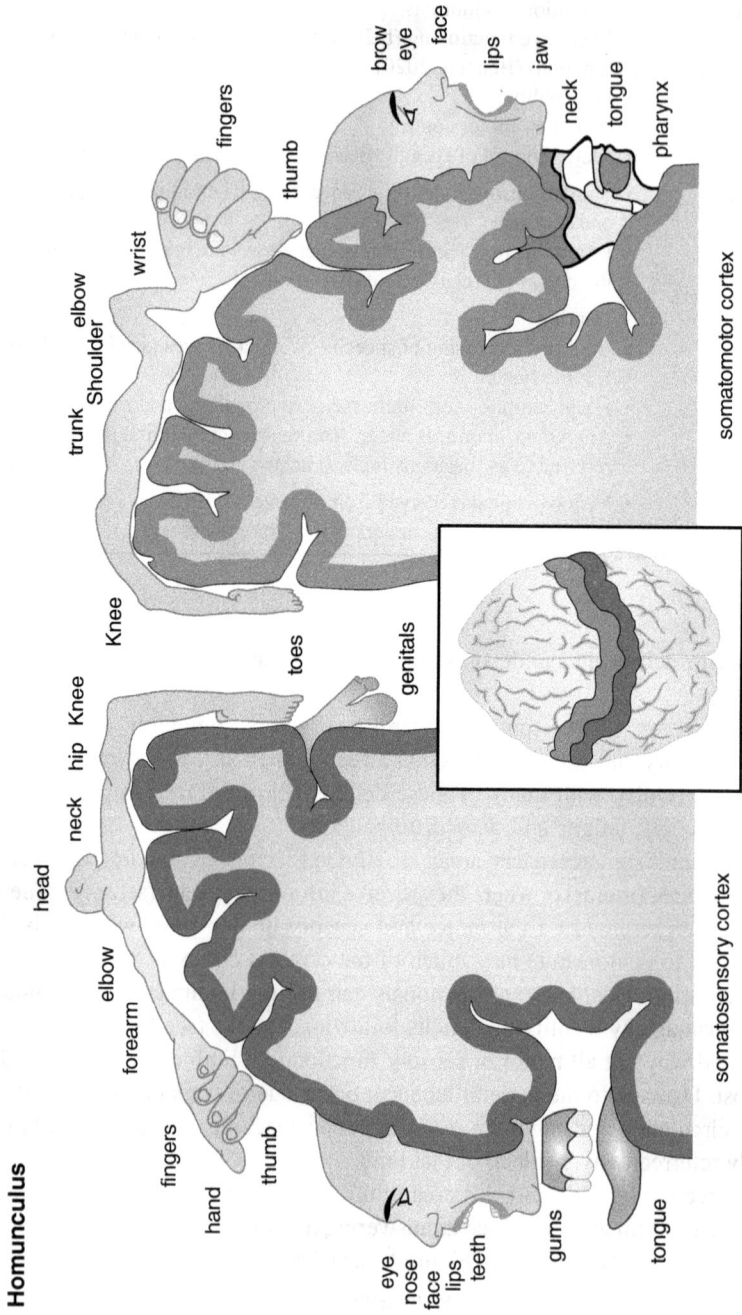

FIGURE 1.11 Image of motor and sensory homunculus.
Source: Baugh (2024).

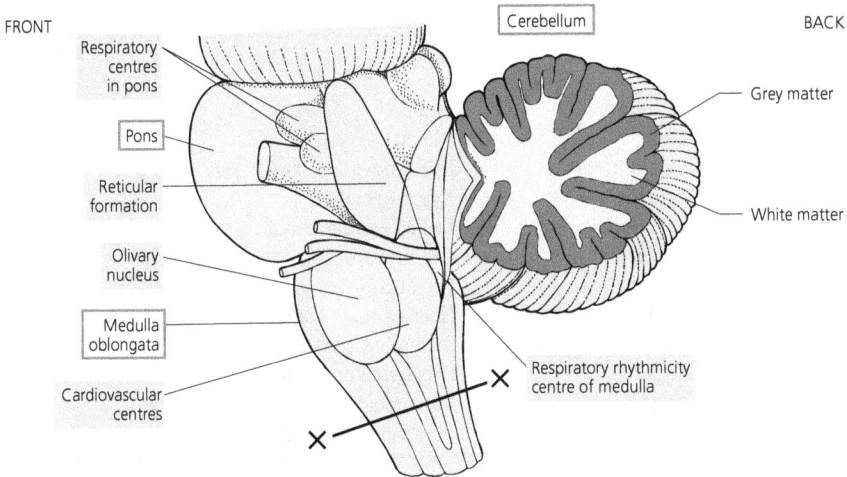

FIGURE 1.12 Key functional areas of the brainstem.
Source: Clancy (2017, p. 177).

significantly improve survivors' functional outcomes and links with better outcome indices for returning to work and social engagement (Morris *et al.*, 2004).

The brainstem connects the brain and spinal cord, with all the descending (information from the brain) and ascending (information to the brain) neuronal tracts passing through it. It also controls the respiratory and cardiac functions of the body. Even if the brainstem is not directly damaged following stroke, a significant increase in ICP may irreversibly damage it, causing difficulties in breathing, cardiac function, pain and conscious level. The cranial nerves (CNs) exit the brainstem in pairs (see Figure 1.12 and Table 1.5). Their function includes the movement of the muscles of the face (CN7) and eyes (CN3, 4 and 6), which can be commonly affected following stroke (McKenna, 2020).

Thalamus

The thalamus is the processing centre for all sensory information (except smell) before the signals are transmitted to the cerebral cortex. It also has a significant role to play in consciousness, pain and awareness, so damage following stroke can lead to reduced conscious levels and reduced or abnormal perception of pain.

Hypothalamus and pituitary gland

The hypothalamus is significant in endocrine function. It mediates the pituitary gland and thermoregulation, releasing important hormones for maintenance of homeostasis, including adrenocorticotropic hormone (ACTH – the precursor to cortisol), anti-diuretic hormone (ADH – controlling urine production) and

TABLE 1.5 Functions of cranial nerves

Number	Nerve	Function
1	Olfactory	Smell
2	Optic	Vision
3	Oculomotor	Eye movements and pupils
4	Trochlear	Eye movement
5	Trigeminal	Facial sensation and chewing
6	Abducens	Eye movements
7	Facial	Facial expressions and taste
8	Auditory	Hearing and balance
9	Glossopharyngeal	Salivation and gag reflex
10	Vagus	Parasympathetic innervations and gag reflex
11	Accessory	Movement of head and shoulders
12	Hypoglossal	Movement of tongue, swallowing and speech

Source: Sturgeon (2018, p. 202).

growth-stimulating hormone (GSH – cellular repair). As a result, damage to the hypothalamus and/or pituitary gland following stroke can have an impact on maintenance of blood pressure, temperature control, sleep and cellular repair.

Summary of the physiological impact of stroke

As an underlying principle, an adequate and significant supply of oxygen and glucose to the brain is required to ensure adequate ATP production for the CNS to function. Disruption to arterial flow, because of any type of stroke, will cause a direct impact on the vascular territory that the blood vessel supplies. It is this that creates the distinct and often individual symptoms of stroke. Whilst the mechanisms of the Circle of Willis and autoregulation attempt to minimise damage and ensure perfusion, structural damage to the arterial system may reduce their ability to do this. To prevent further damage, reperfusion of these territories is a priority, along with prevention of further damage from raised ICP, ischaemia, disruption of CSF pathways or further reduction in CPP elsewhere in the brain.

When considering the pathophysiological impact of stroke, it is important for healthcare professionals to consider the physiological processes underlying symptoms to provide suitable treatment options. There is not only one type of treatment for each stroke type due to the complex and overlapping nature of the processes discussed above. Referring to the physiology of the CNS within this chapter may be useful when proceeding through this book.

Management of ischaemic stroke

Management of ischaemic stroke is aimed at removing the obstruction within the blood vessel and restoring blood flow (revascularisation) to the ischaemic penumbra. In patients who are eligible, this may be achieved via a reperfusion treatment of thrombolysis or thrombectomy.

Thrombolysis involves the injection of a thrombolytic agent, which breaks down and disperses the blood clot. In the UK, the drug of choice is currently Alteplase or Tenectaplase (ISWP, 2023). Thrombolysis with Alteplase is the most common option, administered to between 10 and 11% of patients with acute stroke in the UK and Ireland (ISWP, 2023). Its common use is due to the significant evidence base supporting its effectiveness and side effects. However, Tenectaplase use is becoming more widespread. There are important restrictions which can prevent the administration of thrombolytic agents, including the recommendation that the drug should be given within 4.5 hours of a stroke, although this can be extended up to 9 hours post stroke in some circumstances (ISWP, 2023). However, the earlier a treatment is administered, the better the outcome.

In some cases, in addition to thrombolysis, mechanical thrombectomy is recommended to remove the clot and/or clot remnants from the cerebral vasculature. If thrombolysis is contraindicated, thrombectomy should be considered as a first-line treatment. Mechanical thrombectomy should only be carried out by appropriately trained and experienced specialists in intracranial endovascular interventions, with appropriate facilities and neuroscience support (NICE, 2016). The procedure involves the use of a clot retrieval device, usually inserted into the groin and attached to a guidewire, which is introduced to the site of the occlusion. The clot retriever is then deployed to remove the clot and re-establish blood flow to the affected part of the brain (ISWP, 2023; NICE, 2016).

Following acute ischaemic stroke, patients with large artery occlusions in the anterior circulation should be considered for thrombectomy for up to 24 hours after symptom onset. For patients with acute ischaemic stroke in the posterior circulation (a confirmed intracranial vertebral or basilar artery occlusion), thrombectomy should occur within 12 hours of onset. Again, the earlier the procedure takes place, the better the outcome (ISWP, 2023; NICE, 2016).

Longer-term management includes commencing definitive long-term antithrombotic treatment such as Clopidogrel (NICE, 2023a). If an individual is taking statins prior to their stroke these should be continued, but statins do not need to be commenced immediately after an ischaemic stroke (NICE, 2023a).

Management of haemorrhagic stroke

Initial management of haemorrhagic stroke is usually focussed on blood pressure control with rapid lowering considered for individuals who have a systolic blood pressure between 150 and 220 mmHg (ISWP, 2023; NICE, 2023a). This intervention is not without risk and should be managed by stroke experienced healthcare professionals (NICE, 2023a). Within a stroke specialist unit, the patients' level of consciousness should be monitored closely. If any deterioration is noted, the patient should be referred immediately for brain imaging (ISWP, 2023).

Surgical removal of the clot is not performed routinely but in the event of raised ICP, a decompressive hemicraniectomy may be considered (NICE, 2023a). Healthcare professionals should be aware of the risk of hydrocephalus and monitor for this (ISWP, 2023).

Neuroplasticity

Following stroke, physical and cognitive functions may be impacted, so regaining function is key to a successful recovery and to promote independence (Langhorne *et al.*, 2011). Early rehabilitation is an essential part of the recovery process, but rehabilitation should be considered potentially beneficial at any point after stroke (ISWP, 2023). Neuroplasticity refers to the capacity of the CNS to reorganise and adapt in response to intrinsic and extrinsic stimuli (Mateos-Aparicio and Rodríguez-Moreno, 2019). New neuronal pathways are created in damaged areas both automatically and with rehabilitation exercises, which play a key role in building neural connections. When neurons are used frequently and repetitively, new, strong connections can be made, improving physical function, and potentially enhancing cognitive capabilities (Dimyan and Cohen, 2011). The practice and repetition of tasks for months or even years is a key component of optimal recovery; the more physical therapy that occurs, the greater the neuroplastic and functional outcome. There is evidence that just thinking about the tasks and picturing them can also improve rehabilitation outcomes (ISWP, 2023) See Figure 1.13 for the types of brain plasticity.

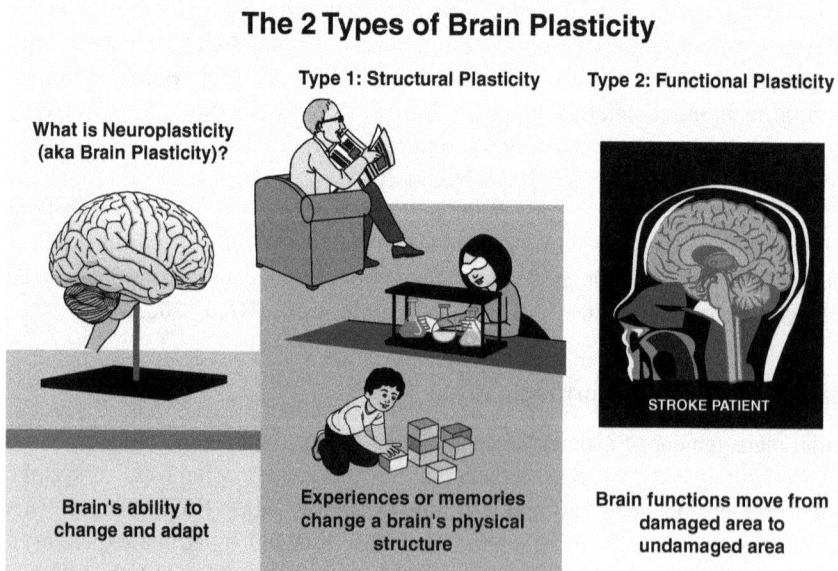

FIGURE 1.13 Types of brain plasticity.

Source: Cherry (2022).

For individuals who need support to practise their rehabilitation activities but who might be on their own for extended periods, encourage them to visualise their exercise such as moving a fork from a plate to their mouth or swinging their legs out of bed to sit up.

Friends and relatives can also remind and encourage stroke survivors to practise rehabilitation exercises or visualisation.

Risk factors for stroke and transient ischaemic attack

Stroke risk factors are well documented and share similarities to risks for coronary heart disease and other vascular diseases. However, studies have shown that many individuals are unaware of their own stroke risk and the contributing cause and so may do little to prevent it occurring.

I think there was more data in the public domain about your risk of heart attacks. I know I am overweight and therefore 'I'm more at risk of heart attack' would have been more in my mind than 'you're more at risk of stroke'.

I was told my cholesterol was borderline, but I do not like taking tablets, so I said I didn't want the statins my doctor suggested. That was about roughly a year before I had my stroke and I've thought back to that time. I wonder if I had been on had a statin on a daily basis, would I still have had my stroke? I don't know. And of course, nobody knows.

(Stuart, 66, ischaemic stroke, 4 years post stroke)

Risk factors for stroke can be non-modifiable – low birth weight, age, sex, ethnicity and genetics, or modifiable. Three key modifiable risk factors for prevention of stroke are management of hypertension, cessation of tobacco smoking and reducing high fasting glucose secondary to diabetes. Environmental risk factors such as high levels of air pollution have also been identified (WSO, 2022; NICE, 2023b). See Figure 1.14 for risk factors.

Following a stroke, individuals remain at heightened risk of recurrent cerebrovascular events, with the greatest vulnerability occurring in the immediate post-stroke period. Up to 25% of people will have a further event within three months; however, half of these will occur within the first 4 days after a stroke. Therefore, secondary prevention, targeting risk factors, should be commenced as soon as possible after a diagnosis (ISWP, 2023). If a patient does not require hospital admission for management of their stroke event, assessment within a TIA clinic is recommended to ensure that appropriate interventions, investigations and treatments can be commenced to reduce further stroke risk (NICE, 2023a).

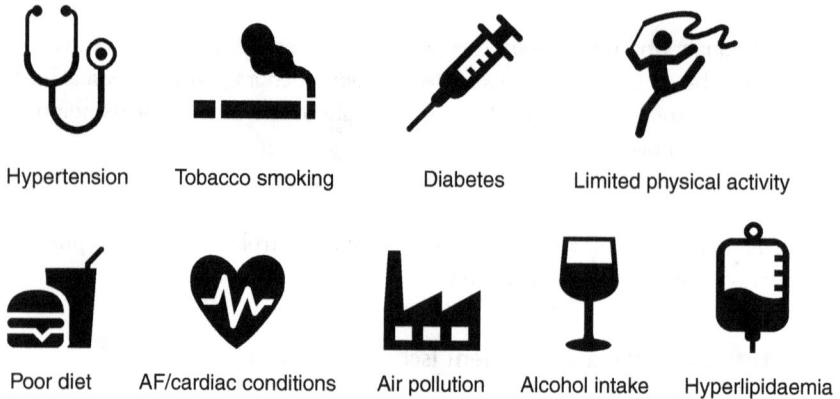

Hypertension   Tobacco smoking   Diabetes   Limited physical activity

Poor diet   AF/cardiac conditions   Air pollution   Alcohol intake   Hyperlipidaemia

FIGURE 1.14   Common risk factors for stroke.

Risk factors for stroke in pregnancy

Risk factors for stroke during pregnancy include advanced maternal age, as well as comorbidities such as smoking, obesity, hypertension and diabetes. It is essential that risks are identified early on in pregnancy and that all healthcare providers are proactive in discussing and managing them, to be able to support individuals in addressing any modifiable factors themselves (Grear and Bushnell, 2013).

> I was not aware of any risk factors at all…. when pregnant I had no warning about a stroke…I was relaxing at home thinking that it's a few weeks away with a mixture of apprehension and excitement. Then I went to make a coffee and was suddenly feeling a strange spike feeling inside my head. Within seconds my left side dropped, and I knew something was very wrong. My voice sounded like an electronic toy with a low battery. I thought at 34 that it was my time to die and felt a feeling of horror that I would not be around for Alice – I knew at 37 weeks she could survive, but was not sure what would happen next. The thought I would be leaving Lucas at 2.5 years old filled me with horror.
>
> *(Nerys, 35, right frontal intracerebral haemorrhage*
> *from a ruptured AVM, 18 months post stroke)*

Hormonal changes like oestrogen and progesterone increase during pregnancy, affecting blood vessel function and blood clotting. These changes may contribute to an increased risk of clot formation, potentially leading to stroke (Grear and Bushnell, 2013). Other risk factors include hypertensive disorders of pregnancy, such as pre-eclampsia, which can increase the risk of stroke due to elevated blood pressure and its impact on blood vessels. Eclampsia is a severe complication of pre-eclampsia which causes seizures, leading to a lack of oxygen to the brain and

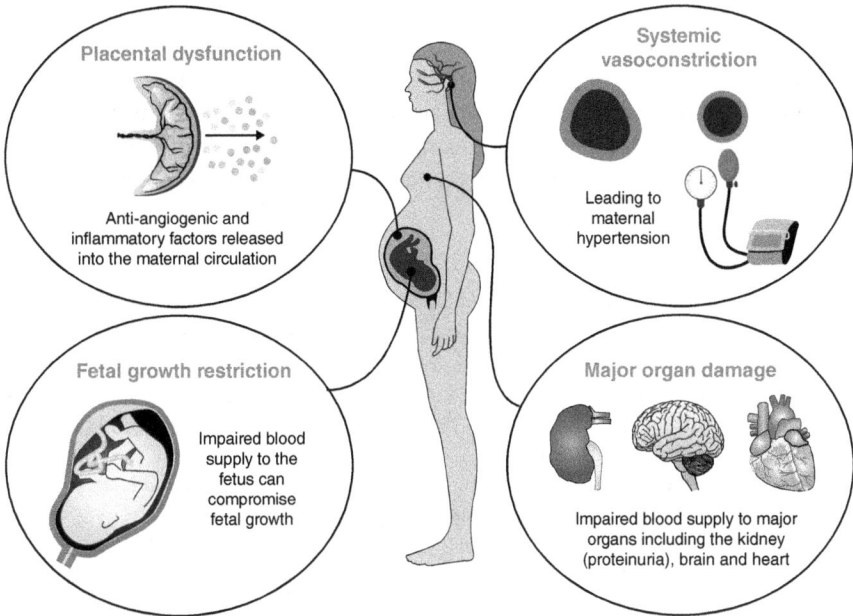

FIGURE 1.15   Pre-eclampsia in pregnancy.

again, potentially resulting in stroke (Liu *et al.*, 2018). See Figure 1.15 showing the effects of pre-eclampsia in pregnancy.

The management of stroke, investigations and assessments should not differ for pregnant women, with treatment being required within 4.5 hours of the stroke onset (Khalid *et al.*, 2020). For procedures such as thrombectomy, a risk–benefit discussion is required due to the risks of uterine bleeding. Unfortunately, many clinical trials generally exclude pregnant women (Vousden *et al.*, 2023), creating a knowledge gap when looking at treatment and prevention measures for medical conditions experienced during pregnancy (Sewell *et al.*, 2022).

- Consider your workplace and your practice:
- Do you effectively educate patients about risk reduction?
- How could you be more proactive in achieving this?
- What resources would you need and how might you procure them?

Conclusion

Stroke is a leading cause of death and disability worldwide, and an understanding of its underlying physiology, associated risk factors and management is important for all healthcare professionals. If a stroke is suspected, prompt interventions provide the opportunity for a reduction in primary injury by limiting ischaemic damage, as well as preventing secondary injury. Symptoms of stroke have a direct relationship to the vascular territory that has been affected, and, as a result, may vary from person to person. These symptoms will be discussed in further detail throughout the book; however, the physiological underpinning of many of them has been introduced here. Patient education regarding risk factors for stroke is important for ongoing management, recovery and for future stroke prevention.

References

Adams HP Jr, Bendixen BH, Kappelle LJ, *et al.* (1993) Classification of subtype of acute ischemic stroke. Definitions for use in a multicentre clinical trial. TOAST. Trial of ORG 10172 in Acute Stroke Treatment. *Stroke* 24:35–41.

Al-Khindi T, Macdonald RL, Schweizer TA (2010) Cognitive and functional outcome after aneurysmal subarachnoid hemorrhage. *Stroke* 41(8):e519–536. Available at: https://pub med.ncbi.nlm.nih.gov/20595669/

Baugh LS (29 January 2024) Homunculus. *Encyclopedia Britannica.* Available at: www.bri tannica.com/science/homunculus-biology

Becske T (2018) Subarachnoid haemorrhage. *Medscape.* Available at: https://emedicine. medscape.com/article/1164341-overview

Bennett N (2020) Diagnostics for patients with neurological disorders, in Hickey JV, Strayer A (eds.) *The Clinical Practice of Neurological and Neurosurgical Nursing.* Eighth edition. Philadelphia, PA: Wolters Kluwer, pp. 227–273.

Castanares-Zapatero D, Hantson P (2011) Pharmacological treatment of delayed cerebral ischemia and vasospasm in subarachnoid hemorrhage. *Ann Intensive Care* 1(1):12. Available at: www.ncbi.nlm.nih.gov/pmc/articles/PMC3224484/

Cauldwell M, Rudd A, Nelson-Piercy C (2018) Management of stroke and pregnancy. *Eur Stroke J* 3(3):227–236. Available at: https://doi.org/10.1177/2396987318769547

Cherry K (2022) What is neuroplasticity? Theories biological psychology. *Verywell Mind.* Available at: www.verywellmind.com/what-is-brain-plasticity-2794886

Clancy J (2017) *Physiology and Anatomy for Nurses and Healthcare Practitioners: A Homeostatic Approach.* Third edition. Oxford: Routledge.

Coppage KH, Hinton AC, Moldenhauer J, *et al.* (2004) Maternal and perinatal outcome in women with a history of stroke. *Am J Obstet Gynecol* 190:1331–1334. Available at: https://doi.org/10.1016/j.ajog.2003.11.002

Coultrap S, Vest R, Ashpole N, *et al.* (2011) CaMKII in cerebral ischemia. *Acta Pharmacol Sin* 32:861–872. Available at: https://doi.org/10.1038/aps.2011.68

Dimyan MA, Cohen LG (2011) Neuroplasticity in the context of motor rehabilitation after stroke. *Nat Rev Neurol* 7(2):76–85. Available at: https://doi.org/10.1038/nrneu rol.2010.200.

Elgendy IY, Bukhari S, Barakat AF, *et al.* (2021) Mechanisms of pregnancy associated stroke. American College of Cardiology Cardiovascular Disease in Women Committee. Maternal Stroke: A Call for Action. *Circulation* 143(7):727–738. Available at: https:// doi.org/10.1161/CIRCULATIONAHA.120.051460.

Grear KE, Bushnell CD (2013) Stroke and pregnancy: Clinical presentation, evaluation, treatment, and epidemiology. *Clin Obstet Gynecol* 56(2):350–359.

Hickey JV (2020a) Overview of neuroanatomy and neurophysiology, in Hickey JV, Strayer A (eds.) *The Clinical Practice of Neurological and Neurosurgical Nursing.* Eighth edition. Philadelphia, PA: Wolters Kluwer, pp. 133–226.

Hickey JV (2020b) Rehabilitation of patients with neurological disorders, in Hickey JV, Strayer A (eds.) *The Clinical Practice of Neurological and Neurosurgical Nursing.* Eighth edition. Philadelphia, PA: Wolters Kluwer, pp. 669–736.

Hickey JV, Livesay SL (2020) Intracerebral haemorrhagic stroke, in Hickey JV, Strayer A (eds.) *The Clinical Practice of Neurological and Neurosurgical Nursing.* Eighth edition. Philadelphia, PA: Wolters Kluwer, pp. 1204–1238.

Intercollegiate Stroke Working Party (ISWP) (2023) *National Clinical Guideline for Stroke for the UK and Ireland.* London. Available at: www.strokeguideline.org

Khalid A, Hadbavna A, Williams D, Byrne B (2020) A review of stroke in pregnancy: Incidence, investigations and management. The Obstetrician & Gynaecologist 22:21–33. https://doi.org/10.1111/tog.12624

Langhorne P, Bernhardt J, Kwakkel G (2011) Stroke rehabilitation. *The Lancet* 377(9778):1693–1702. Available at: https://doi.org/10.1016/S0140-6736(11)60325-5; www.sciencedirect.com/science/article/pii/S0140673611603255

Liu S, Chan W, Ray JG, *et al.* (2018) Stroke and cerebrovascular disease in pregnancy: Incidence, temporal trends, and risk factors. *Stroke* 50:13–20. Available at: www.ahajournals.org/doi/full/10.1161/STROKEAHA.118.023118

Luoma A, Reddy U (2013) Acute management of aneurysmal subarachnoid haemorrhage. *CEACCP* 13(2):52–58. Available at: https://doi.org/10.1093/bjaceaccp/mks054

Mateos-Aparicio P, Rodríguez-Moreno A (2019) The impact of studying brain plasticity. *Front Cell Neurosci* 13:66.

McKenna GM (2020). Cranial nerve diseases, in Hickey JV, Strayer A (eds.) *The Clinical Practice of Neurological and Neurosurgical Nursing.* Eighth edition. Philadelphia, PA: Wolters Kluwer, pp. 993–1107.

Miller EC, Leffert L (2020) Stroke in pregnancy: A focused update. *Anesth Analg* 130(4):1085–1096. Available at: https://doi.org/10.1213/ANE.0000000000004203.

Morris P, Wilson L, Dunn L (2004) Anxiety and depression after spontaneous subarachnoid haemorrhage. *Neurosurgery* 54(1):47–52. Available at: https://pubmed.ncbi.nlm.nih.gov/14683540/

National Institute for Health and Care Excellence (NICE) (2016) *Interventional Procedures Guidance [IPG548]. Mechanical Clot Retrieval for Treating Acute Ischaemic Stroke.* NICE. Available at: www.nice.org.uk/guidance/ipg548

National Institute for Health and Care Excellence (NICE) (2023a) *Clinical Guideline [NG128]. Stroke and Transient Ischaemic Attack in over 16s: Diagnosis and Initial Management.* NICE. Available at: www.nice.org.uk/guidance/NG128 (accessed 9 August 2024).

National Institute for Health and Care Excellence (NICE) (2023b). *Clinical Guideline [CG181]. Cardiovascular Disease: Risk Assessment and Reduction, Including Lipid Modification.* NICE. Available at: www.nice.org.uk/guidance/CG181

Persson HC, Tornbom K, Sunnerhagen KS, *et al.* (2017) Consequences and coping strategies six years after a subarachnoid hemorrhage – a qualitative study. *PLoS ONE* 12(8):e0181006. Available at: https://pubmed.ncbi.nlm.nih.gov/28854198/

Public Health England (PHE) (2018) *New Figures Show Larger Proportion of Strokes in the Middle Aged.* GOV.UK. Available at: www.gov.uk/government/news/new-figures-show-larger-proportion-of-strokes-in-the-middle-aged

Sewell CA, Sheehan SM, Gill MS, *et al.* (2022) Scientific, ethical, and legal considerations for the inclusion of pregnant people in clinical trials. *Am J Obstet Gynecol* 227(6):805–811. Available at: https://doi.org/10.1016/j.ajog.2022.07.037; www.ncbi.nlm.nih.gov/pmc/articles/PMC9351207/

Singhal AB, Biller J, Elkind MS, *et al.* (2013) Recognition and management of stroke in young adults and adolescents. *Neurology* 81(12):1089–1097.

Sturgeon D (2018) *Introduction to Anatomy and Physiology for Healthcare Students.* London: Routledge.

Tonetti D, Kano H, Bowden G, *et al.* (2014) Hemorrhage during pregnancy in the latency interval after stereotactic radiosurgery for arteriovenous malformations. *J Neurosurg* 121(Suppl):226–231.

van Gijn J, Kerr RS, Rinkel GJ (2007) Subarachnoid haemorrhage. *Lancet* 369(9558):306. Available at: https://pubmed.ncbi.nlm.nih.gov/17258671/

Vousden N, Haynes R, Findlay S, *et al.* (2023). Facilitating participation in clinical trials during pregnancy. *BMJ* 380:e071278. Available at: www.bmj.com/content/380/bmj-2022-071278

World Health Organization (WHO) (1978) *Cerebrovascular Diseases: A Clinical and Research Classification.* Geneva: World Health Organization. Available at: https://apps.who.int/iris/bitstream/handle/10665/37194/WHO_OFFSET_43.pdf?sequence=1&isAllowed=y

World Health Organization (WHO) (2020) *The Top 10 Causes of Death.* WHO. Available at: www.who.int/news-room/fact-sheets/detail/the-top-10-causes-of-death

World Stroke Organization (WSO) (2022) *Global Stroke Fact Sheet.* Available at: www.world-stroke.org/news-and-blog/news/wso-global-stroke-fact-sheet-2022

2

MAINTAINING INDEPENDENCE AND KEEPING SAFE

Fiona Chalk, Jennifer Huffadine and Lyndsey Shawe

In collaboration with the Oxford Stroke Patient Group

Learning objectives

- To understand the meaning of maintaining independence and keeping safe.
- To be aware of the need for individualised care and rehabilitation programmes.
- To gain an insight into some of the different challenges and solutions to facilitate maintaining safety and promoting independence.
- To recognise that there is a balance between managing risks to keep the individual safe whilst promoting rehabilitation progression.

Background

Often patients state, 'I just want to be independent again', while the patient's family members state 'I just want them to be safe'. This chapter will explore these two, sometimes conflicting, ideas.

What does independence mean?

> Independence is everything.
>
> *(Oxford Stroke Patient Group member)*

To be independent means to be self-sufficient, self-reliant and not under the influence or control of others (Cambridge Dictionary, no date). Independence can relate to an individual's physical, mental, emotional and financial ability, stability or control.

DOI: 10.4324/9781003426196-3

Despite this definition, the word independence can mean different things to different people. Each person will put their individual emphasis, or level of importance, on different elements of independence and these priorities will likely change at varying points in their life. For example, some people may see independence as a measure of how much they can physically do for themselves in their everyday life. Others may not place as much importance on being able to physically carry out tasks and instead feel that independence comes from being able to think or speak for themselves and hold a level of control over what happens in their life. Another example is that some people feel comfortable receiving financial assistance or being financially reliant on someone else, whilst some others feel that it is of utmost importance to be completely financially independent. It is important to remember that there is no 'right and wrong' in how someone interprets independence; only differences in how people choose to live their lives.

What does independence mean to you, and what are your priorities when you consider physical, mental, emotional or financial independence?

Following a stroke, an individual's level of independence is often a fluctuating journey. Immediately after the stroke, independence is often temporarily lost, particularly if admission to hospital is required. A hospital admission can remove a lot of a person's independence. Hospital staff and ward routines may impact what a patient eats, when they sleep, and when and which medications they take, and patients may have tasks completed for them that they would normally complete themselves. A stroke can also remove a person's independence by limiting function due to issues with sensation, proprioception, coordination, executive functioning, vision, communication or muscle weakness (NHS, 2022). This initial loss of independence (combined with the unexpected nature of having a stroke and the symptoms the stroke may cause) often comes as a big shock and requires a period of adjustment from both the patient and their family and friends.

Following the acute management stage, the patient then progresses into the rehabilitation stage, where the aim is to regain as much independence as possible, within the limitations of the neurological deficits caused by the stroke. Following a period of rehabilitation, the patient and their family, friends, or caregivers will then need to adjust to the new levels of independence and functional abilities. Almost all stroke patients show considerable levels of recovery; however, only 61.4% achieve functional independence 6 months post stroke (Yun *et al.*, 2020). In 2016, the Stroke Association's State of the Nation report outlined that stroke is one of the largest causes of disability; half of all stroke survivors have a disability, and over a third of stroke survivors in the UK are dependent on others, with one in five cared for by family or friends (Stroke Association, 2016).

During the rehabilitation phase, a key task of utmost importance is to get to know the patient, understand the level of independence they had pre-stroke and understand their goals regarding their future levels of independence. The

2023 Intercollegiate Stroke Working Party (ISWP) guidelines acknowledge the importance of goal setting being led by the patient to ensure that goals are meaningful and have personal value to the patient.

It is also important to understand how a patient wishes to achieve their goal or desired level of independence. Are they fixed on being able to complete the task in the same way as prior to their stroke, or are they open to adaptations, assistive technology or physical compensation strategies to help them complete the task? For example, a patient has the goal of being able to turn a lamp on independently. One way to achieve this goal is to be able to turn it on using the switch as they did prior to their stroke. Another way is to be able to use a larger switch or a touch-activated lamp. An alternative adaptation would be to use assistive technology in the form of a smart lamp or smart plug so that the patient can use their smartphone or ask a smart speaker to turn the lamp on. All of these suggestions successfully achieve the goal of being able to turn the lamp on independently. Talking with the stroke survivor and assessing their functional abilities will help healthcare professionals understand how best to achieve the goal and meet the patient's expectations of 'independence'.

Stroke guidelines around independence

The 2023 ISWP National Clinical Guideline for Stroke and the 2023 NICE Guidelines for Stroke Rehabilitation (NICE, 2023) both mention that stroke can influence a person's abilities to independently complete activities of daily living, and this should therefore be an important basis for their rehabilitation programme.

The NICE (2023) guidelines advise that patients with difficulties in activities of daily living should have regular monitoring and treatment by suitably skilled occupational therapists who play an important part in stroke recovery and rehabilitation. The occupational therapist helps the individual to regain the skills needed for day-to-day activities and the things they want to do (occupations) (Stroke Association, 2022a).

The ISWP (2023) guidelines acknowledge that completing personal activities of daily living such as washing, dressing, bathing, going to the toilet and eating and drinking can be difficult following a stroke due to physical and cognitive impairments. The resultant loss of function can have implications on a person's ability to live independently at home and is therefore a key part of stroke rehabilitation. The guidelines go on to make some recommendations, including:

- People with stroke should be formally assessed for their safety and independence in all relevant personal activities of daily living by an appropriate clinician and should be offered specific treatments to address issues.
- Assessments should include consideration of the impact of hidden deficits affecting function, including neglect or inattention (the brain not processing information, for example from one side), executive dysfunction (impairment in processing how to do something), and visual impairments.

The ISWP (2023) guidelines acknowledge that there is minimal recent research in this area. The main evidence is summarised in a Cochrane systematic review which found that people with stroke who receive occupational therapy targeting personal activities of daily living perform better and have a reduced risk of a poor outcome compared to those without occupational therapy input.

What does maintaining safety mean?

It is about what is realistic and important for that person. *(Oxford Stroke Patient Group member)*

Maslow's hierarchy of needs theory originally described what motivates people but has since been used to outline the priority that humans have for the basic physiological needs such as food, water and warmth, and the need for safety as utmost importance (see Figure 2.1). If these requirements are met satisfactorily, then psychological needs are of next importance. Lastly, if all previously mentioned needs are met, then self-fulfilment needs can be considered, including the sense of independence (American Stroke Association, 2021). However, the individual may not prioritise their needs in the same order as outlined in the theory.

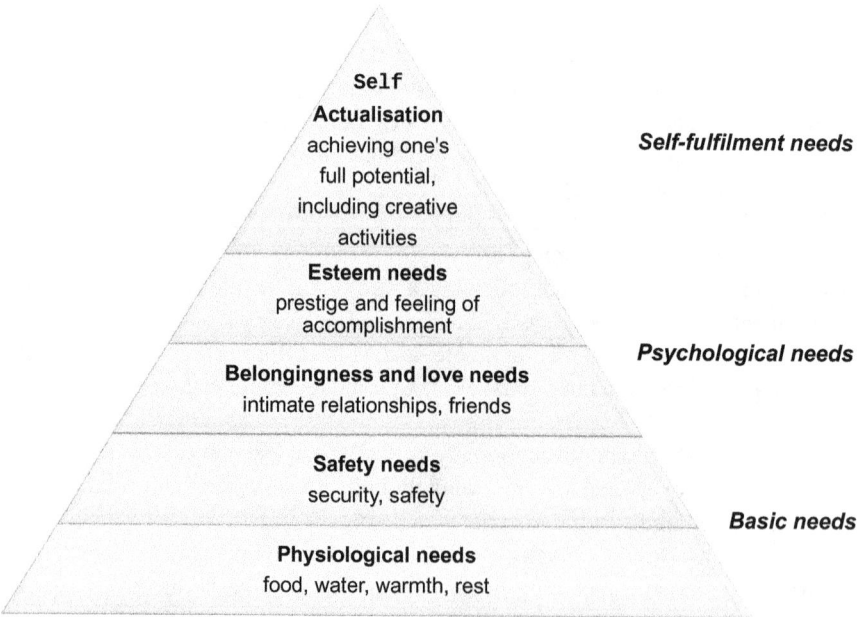

Self Actualisation
achieving one's full potential, including creative activities

Self-fulfilment needs

Esteem needs
prestige and feeling of accomplishment

Belongingness and love needs
intimate relationships, friends

Psychological needs

Safety needs
security, safety

Physiological needs
food, water, warmth, rest

Basic needs

FIGURE 2.1 Overview of Maslow's hierarchy of needs.

As an individual's priorities, needs and motivation will vary, these should be explored with the individual (and their family) as early as possible and regularly reviewed.

Promoting safety includes ensuring physical, mental and emotional wellbeing, ensuring effective person-centred care (Martín-Sanz, 2022). Each of these three factors is important and can both overlap and interact with each other. Supporting physical health may mean minimising the risk of falls, ensuring correct medication management and enabling access to exercise. While supporting mental health may mean ensuring they get sufficient social opportunities, mental stimulation and access to interests or hobbies. Emotional wellbeing may mean ensuring the patient has sufficient support from family, friends or professionals as well as opportunities to express and explore emotions. Whilst all three elements of keeping someone well are important, they are not independent of each other. This means that at times one may need to be prioritised over another. For example, to ensure mental wellbeing, accessing outdoor walks in the local park might be important to a particular individual. However, this puts them at risk physically as they are at an increased risk of falling when mobilising outdoors. The stroke survivor in this example has decided that they would like to prioritise their mental wellbeing over the potential physical risks. There are different ways of improving someone's safety depending on the risks to that person. Risks may be mitigated by use of equipment, altering the environment, adding in carer's support, providing a support network or with medical management.

What *barriers* to safety have you experienced? What *enablers* can you utilise to mitigate risks?

When considering the safety of stroke patients, safeguarding also needs to be considered. Safeguarding means protecting a person's health, wellbeing and human rights; enabling them to live free from harm, abuse and neglect (NHS England, no date a). It is an integral part of providing high-quality health care. NHS England Safeguarding identifies adults such as those receiving care in their own home and people with physical, sensory and mental impairments as being those at most risk and therefore in most need of protection. Stroke survivors will often fall into this category. All staff, whether they work in a hospital, a care home, general practice, community care, in the public or private sector have a responsibility to safeguard children and adults at risk of abuse or neglect (NHS England, no date a).

Safety versus rehabilitation

Keeping someone safe whilst ensuring rehabilitation continues to progress effectively can sometimes be difficult and conflicting. In order for someone to keep progressing, they need to be practising things that are just outside of their current abilities; often this means that it is not the safest way for them to be doing the activity. For example, someone is able to walk safely with a walking stick on their own, but their goal is to be able to walk unaided (without the walking

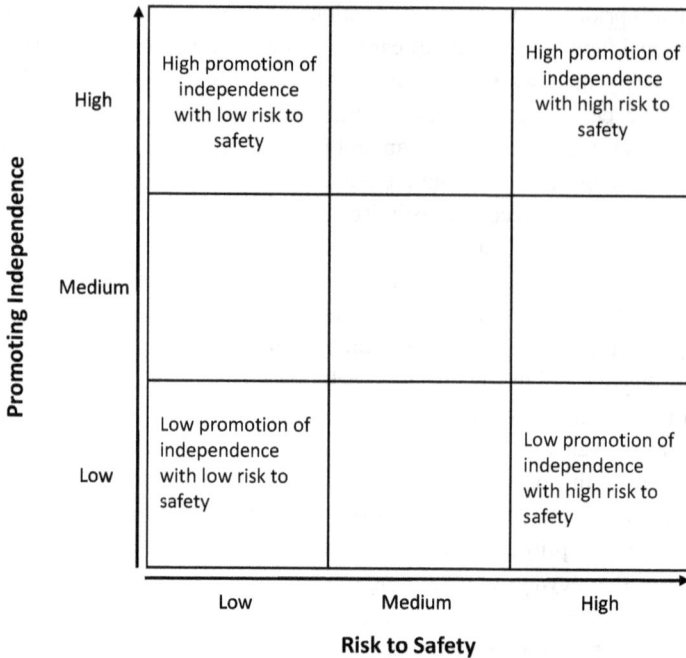

FIGURE 2.2 Link between promotion of independence and risk to safety.

stick) on their own. To achieve their goal, they will need to practise walking unaided. This comes with an increased risk of falls (compared to walking with the stick), but without practising walking unaided, they will not achieve their goal. Therefore, the patient's rehabilitation plan needs to be formed in a way that helps to minimise risks whilst still being effective to allow the individual to reach the desired goal.

Figure 2.2 shows how the lowest risk to safety often correlates to the lowest level of independence promotion, and the highest risk to safety is often associated with high promotion of independence. With careful risk management, independence can be promoted whilst minimising the risk to safety.

Figure 2.3 provides some ideas relating to risk management to consider when developing a rehabilitation plan: one suggestion is to complete a falls risk assessment. Stroke is a risk factor for falls (NICE, 2019) and falls occur in up to 73% of people within the first year after severe stroke (ISWP, 2023). About 40–60% of falls result in major lacerations, traumatic brain injuries, or fractures. Other complications of falls include distress, pain, loss of self-confidence, reduced quality of life, loss of independence, and mortality (NICE, 2019). NICE (2019) recommends that people at risk of falls should receive a multifactorial risk assessment by an appropriately skilled and experienced clinician, which should include assessment for gait and balance abnormalities.

Complete a falls risk assessment, a general risk assessment or a risk assessment related to a particular issue or concern.

Grade the difficulty of the task (i.e. small stepping stones towards the bigger goal).

Grade the level of support/supervision provided (i.e. gradually decreasing the support).

Ensure appropriate equipment choice.

Ensure appropriate level of support (to ensure safety, confidence but not 'over support'.

Only progress rehabilitation when the patient is mentally, emotionally and physically ready for the next step. Going back a step is always an option before progressing forwards again.

When identifying risks, try to ensure that they are small, measured risks that are unlikely to cause harm.

Try to ensure that a patient's progress is not being hindered by being overly risk adverse, ensure they remain challenged and moving forwards with their rehabilitation whilst being as safe as possible.

FIGURE 2.3   Risk management ideas to consider when developing rehabilitation plans.

Equipment and adaptations within the home environment

Equipment and home adaptations are a common way of minimising risks and maximising safety. Prior to discharge home from the stroke ward or rehabilitation unit, the occupational therapist will discuss potential changes that could be made to the home environment to reduce risks and help promote independence (Stroke Association, 2024). Some patients may have a home visit where they return to where they live for a short period of time. This will give the patient the chance to see how they will manage to get in and out of the property and transfer on and off the bed, chair and toilet and if applicable allows them to try the stairs and complete kitchen tasks. The occupational therapist will then be able to make recommendations for equipment and potential changes to the property or room layout which can be carried out prior to discharge home. Without a home visit, the occupational therapist will still be able to assess the patient in the hospital and gain some perspective on how they might cope at home. The occupational therapist will discuss with the patient and their support network what the home environment is like, how the individual managed to complete tasks before their stroke and how completion of tasks may differ post stroke (Stroke Association, 2024). This can be a challenging task for patients without a support network or with communication difficulties, and creativity might be required, as discussed in Chapter 3.

A quicker and easier alternative to a home visit is an access visit, where the occupational therapist will go out to assess the home environment and establish if there is enough space for new equipment that is required, such as a hospital bed, or wheelchair access. The occupational therapist, often alongside a physiotherapist, will advise the stroke survivor and provide the essential equipment either to take home from hospital or for delivery. Home visits and access visits used to be much more common; however, due to pressures for the freeing up of hospital beds and decreased staffing, they tend only to be organised where someone has major changes in their mobility or ability to transfer (Read *et al.*, 2020).

The ISWP guidelines (2023) state that the expectation is for patients to be discharged from hospital as early as possible, not only to avoid hospital-based complications, including risk of infection, but also to support the individual's preference. Recovery at home is comparable to remaining in hospital (NICE, 2023). A variety of approaches exist to support earlier discharges from hospital, dependent on geographical location. Early supported discharge teams exist to help facilitate a timely discharge and ensure someone is properly supported when they return home (ISWP, 2023). Another approach is the 'Discharge to Assess' pathway, which is also becoming more common. This is an approach used when patients no longer require hospital-based services but may still require care services and are supported to be discharged to their own home or appropriate community setting with short-term, funded support (Department of Health, 2024).

There are common changes suggested within the home environment to support independence and promote safety. These can include lifting or securing loose rugs and wires and moving furniture so that someone can move more easily around their home, particularly if they use a walking aid. Sometimes individuals may have previously used furniture to steady themselves when walking rather than using an aid (often called 'furniture walking'). If this is something that is their norm, then removing or moving furniture may cause more of a hazard. It is essential that the healthcare professionals work in collaboration with stroke survivors and their families to make suggestions for changes rather than imposing their own views about what is needed. There is a need for healthcare professionals to be mindful that any changes impacting someone's home could be a difficult and emotive concept for the person and their family. It is common to have memory and visual changes following stroke, and therefore, it can be helpful to keep the person's home surroundings as familiar as possible to reduce confusion and disorientation. Where space is limited, a potential compromise may be to convert a sitting room into a temporary bedroom for someone who is unable to manage stairs on discharge home.

Fatigue is common after stroke, and the home environment can be altered to ensure energy is conserved. This could mean arranging the items required for making a cup of tea so they are within easy reach rather than having to walk from one side of the kitchen to the other several times. Conversely, if the person's goal is to improve their mobility, it may be useful to position items further away to increase opportunities for mobilisation.

Many hospitals have a policy of only providing equipment essential for discharge. This could include a mobility aid as well as equipment to help someone transfer on and off the bed, chair and toilet. Getting in and out of the bath or shower would not normally be considered essential for discharge. The patient may be advised to have a strip wash initially until an assessment can be completed in their home environment by a community team who can then order further equipment as required. Onward referrals can be made if longer-term adaptations to the property are indicated, such as a level access shower or ramps to get in and out of the house. A disabled facilities grant may be available but is dependent on meeting certain eligibility criteria.

Different organisations, including hospital teams, early supported discharge services and social services, have their own eligibility criteria for what equipment can be provided and how quickly it is available. Other restrictions may apply, such as only providing one of a particular item, for example, a perching stool that is used to sit on when washing/dressing and then also in the kitchen. This may mean a family member or carer having to move the equipment from room to room as required and sometimes up and downstairs. Alongside variations between teams, there will also be differences in what can be provided depending on the geographical area (Royal College of Occupational Therapists, 2022), although work is being done across health and social care to agree on national standards and guidelines for more equitable provision (Scottish Government, 2023). General principles will apply, such as acute hospitals providing what is essential for discharge and referrals being made to community teams for longer-term equipment needs.

There is an increasing range of aids and technology available. This may be funded by healthcare, social care, charities or can be privately funded. It might be possible for people to try before they buy. Some aids are quite low cost, such as plate guards to prevent food slipping off the plate when feeding one-handed. Other aids are more expensive, such as a mobile arm support, which may help to take the weight of a weak arm to enable someone to feed themselves, particularly if their other side is also weak, perhaps from a previous stroke. Smart devices can be an option and can be set up to enable voice activation to facilitate tasks such as turning lights on and off, opening and shutting curtains and providing reminders to take medicines. Technology continues to improve rapidly, and it is worth searching online for what is currently available alongside contacting local organisations and charities with expertise in the area of assistive technology. Whilst there are specific charities for stroke (such as the Stroke Association, or Chest, Heart and Stroke

Scotland), other charities can be helpful for specific impairments, such as the Royal National Institute of Blind People, which can provide resources such as audiobooks and raised dots to mark settings on an oven or microwave.

Many people will have rehabilitation following stroke and see some recovery and improvement in function. It is therefore important to consider that equipment needs may change over time. This is worth keeping in mind, particularly when considering self-funding equipment. Table 2.1 provides a range of suggestions for aids that could support function post stroke to maximise safety and independence.

Look at Table 2.1 and consider all the different aids available. How would you feel about adding these changes to your home environment?

TABLE 2.1 Overview of suggested aids to support function

Functional activity	Aids available
Mobility	Walking stick
	Quad/Tri stick
	Zimmer frame +/− wheels
	3- or 4-wheeled walker
	Wheelchair +/− accessories
	Ramps
	Grab rails
	Stair rails
Transfers	Hoist
	Stand aid
	Transfer aids
	Slide Board
	Chair/bed raisers
	Bed lever
	Pillow lifter
	Profiling bed
	Slide sheet
	Leg lifter
Toileting	Urine bottle
	Static/wheeled commode
	Raised toilet seat +/− frame
	Catheter
	Urinary sheath
	Bidet toilet
Washing and dressing	Bath board/lift
	Shower stool/chair
	Perching stool
	Long-handled sponge
	Button hook
	Long-handled shoehorn
	Elasticated shoelaces
	Helping hand

TABLE 2.1 (Continued)

Functional activity	Aids available
Kitchen activities and eating/drinking	Kitchen trolley
	Perching stool
	Spike board
	Kettle tipper
	One-handed can opener
	Adaptive cutlery
	Plate guard
	Adapted drinking cups
	Over bed table
Pressure relief	Profiling bed
	Pressure relieving mattress
	Pressure relieving cushion
	Heel protection boots
Improving safety	Pill dispenser
	Memory aids, e.g., diary/calendar
	Bed/chair sensor
	Key safe
	Pendant alarm
	Smart speaker
	Camera systems

Involving patients in decision-making

> They need to ask the patient 'how do you want to do it?'
> *(Oxford Stroke Patient Group member)*

For healthcare professionals, courtesy and respect for the individual, shared decision-making and supporting patient choice are essential approaches (NHS England and NHS Improvement, 2019; NICE, 2024). Inclusion of the individual as part of interdisciplinary planning at any stage following a stroke is essential, as shared decision-making is at the centre of person-centred stroke-related goals, patient choice and control (NICE, 2023). This also reflects the 'No decision about me, without me' approach from the Department of Health (2012). This should result in facilitated collaborative decision-making that ensures the stroke-skilled multidisciplinary team works with the person and their family towards achievable, individualised, meaningful goals (ISWP, 2023). It is also acknowledged that shared decision-making is a key component of universal personalised care (NHS England, no date b) and that the stroke survivor's goals should assist in determining the rehabilitation pathway (ISWP, 2023).

One of the priorities of the NHS Long Term Plan is for people to gain control over their own health and have more personalised care (Department of Health and Social Care, 2025). It is recommended that stroke patients are actively involved in their rehabilitation and that their feelings, wishes and expectations for recovery are understood and acknowledged (ISWP, 2023). It is expected that specialist multidisciplinary teams made up of skilled professionals will work together to deliver goal-directed rehabilitation. This is with the aim of helping stroke survivors to relearn any lost skills, improve their quality of life and maximise independence (NICE, 2023). However, the stroke survivor's preferences may differ from the healthcare professional's opinions and ideas regarding the approach to recovery.

> Therapists have to be realistic – what will the person really do when staff are not there? So, for example if therapist is saying wear this particular shoe because it is best and safest, but they suspect that when they are gone the person will revert to their comfy shoe, then the therapist should deal with the reality and make that the best it can be.
>
> *(Oxford Stroke Patient Group member)*

It is important that the healthcare professional takes time to understand the person behind the 'patient'. A person-centred approach is required to ensure the individual's preferences are part of the assessment and discharge plan. In the acute setting, discharge is often the priority to maintain patient flow, where patients typically spend 72 hours on a hyperacute stroke unit (Stroke Association, 2022b). There is therefore often insufficient time to fully explore a patient's wishes. Following discharge, there is more opportunity for the healthcare professional to get to know the patient in their home environment and be able to create more meaningful goals with that person. However, there may still be some time pressures dependent on local service provision.

Guidelines state that patients should be given the opportunity to participate in goal setting unless they prefer not to or are unable to participate due to cognitive and language impairments (ISWP, 2023). NICE (2023) outlines that healthcare professionals need to enable the post-stroke individual with communication difficulties to express their wishes and support them to understand and participate in everyday and major life decisions. Speech and language therapists can help in facilitating communication and providing choices in alternate forms such as the use of pictures or in written form. The National Stroke Service Model outlines that patients should be given the opportunity to take ownership of their rehabilitation through goal setting and developing a personalised plan (NHS, 2021).

The ISWP (2023) states that during goal-setting meetings, healthcare professionals should ensure that each individual is provided with an accessible-format explanation of their goal-setting process and information needed for their rehabilitation. Additionally, after each goal-setting meeting, the individual should be provided with copies of their agreed goals. Communication of risks, benefits and consequences should also be explored as part of shared decision-making (NICE, 2023).

Advocacy

Practitioners should ensure that stroke survivors, particularly those with established capacity impairments, are aware of advocacy services (ISWP, 2023). Local authorities are required to offer independent advocacy services (NICE, 2018). This provision should include support to enable decision-making about fundamental parts of life, including medical treatment, property and personal welfare, and facilitating involvement in decisions made in the stroke survivor's best interests under the Mental Capacity Act (NICE, 2018). However, every healthcare professional should also act as an advocate for the stroke survivor ensuring effective support for shared decision-making.

A patient decides to not follow your advice relating to an activity. You are concerned about the safety implications of this, but their capacity is not in question. How do you continue to offer support?

Duty of care

Healthcare professionals have a duty of care to ensure capacity or lack of capacity is established. Capacity can fluctuate for a variety of reasons in the stroke survivor, so each time a decision needs to be made, capacity should be re-established. Once capacity to make a particular decision has been decided, then the patient may choose to go against what has been advised. If the patient has been deemed not to have capacity to make a particular decision, the healthcare professional has a duty to take steps to increase the person's safety. The law imposes a duty of care on all healthcare professionals in situations where any practitioner might cause harm to patients through their actions or omissions, as a reasonable standard of care is required. This exists when the practitioner has assumed responsibility for the patient's care and is not optional (Chartered Society of Physiotherapy, 2022; Royal College of Nursing, 2023).

Family involvement in decision-making/capacity compromised

The benefits of family involvement in decision-making have been acknowledged, as this can help achieve more satisfactory outcomes. This is highlighted specifically in the context of severe stroke (Visvanathan *et al.*, 2017). If an individual lacks capacity and a family member has power of attorney, then their inclusion in discussions and planning is as important as the individual's. However, even if the stroke survivor lacks capacity for any reason, whether short or long term, every attempt should still be made to involve that individual as much as possible in the decision-making process (ISWP, 2023).

Support for the family of stroke survivors is essential, and the ISWP (2023) outlines that long-term support services should ensure that the family/carers of people with stroke:

- are aware that their needs can be assessed separately;
- are able to access the advice, support and help they need;
- are provided with information, equipment and appropriate training (e.g. manual handling) to enable them to care for a person with stroke;
- have their need for information and support reassessed whenever there is a significant change in circumstances (e.g. if the health of the family member/carer or the individual changes).

Medication management

The stroke survivor will potentially continue to deal with a range of issues, including physical disabilities and cognitive issues for the rest of their life (Yetzer et al., 2017). Any of these issues have the potential to impact medication safety for a variety of reasons.

Compliance with a medication regimen for the individual following a stroke can be important for a range of reasons, including:

- Treatment of conditions resulting from stroke complications, including spasticity, nausea, urinary and chest infections, and support for continence
- Secondary prevention post stroke
- Continuing management of long-term conditions that contributed to the individual's stroke risk, including atrial fibrillation (AF), high cholesterol and diabetes
- Short- and long-term pain management (ISWP, 2023).

Management of these issues through a variety of approaches is important to promote independence and maintain safety for an individual. Pharmacological support approaches are the most common intervention in health care. Medication administration will require the stroke survivor to have a range of knowledge and skills to ensure medicine adherence and/or external support, depending on post-stroke impairments (Yetzer et al., 2017).

Behaviour associated with medicine taking is complex and individual, and there are many reasons for lack of adherence. Non-intentional non-adherence with medicines is where there are reasons or factors beyond the individuals control that impact medicine taking. Intentional non-adherence with medicines occurs when the individual makes a deliberate decision not to follow the prescribed drug regime (De Simoni, Mant and Sutton, 2015). Issues with medicine adherence are acknowledged within stroke literature, with adherence to secondary prevention medicines in the first years following stroke identified as a significant issue (Glader *et al.*, 2010).

> It's a disaster for me ... because so far I have had a couple of days on beta blockers where I just felt really, really weird and really strange and a bit like I had too much to drink and felt tipsy, but not really aware of my surroundings and uncomfortable in my own body... it is really hard sometimes.
>
> *(Jo, 47, embolic stroke as a result of endocarditis, 20 years post stroke)*

There are potential challenges to adherence due to side effects of a change in secondary prevention medications. In those with cognitive issues following stroke, it is also acknowledged that medicine adherence is more likely to be adversely impacted (Rohde *et al.*, 2017). Specific factors that can predict medicine adherence in the stroke survivor include:

- Knowledge
- Beliefs about medicines, including overuse
- Anger
- Lack of support for medicine taking
- Severity of stroke and specific neurological defects (e.g. hemiplegia, swallowing impairment and short-term memory issues)
- Concerns about treatment
- Polypharmacy (managing a complex range of medications)
- Disruptive side effects (Arkan *et al.*, 2022; Gibson, Coupe and Watkins, 2021).

Despite the commonality and necessity of inclusion of family or carers in education to support medicine adherence (Gibson, Coupe and Watkins, 2021), there may also be issues with adherence relating to the carer's ability or willingness to support. However, evidence is lacking on how carers may affect adherence in stroke survivors reliant on support (Gibson, Coupe and Watkins, 2021). For example, a carer could withhold medicine or give a lower dose, or a carer could forget to have a prescription refilled or not give the medicines at the right time.

Polypharmacy is a growing complex issue that affects many people when using a variety of medicines. Polypharmacy is not simply about the number of medicines needed, it can occur because medicines continue to be prescribed when no longer needed, when the potential for harm from medicines outweighs the potential benefit, or when the practicalities of medicines used cause harm or distress or become unmanageable (Royal Pharmaceutical Society, 2023). Polypharmacy and specifically use of potentially inappropriate medications is also a common issue following a stroke, with this particularly the case for older people post stroke, with the potential for negative impact on activities of daily living (Matsumoto *et al.,* 2022). It is established that stroke survivors have a heightened risk of experiencing polypharmacy due to the importance of controlling blood pressure, cholesterol levels and blood glucose levels. Additionally, stroke survivors are likely to have a range of long-term conditions, including hypertension, diabetes and high cholesterol as part of cardiovascular disease, that may have contributed to their risk of stroke (Matsumoto *et al.,* 2022).

> You read the leaflet, you read the instructions on the box, and go do what it says ... actually in reality sometimes it's really hard to manage your own meds when you've got lots of other meds as well.
>
> *(Jo, 47, embolic stroke as a result of endocarditis, 20 years post stroke)*

Due to the range of medicines required following a stroke, a regular review of medication is important. Common medicines include analgesia, psychotropics, anti-hypertensives and beta blockers (Matsumoto *et al.,* 2022), which may have side effects that can cause dizziness and weakness, which could contribute to an already increased risk of falls (ISWP, 2023).

Pain is a common issue experienced by stroke survivors, including post-stroke pain. Musculoskeletal pain is also experienced following a stroke due to prolonged immobility and posture issues that can not only be the direct cause of pain, but also exacerbate pre-existing long-term conditions, e.g., osteoarthritis (ISWP, 2023). Any of these situations can lead to complex and long-term management of pain needs. Some stroke survivors report issues with pain flares despite the range of non-pharmacological and pharmacological approaches utilised.

> I've learnt that when I'm having really bad pain flares that I need to have a record by my bed and just write down the time I took my last meds ... because quite often the pain medication runs out before the hours when you are allowed to take meds again.
>
> *(Jo, 47, embolic stroke as a result of endocarditis, 20 years post stroke)*

Effective assessment to identify any impairments and abilities enables the healthcare professional to support the individual, their family, and any care providers in techniques, methods, and aids for safe medicines management (ISWP, 2023). Careful documentation should provide key information about the individual outlining abilities, knowledge and challenges with medicines management. This ensures effective follow-up across health care providers and continuity of support (Yetzer *et al.,* 2015).

Clear, accessible information on medication regimen and associated common side effects	Setting alarms or using reminder lists	Documentation and monitoring of administration and adherence
Ensuring effective, updated information is provided to the individual and/or their family/carers following any review, hospital admission or appointment	Effective engagement with family and carers who will provide medication support, if indicated	Provision of medication in a form that can support the individual's needs: tablets, liquids or dispersible tablets, skin patches, sub lingual/buccal, sub-cutaneous injectables
Regular review by GP, community pharmacist and any specialist services providing the individual with ongoing support, including structured medicines reviews to ensure medicine prescriptions are still appropriate	Provision of support, dependent on issues such as dexterity and cognition that can include – safe storage, dossette box, medicines dispensing devices, large print labels, non-child proof lids (if safe to do so)	

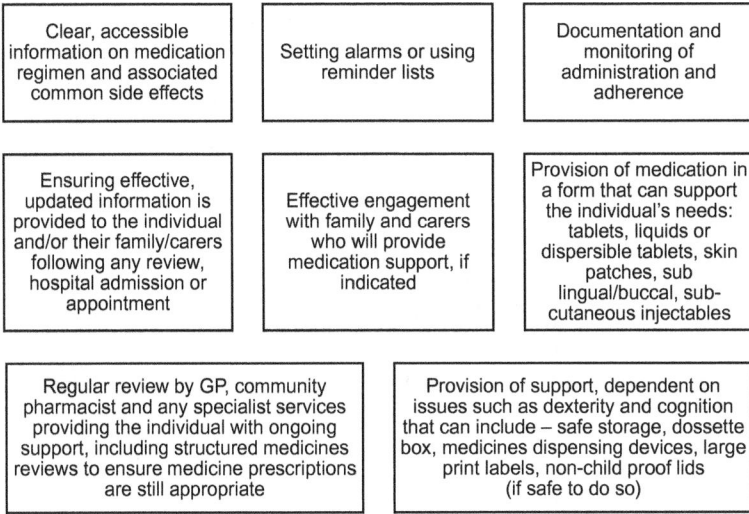

FIGURE 2.4 Education approaches to support medication safety and adherence.

Sources: Matsumoto *et al.*, (2022), NHS England (no date c), ISWP (2023).

Education to support the stroke survivor and their family is a key element for rehabilitation (ISWP, 2023). Figure 2.4 provides an overview of the education that should be provided by healthcare professionals to support medication safety and adherence for the individual post stroke.

I have learnt the hard way that actually you need more education... In the past I've made mistakes [with medications] and then you've got the fear that that's going to have long term effects or you're actually gonna overdose.

(Jo, 47, embolic stroke as a result of endocarditis, 20 years post stroke)

Quality of life post stroke is acknowledged as correlating with medicine adherence beyond simple morbidity and mortality statistics (Cevik, Tekir and Kaya, 2018). Therefore, medicine adherence issues could highlight the potential for poor outcomes before they are obvious and assist healthcare professionals in identifying and addressing wider issues for the stroke survivor. Problems can occur, including emergency admission to hospital related to medicine non-adherence or errors in administration, making this an important issue. However, all decisions relating to stroke recovery, rehabilitation and risk prevention through medicine use and adherence should follow the principles of shared decision-making. This can promote support from family and carers and improves the individual's engagement to ensure plans made are effective for that individual, improving the likelihood of medicine safety and adherence.

Anyone can check with the stroke survivor to ascertain if they have any concerns about their medicines and how the medicines are impacting them on a day-to-day basis, it doesn't need to be the prescriber or a pharmacist.

As a practitioner, reflect on whether your approach to the post-stroke patient supports the need for independence and safety effectively.

You could consider:

- Are your goals the same as the patient's goals?
- What is important to that person?
- What is realistic for that person?
- What limitations exist for that individual? For example financial, environmental, functional ability

Conclusion

This chapter has outlined a range of issues relating to independence and safety. Rehabilitation priorities should reflect a person-centred approach, focusing on engagement with the individual and their families or care-givers through shared decision-making. It should be recognised that independence means different things to different people, and maintaining safety encompasses physical, mental, and emotional wellbeing. Care and rehabilitation plans must be individualised to maximise each person's independence and safety.

Healthcare professionals should be aware of the variety of aids, equipment, and home adaptations available to support safety, rehabilitation, and independence. The management of medications following a stroke involves complex considerations that must take into account the individual's preferences and specific needs. In all aspects of post-stroke management, he individual's choices should be respected, even when they may not align with what is considered the optimal approach for safety.

References

American Stroke Association (2021) *Rebuilding identity: a critical step in recovery.* Available at: www.stroke.org/en/stroke-connection/stroke-onward/rebuilding-identity--a-critical-step-in-recovery

Arkan, G., Sarigol Ordin, Y., Ozturk, V., and Ala, R. (2022) 'Investigation of medication adherence and factors affecting it in patients with stroke', *Journal of Neuroscience Nursing*, 54(1), pp. 35–41. https://doi.org/10.1097/JNN.0000000000000621

Cambridge Dictionary (no date) *Meaning of independence in English.* Available at: https://dictionary.cambridge.org/us/dictionary/english/independence

Cevik, C., Tekir, O., and Kaya, A. (2018) 'Stroke patients' quality of life and compliance with the treatment', *Acta Medica Mediterranea*, 34, pp. 839–846. https://doi.org/10.19193/0393-6384_2018_3_128

Chartered Society of Physiotherapy (2022) *Duty of care.* Available at: www.csp.org.uk/publi cations/duty-care

Department of Health (2012) *Liberating the NHS: no decision about me, without me.* Available at: www.gov.uk/government/publications/government-response-to-the-consu ltation-on-proposals-for-greater-patient-involvement-and-more-choice

Department of Health (2024) *Statutory guidance – hospital discharge and community support guidance.* Available at: www.gov.uk/government/publications/hospital-discha rge-and-community-support-guidance/hospital-discharge-and-community-support- guidance

Department of Health and Social Care (2025) *Fit for the future: 10 year health plan for England.* Available at: www.gov.uk/government/publications/10-year-health-plan-for- england-fit-for-the-future

De Simoni, A., Mant, J., and Sutton, S. (2015) 'Adherence to medication in stroke survivors dependent on caregivers', *British Journal of General Practice*, 65(640), pp. e789–e791. https://doi.org/10.3399/bjgp15X687589

Gibson, J., Coupe, J., and Watkins, C. (2021) 'Medication adherence early after stroke: using the perceptions and practicalities framework to explore stroke survivors', informal carers' and nurses' experiences of barriers and solutions', *Journal of Research in Nursing*, 26(6), pp. 499–514. https://doi.org/10.1177/1744987121993505

Glader, E., Sjölander, M., Kriksson, M., and Lundberg, M. (2010) 'Persistent use of secondary preventive drugs declines rapidly during the first 2 years after stroke', *Stroke*, 41, pp. 397–401. https://doi.org/10.1161/STROKEAHA.109.566950

Intercollegiate Stroke Working Party (ISWP) (2023) *National clinical guideline for stroke for the United Kingdom and Northern Ireland.* 5th Edition. London. Available at: www. strokeguideline.org

Martín-Sanz, M.B., Salazar-de-la-Guerra, R.M., Cuenca-Zaldivar, J.N., Salcedo-Perez- Juana, M., Garcia-Bravo, C., and Palacios-Ceña, D. (2022) 'Person-centred care in individuals with stroke: a qualitative study using in-depth interviews', *Annals of Medicine*, 54(1), pp. 2167–2180. https://doi.org/10.1080/07853890.2022.2105393

Matsumoto, A., Yoshimura, Y., Nagano, F., Bise, T., Kido, Y., Shmazu, S., and Sharaishi, A. (2022) 'Polypharmacy and potentially inappropriate medications in stroke rehabilitation: prevalence and association with outcomes', *International Journal of Clinical Pharmacy*, 44(3), pp. 749–761. https://doi.org/10.1007/s11096-022-01416-5

NHS (2021) *National Stroke Service Model.* Available at: www.england.nhs.uk/wp-content/ uploads/2021/05/stroke-service-model-may-2021.pdf

NHS (2022) *Recovery from a stroke.* Available at: www.nhs.uk/conditions/stroke/recov ery/#:~:text=The%20injury%20to%20the%20brain,the%20symptoms%20and%20th eir%20severity

NHS England (no date a) *About NHS England safeguarding.* Available at: www.england. nhs.uk/safeguarding/about/#:~:text=Safeguarding%20means%20protecting%20a%20 citizen's,providing%20high%2Dquality%20health%20care

NHS England (no date b) *Shared decision-making.* Available at: www.england.nhs.uk/perso nalisedcare/shared-decision-making/

NHS England (no date c) *Structured medication reviews and medicines optimisation.* Available at: www.england.nhs.uk/primary-care/pharmacy/smr/

NHS England and NHS Improvement (2019) *Shared decision-making: summary guide.* Available at: www.england.nhs.uk/publication/shared-decision-making-summary- guide/

NICE (2018) *Decision-making and mental capacity.* Available at: www.nice.org.uk/guida nce/ng108

NICE (2019) *Falls risk assessment.* Available at: https://cks.nice.org.uk/topics/falls-risk-ass essment/ (accessed 18 January 2024).

NICE (2023) *Stroke rehabilitation in adults.* Available at: www.nice.org.uk/guidance/ng236

NICE (2024) *Shared decision making.* Available at: www.nice.org.uk/about/what-we-do/ our-programmes/nice-guidance/nice-guidelines/shared-decision-making

Read, J., Jones, N., Fegan, C., Cudd, P., Simpson, E., Mazumdar, S., and Ciravegna, F. (2020) 'Remote home visit: exploring the feasibility, acceptability and potential benefits of using digital technology to undertake occupational therapy home assessments', *British Journal of Occupational Therapy*, 83(10), pp. 648–658. https://doi.org/10.1177/03080 22620921111

Rohde, D., Williams, D., Gaynor, E., Bennett, K., Dolan, E., Callaly, E., Large, M., and Hickey, A. (2017) 'Secondary prevention and cognitive function after stroke: a study protocol for a 5-year follow-up of the ASPIRE-S cohort', *BMJ Open*, 7(3), p. e014819. https://doi.org/10.1136/bmjopen-2016-014819

Royal College of Nursing (RCN) (2023) *Duty of care.* Available at: www.rcn.org.uk/Get-Help/RCN-advice/duty-of-care

Royal College of Occupational Therapists (2022) *Guidance on the provision of community equipment and housing adaptations – 20 21-22- RCOT response.* Available at: www.rcot.co.uk/practice-resources/policy-legislation/consultations/clo sed/scotland

Royal Pharmaceutical Society (2023) *Polypharmacy: getting our medicines right.* Available at: www.rpharms.com/recognition/setting-professional-standards/polypharmacy-getting-our-medicines-right#key

Scottish Government (2023) *Equipment and adaptations: guidance on provision.* Available at: www.gov.scot/publications/guidance-provision-equipment-adaptations-2/

Stroke Association (2016) *State of the Nation.* Available at: www.stroke.org.uk/sites/default/ files/state_of_the_nation_2016_110116_0.pdf

Stroke Association (2022a) *Occupational therapy after stroke.* Available at: www.stroke. org.uk/resources/occupational-therapy-after-stroke

Stroke Association (2022b) *Transforming and reorganising acute stroke services – rebuilding lives after stroke.* Available at: www.stroke.org.uk/sites/default/files/new_pd fs_2019/our_policy_position/psp_-_reorganising_acute_stroke_services_0.pdf

Stroke Association (2024) *Occupational therapy.* Available at: www.stroke.org.uk/life-after-stroke/occupational-therapy

Visvanathan, A., Dennis, M., Mead, G., Whiteley, W. N., Lawton, J., and Doubal, F. N. (2017) 'Shared decision making after severe stroke—How can we improve patient and family involvement in treatment decisions?', *International Journal of Stroke*, 12(9), pp. 920–922.

Yetzer, E., Blake, K., Goetsch, N., Shook, M., and St. Paul, M. (2015) 'SAFE medication management for patients with physical impairments of stroke, part one', *Rehabilitation Nursing*, 40, pp. 260–266. https://doi.org/10.1002/rnj.194

Yetzer, E., Blake, K., Goetsch, N., Shook, M., and St. Paul, M. (2017) 'SAFE medication management for patients with physical impairments of stroke, part two', *Rehabilitation Nursing*, 42(5), pp. 282–289. https://doi.org/10.1002/rnj.286

Yun, S.M., Lee, S.Y., Sohn, M.K., Lee, J., Kim, D.Y., Lee, S.G., Shin, Y.I., Lee, Y.S., Joo, M.C., Lee, S.Y., Han, J., Ahn, J., Oh, G.J., Lee, Y.H., Chang, W.H., and Kim, Y.H. (2020) 'Factors associated with changes in functional independence after six months of ischemic stroke', *Brain & Neurorehabilitation*, 13(3), e19. https://doi.org/10.12786/bn.2020.13.e19

3

COMMUNICATION

Claire Hartley

In collaboration with the South Birmingham (BCU) Conversation Group and Family Group

Learning objectives

- To understand how communication can be affected after a stroke.
- To examine ways to communicate more effectively with stroke survivors who have a communication disability.
- To gain an insight into the impact of communication disability on life after a stroke.
- To develop knowledge and skills to promote best practice in all aspects of communication with stroke survivors and their relatives.

Background

Approximately two-thirds of stroke survivors have communication problems directly after their stroke (Stroke Association, 2021). Long-term (chronic or life-altering) difficulties are experienced by a third of these survivors (Stroke Association, 2021). Additionally, stroke survivors with communication difficulties are more likely to experience depression than those without (Kauhanen *et al.*, 2000). National Institute for Health and Care Excellence (NICE, 2023) recommends that a screen for communication difficulties is completed within 72 hours of the onset of a stroke. No matter the clinical setting, healthcare professionals are likely to meet stroke survivors with communication disabilities.

This chapter will provide readers with an overview of what is considered best practice around communication in healthcare after a stroke, with a particular focus on stroke survivors who are living with a communication difference/disability. The views shared here represent those of Experts by Experience (EbyE) and their family members but may not be everyone's experience due to the unique nature of

DOI: 10.4324/9781003426196-4

stroke and recovery. It is hoped that by sharing our stories, we can help the reader to understand the impact of communication disability and the role that healthcare professionals can have in improving stroke care for this population. We hope to use our experiences to inspire and give hope.

> You have to have hope, because without hope what is there?
> *(Karen, family member)*

Through sharing our resources and stories and trying out our practical tips, healthcare professionals can make life a little easier for a stroke survivor and improve the care they receive.

Take an honest look at what you already know and the skills you already have in working with people with communication difficulties. Any steps taken from here will improve your practice. Consider the following questions:

- How might someone's communication be affected following a stroke?
- What are your current skills that help patients communicate with you?
- What do you do now that helps your patients to have a conversation with you?

Communication fundamentals

Everyone has different communication strengths and challenges. Stroke survivors are no exception, and the addition of post-stroke communication disability will impact this further. It is recommended that healthcare professionals consider the communication needs of *everyone* they meet, maximising the potential for success by being mindful of differences as well as disability. Being unwell, in hospital, feeling scared and vulnerable are enough of a challenge without increased communication support needs. These arise not just because of communication disability but also due to age-related hearing loss, visual difficulties or other medical conditions, for example, previous stroke, head and neck cancer, cerebral palsy or Downs syndrome. Additionally, the individual might speak a different language to that in which care is provided. Zingelman *et al.* (2024) identified that two-thirds of patients needed increased communication support to participate in their healthcare activities.

Swaydon *et al.* (2012) in a study of doctor–patient interaction found that sitting instead of standing at someone's bedside leads to increased satisfaction. Participants perceived that those doctors had spent three times as long with them compared to the control group, despite the time difference being minimal. Sitting also makes it easier to see each other's face, use resources to support conversations and promote a more relaxed interaction. Care should also be taken to maximise the stroke survivor's communication abilities, and following this study, pulling up a chair is included (see Table 3.1). This can support access to therapies, care and

TABLE 3.1 Communication fundamentals checklist

Vision

Does the person normally wear glasses/contact lenses, especially for reading?
Are they currently wearing their glasses?
Are the glasses clean?
Do they need an assessment of their vision? (NICE, 2023, recommendation
   1.8.1 offer a specialist orthoptist assessment as soon as possible)

Hearing

Do they usually wear hearing aid(s)?
Are the hearing aids in and switched on?
Are the hearing aids working? (For example, do they need batteries/charging?)
Screen for hearing problems completed (NICE, 2023, recommendation 1.9.1)

Mouth

Is their mouth clear of debris and moist?
Do they have a denture (full, partial)?
Is the denture in?
Does it fit? Do they need denture adhesive?

Positioning

Pull up a chair and sit together.
Sit at equal eye level if possible.

---

decision-making. This is particularly pertinent in the acute care setting where the stroke survivor may not be personally responsible for all their belongings or may have attended as an emergency and not brought all of their usual communication aids with them.

Typical communication

Communication is a wonderful, complex, human activity that allows us to express ideas and feelings, make decisions, build and maintain relationships and access education, occupation and health and social care. The way in which we understand typical communication is still evolving due to modern imaging techniques and research studies looking at language recovery after stroke. This includes new models of language processing, such as Hickok and Poeppel's dual stream model (Nasios *et al.*, 2019). Figure 3.1 shows a much-simplified illustration of what is sometimes known as the brain-language network, as a contrast to the perhaps more well-known Broca–Wernicke–Lictheim–Gerschind model (Nasios *et al.*, 2019).

Once the thalamus sends the speech motor plan via the central nervous system, a complex process of movement occurs to produce normal-sounding speech. This process is illustrated in Figure 3.2.

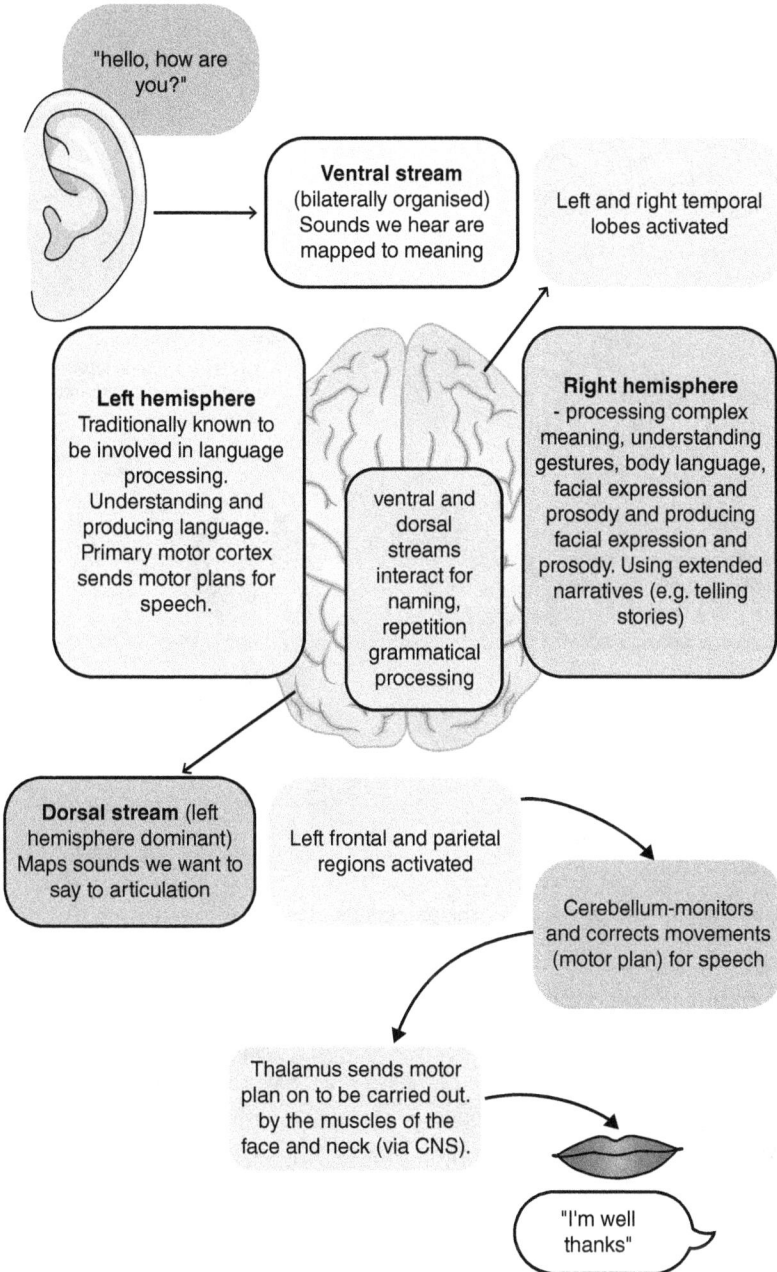

FIGURE 3.1 Brain-language network.

Sources: Using ideas from Nasios *et al.* (2019) and Manasco (2021).

Movement of the lips, tongue, jaw & soft palate, changes the shape & volume of the oral cavity to produce range of sounds.

The nasal cavities and sinuses amplify sound vibration

Varying intensity & frequency of vocal fold vibration changes loudness & pitch respectively. This, along with changes in rate & rhythm give rise to prosody used to signify sarcasm, different meanings etc.

Vocal folds come together vibrating to provide voicing for sounds e.g. vowels and b, d, g, dg z in English

Respiration-generates airflow & provides power for speech

Phrenic nerve innervates diaphragm, controlling respiration

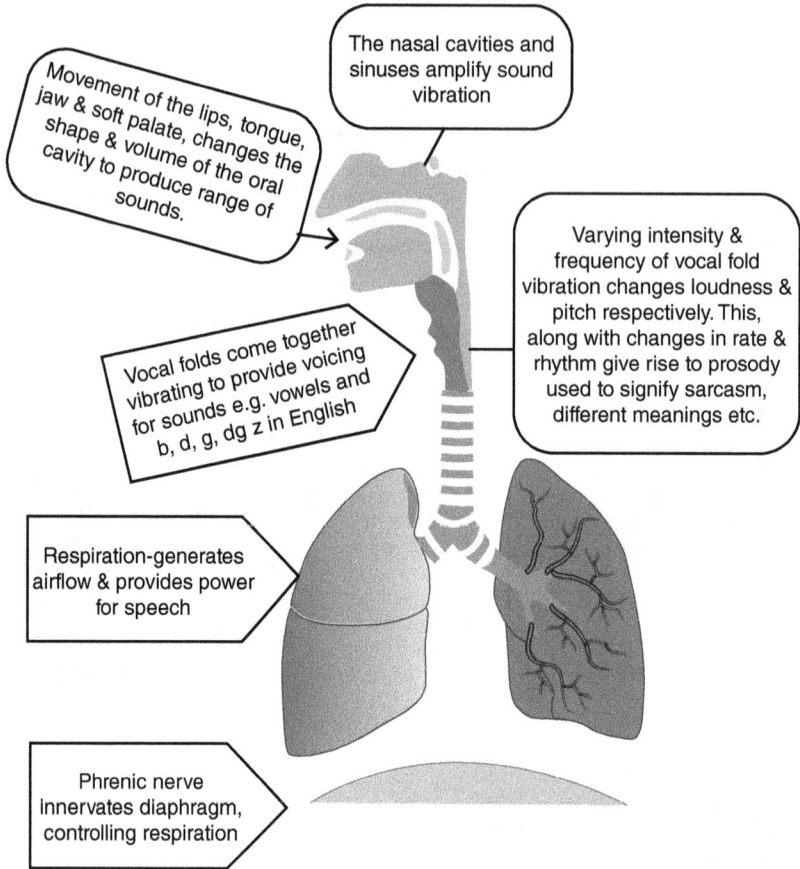

FIGURE 3.2   Speech production – the process involved in articulating words.

Communication disability after stroke

The neurological consequences of stroke can cause difficulty with speech, language or both at the same time. Speech is how we say the words, and if there is difficulty, this is a speech disorder. Language is associated with our ability to understand others, express ideas and convey them, and several areas of the brain play a critical part in normal function (Stroke Association, 2021).

> It is depressing as I know what to say; my brain is the size of a planet, but my delivery is flawed – classic aphasia I think.
>
> *(Jeremy, 69, haemorrhagic stroke, 12 years post stroke)*

Speech and language therapists (SLT) work with this population to identify the nature of the difficulty and provide the stroke survivor with a diagnosis of one or more of the following communication disabilities. When working with communication disability, the SLT will support the individual, as well as significant others in their life. They may, for example, train communication partners (their family or friends) as well as the stroke survivor, giving advice on how best to maximise communication. They will also support staff working with the stroke survivor as well as advocating for individuals to get the support they need.

The specific communication disabilities are:

• Aphasia
• Cognitive-communication disorder
• Dysarthria
• Apraxia of speech

Aphasia (pronounced a-fay-zee-uh or a-fay-zyuh)

In the United Kingdom, the term dysphasia is sometimes used, although international consensus has called for the use of the term *aphasia* to reduce confusion and improve awareness of the disability (Worrall *et al.*, 2016). Around 350,000 people in the United Kingdom have aphasia (Say Aphasia, 2023). In aphasia, the neurological damage caused by the stroke impacts areas of the complex brain-language network, and consequently, the stroke survivor develops an acquired *language difficulty* affecting their ability to use language in every form (see Table 3.2).

A stroke survivor describes his initial experience of aphasia following his stroke:

Locked in because getting out (gestures movement from mouth outwards) no way (waves hand across mouth to indicate no) but in my head fine, but slowly, slowly (cycles hand round in a circle to demonstrate slow movement) … it was really good, 6 months, a year, every day [meaning that he was getting better and better].

(Damian, 55, ischaemic stroke, 8 years post stroke)

I was terrified at that stage because I was on my own. I didn't understand what was happening.

(Jan, 80, ischaemic stroke,14 years post stroke)

People with aphasia will have different strengths, needs or impairments in the different domains of language. Everyone with aphasia is different. The impact of aphasia means people with aphasia can find it difficult to participate in everyday

TABLE 3.2 The different domains/forms of language affected

	Difficulty understanding what people say Described as comprehension or receptive language difficulties
Sometimes people with aphasia will talk about *not hearing it* or *not getting it*. Family and the person themselves may think they have hearing difficulties, but it is often comprehension challenges. People with aphasia need more time to process and understand something that is said to them.	
	Difficulty finding the right words Described as anomia
	Difficulty putting sentences or longer stories together or having a conversation. Described as discourse or narrative difficulties
Producing sentences, stories or understanding 'turns' in conversation requires the speaker to find the words needed, combine them in the right order, with any grammatical markers needed, such as adding a plural or using the past tense (referred to as morphology and syntax).	
	Difficulty reading (aloud or in their head and understanding what they have read) Described as alexia
	Difficulty writing (spelling words correctly and putting words into sentences) Described as agraphia
	Difficulty understanding and using numbers in communication Described as dyscalculia
Numbers require complete accuracy, which makes them particularly challenging for some people with aphasia. For example, getting one digit wrong in a phone number means the person cannot call you. Misunderstand the date for an appointment, and you become a 'did not attend'.	

communicative acts such as conversations with friends, reading a menu, ordering food in a café or writing a birthday card or text message. Aphasia does not affect a person's intelligence. If communication partners do not make accommodations, people with aphasia can struggle to reveal their competent selves (Kagan, 1998), but with support to use additional communication methods, people can be highly successful. Unfortunately, people with aphasia are frequently treated as if they are not intelligent individuals as Jo and Kelly explain:

> That stupidness that you feel – that judgement. You have that, you feel awkward.
>
> *(Kelly, 55, ischaemic stroke, 7 years post stroke)*

> I felt sometimes quite frustrated that people assumed that I didn't understand what was going on because I couldn't verbalise my responses. There were times when people (nurses and doctors) would wait and ask Mum and Dad questions, and they were things I could have answered in a written response myself and that was quite frustrating.
>
> *(Jo, 47, embolic stroke as a result of endocarditi, 20 years post stroke)*

Types of aphasia

There are labels attached to aphasia, including global, fluent, or Broca's. There are in fact 30 different classification systems for aphasia (documented in Copland *et al.*, 2018), some of which are based on outdated science, others which are emerging, none of which are perfect. As experts in the field of aphasiology, Copland and colleagues state that for the moment, people with aphasia are 'best served by careful description of their signs and symptoms' (LaPointe and Stierwalt, 2018, p.31) rather than shorthand, inadequate labels. Whilst most healthcare professionals will have met someone with aphasia, it is unlikely they will be aware of the full range of aphasia symptoms. The next activity is offered to illustrate this.

Look at the following videos of two different people with aphasia. Their aphasia is described using the fluent/non-fluent classification. They are offered to explore the significantly different language symptoms experienced by someone with aphasia.

Fluent Aphasia: Meet Byron. Visit www.youtube.com/watch?v=3oef68YabD0 Someone with a fluent aphasia can say a lot, but the meaning can be unclear to the listener. The person with aphasia typically finds understanding what is said to them difficult (receptive language).

Non-fluent Aphasia: Meet Mike. www.youtube.com/watch?v=JWC-cVQmEmY Someone with a non-fluent aphasia can usually understand quite well but will struggle to find the words they want to say, and there can be frequent hesitations. They may sound 'telegrammatic' – only key words are said with the 'joining words' missing. Consider:

What helps me understand the intended meaning?
- How might I check that I have understood their view if I am working with this person in practice?
- What support or advice might I request from a SLT when working with this person?

One of the most common features of aphasia is word retrieval difficulties, also known as anomia. This results in challenges finding and using the words needed, or a slower ability to do this – often a stroke survivor will get the word eventually, but it might take some time, or they may need to focus completely on this, for example, closing their eyes to help. Others might find that the word comes if they start to write the first letter, or it may come in the middle of the night, so they keep a notebook at the side of the bed for this eventuality. Sometimes instead of the word the person wants to say, they may produce something else instead (known as a paraphasia), which can derail the conversation and result in a communication partner not understanding the intended meaning of the conversation. Or the word may not come at all, resulting in a gap in conversation and a point at which the person with aphasia may give up. Some people with aphasia are fully aware of these kinds of errors or paraphasia, but may not be able to correct them, and others may not notice them.

It is helpful for healthcare practitioners to know these coping strategies to encourage them or offer them as communication aids. The most common errors and challenges in the language of people with aphasia are outlined in Table 3.3.

Aphasia, regardless of recovery, can make a lot of everyday activities challenging, and this challenge may continue for months or years after the stroke. Strategies, therefore, need to be put in place to facilitate effective communication and to ensure that the person who has communication difficulties is supported and safe when conducting everyday activities. Jo and Kelly both describe seeking support from family or trusted friends, particularly around financial or legal issues (e.g., contracts and mortgages). Legal language is typically complex, and legal documents are rarely provided in an easy-read format. Whilst they are both financially independent and successful adults, they still ask someone to double-check that they have fully understood complex written information for decision-making. Despite these challenges, there is joy to be found in living with aphasia; people do it successfully every day.

If you are supporting someone who has had a stroke, share the message that things continue to improve. Explore and consider ways to offer support with communication.

TABLE 3.3 Types of errors heard

Verbal (or semantic) paraphasia	A word similar in meaning is said instead of the intended word. This can be closely related or more distantly related, or completely unrelated.	Close: Saying 'wife' when you meant 'husband' Distant: Saying 'horse' when you meant 'race' or when Byron from the video says, 'Are you pretty?' meaning 'are you well/good' Unrelated: Saying 'slipper' when you meant 'coffee'
Phonemic (or literal) paraphasia	An error is made in how the word sounds. At least 50% of the word is the same as the intended word. Sounds or syllables from the word may be transposed.	For example, saying 'lar' when you meant 'car' 'ephelant' when you meant 'elephant'
Neologistic paraphasia	The word produced is unrelated to the word they wanted to say (either in meaning or in sound). The person produces a made-up word (a non-word), which does not have any meaning for them.	For example, calling milk 'blatch'
Perseveration	Words or phrases are said repeatedly and unintentionally. Sometimes this can make up most of what someone says.	For example, Jeremy describes saying two words 'Vince' and 'Max' initially after his stroke – these words kept coming out even though he did not know a Vince or a Max, and they were not intentional.
Circumlocution	The stroke survivor can produce a description of the word by talking around it, but not the word itself. This can be a helpful strategy and is often encouraged by speech and language therapists.	For example, saying 'the nurse who looks after babies' for 'a midwife'

Source: With reference to Lingraphica (2024).

Aphasia and bilingualism/multilingualism

Whilst it is challenging to source exact statistics about the number of people across the world who speak more than one language, multilingualism is common (Norvik and Goral, 2020). It is a must, therefore, to consider the languages the stroke survivor speaks, reads and writes as part of routine care. This is even more important for a stroke survivor living with aphasia. If an individual speaks several languages, aphasia can affect any of them; the extent of this will vary from person to person and may also be related to when the individual learnt that language as well as their pre-stroke language use and proficiency. Adults will lose proficiency in languages they are not using. In *parallel aphasia impairment*, both or all the languages spoken by the stroke survivor are affected equally; in *differential impairment*, one language is affected more than the other (Hallowell, 2017).

PJ explains the significant impact of aphasia on communication between him and his wife. He speaks Creole and English; his wife speaks Swahili and English. PJ could speak Creole more easily after his stroke, although it was still affected by the aphasia. The aphasia affected his English more.

My wife is talking Kenyan (Swahili)... I don't know what she's talking about (PJ doesn't speak Swahili). She can talk in English but me, now I'm talking (English) slowly, slowly. She can talk English, she can talk Kenyan but me is Creole, Creole, Creole.

(PJ, 57, ischaemic stroke, 4 years post stroke)

For PJ and his wife, their shared language of English was significantly affected, making day-to-day conversations really challenging. PJ says that in the early days, he sometimes had to ring his brother (also a Creole speaker) who could then translate and make sense of what he was trying to say. His brother would then ring PJ's wife to explain it to her using English.

It is important for rehabilitation to establish a language profile for the stroke survivor, exploring languages spoken, understood and used for reading and writing. It is also helpful to establish the survivor's proficiency in these languages and the value they place on them (Norvik and Goral, 2020). The way in which the languages are used, and with whom, needs to be understood. For example, someone may use a language with their elderly parents but not with anyone else – if they cannot speak this language, then their relationship with their parents is significantly affected. It is best practice that SLTs work with interpreters and bilingual coworkers wherever possible to support aphasia therapy in different languages.

When you are working with someone who speaks more than one language, do you consider how the stroke has affected their different languages? What might the impact be on their relationships and their ability to stay connected with family and friends? What ONE change could you make to improve your practice?

The impact of aphasia

Post-stroke aphasia is associated with poorer quality of life (Hilari, 2011) and greater difficulty maintaining friendships (Northcott and Hilari, 2011). Patients with aphasia report losing contact with friends (Hilari, 2011), with friendship numbers diminishing, as people stay away as they find it difficult to deal with the situation (Dalemans *et al.*, 2010):

> (My friend) was great, in the hospital all the time, in the hospital every day, back home nothing – where she gone? I realised she can't communicate (with) me, she had no tools. I just don't know what to do, I don't know what to say, I am the same person (but) it is going to take a little while.
>
> *(Kelly, 55, ischaemic stroke, 7 years post stroke)*

Kauhanen *et al.* (2000) found that 12 months after a stroke, 62% of people with aphasia were experiencing depression. There is also a higher rate of anxiety for stroke survivors with aphasia as compared to those without (Morris *et al.*, 2017), which appears to be associated with younger age at the time of the stroke and the severity level of the aphasia.

(Non-aphasic) Cognitive-communication disorder

Between 31% (Duffy *et al.*, 2018) and 56% (Dhufaigh *et al.*, 2019) of people with right-hemisphere stroke experience cognitive-communication disorder (CCD), with one study hypothesising it could be as high as 80% (Côté *et al.*, 2007). CCD is more subtle in its features than aphasia, so it is unlikely that all stroke survivors with CCD present for rehabilitation. Indeed, the National Clinical Guidelines for Stroke (National Clinical Guideline for Stroke for the UK and Ireland, 2023) do not list CCD in the guidelines at all, suggesting this group of stroke survivors remains less well attended to.

People with CCD have difficulty expressing or understanding 'what someone means as opposed to what they say' (Blake, 2022, p. 406) as well as difficulties communicating effectively and efficiently (Blake, 2021). People with CCD also have difficulties with language because of changes to the components of cognition: memory, attention and executive function (Purdy, 2018) as a result of the stroke.

Whilst CCD arises as a result of a right-hemisphere stroke, *not all* right-hemisphere strokes result in CCD (Côté *et al.*, 2007). Post-stroke CCD is under-researched and complex, with many conflicting conclusions in the literature (Blake, 2021). Impact on the right-hemisphere language skills (see Figure 3.1) results in difficulties in understanding and using language in some more complex and subtle ways:

Difficulties understanding language: People with CCD have difficulties where words have multiple meanings, in particular with the less common of those meanings. People may also find it difficult to use the context of the conversation to interpret the intention of the speaker, for example, when understanding a joke or sarcasm. Jokes often rely on multiple meanings of words and revising of initial interpretations of statements to find the humour. Intention in texts or emails (Blake, 2021) (because it is not accompanied by non-verbal communication) may be missed; emojis can help with this.

Difficulties producing discourse: Examples can include narrative/discourse/story-telling skills. For example, imagine someone telling a story in a conversation about their holiday – they might not give enough specific information for the listener to understand where they went and with whom, or they might move from the holiday conversation to another story without bridging the two. Sometimes taking turns in conversation can also be more challenging, along with looking at the speaker and demonstrating attention (Blake, 2021).

Expressing or understanding emotional meaning using prosody: Prosody is the rate, rhythm and tone of our speech and a way we convey meaning, for example, conveying or understanding the anger in a statement like 'Don't speak to me like that!' (Sheppard *et al.*, 2022).

What is most important when exploring communication after a right-hemisphere stroke is to find out how differences in communication noted by the healthcare team differ from the stroke survivor's pre-stroke communication (Ferré and Joanette, 2016) because these areas are part of 'the range of acceptable communication behaviours in the general population' (Blake, 2021, p. 572). A great example of this is eye contact – everyone differs in how much they look at people when they are talking. What was typical for this person before their stroke?

Impact of CCD

In one study, 88% of those with CCD reported changes to vocational roles and duties, and 85.7% reported that the amount and frequency of leisure activities they participated in had reduced. This was statistically significantly different to those stroke survivors without CCD. They also experienced a greater frequency of change in relationships with their spouses, friends and other family members (Hewetson *et al.*, 2018).

Motor speech difficulties

The following difficulties are classed as motor speech difficulties. These stroke survivors do not have difficulty using their left and right-hemisphere language skills but have challenges with their motor speech planning and production (see Figures 3.1 and 3.2).

Dysarthria

Between 30,000 and 45,000 people are estimated to be diagnosed with dysarthria after a stroke each year in the United Kingdom (Brady *et al.*, 2011a).

Dysarthria is a group of speech difficulties due to a disruption in neuromuscular control and execution (Duffy, 2020). The stroke results in abnormalities in strength, range, tone, speed and accuracy of movement (Duffy, 2020) for the five components/dimensions of speech production shown in Figure 3.2:

- Respiration (power for speech)
- Phonation (raw sound)
- Resonance (tonal qualities)
- Articulation (speech sounds)
- Prosody (musical qualities) (Duffy, 2020; Rouse, 2016).

The most common dysarthria following stroke is unilateral upper motor neurone dysarthria (Duffy, 2020). The survivor can think of the words they want to say and put these into sentences but struggles to produce clear speech and may have difficulty being understood. People may speak more slowly, quietly, may be monotone, or the sounds might be unclear. When dysarthria is severe, speaking may be very difficult indeed, with the inability to produce any speech or speech produced being extremely difficult to understand. These difficulties can persist long after discharge from a stroke service (Brady *et al.*, 2011a).

People with dysarthria have preserved reading and writing skills as it is a speech, not language difficulty; so, this can provide an avenue for communication. However, it must be remembered that many stroke survivors might struggle to hold a pen or may be using their non-dominant hand to write, which in itself can make the writing hard to read and further limit solutions for communication. Apps and accessibility options on tablets/phones that use text-to-speech options make use of this preserved writing ability. Mitchell *et al.* (2021) found that 28% of stroke survivors have aphasia and dysarthria combined, making communication additionally challenging.

Impact of dysarthria

People with dysarthria are working hard, putting substantial effort into communication to make sure it is effective (Brady *et al.*, 2011b). This includes overt strategies such as slowing their speech, speaking more loudly and saying sounds very deliberately, as well as more covert strategies such as planning and rehearsing ahead of time to enable understandable speech (Brady *et al.*, 2011b).

People also describe constantly monitoring their speech, so they can adjust as they speak (Brady *et al.*, 2011b). These adjustments include repairing a breakdown by saying it again, substituting words or using nonverbal strategies like writing it down or using an alphabet chart.

People with dysarthria also experience:

- *Changes in self and social identity*: These seem related to feeling different, sounding different (for example, their voice), experiencing a changed role in the family and being treated differently by others (Dickson *et al.*, 2008; Brady *et al.*, 2011a).
- *Social isolation:* Avoiding socialising due to worries about being understood or keeping up with the conversation so they feel left out (Dickson *et al.*, 2008; Walshe, 2011).
- *Emotional distress*: The emotional impact can be 'disproportionate to the physiological severity of dysarthria' (Dickson *et al.*, 2008, p. 146).
- Stigmatisation, for example, sounding drunk (Dickson *et al.*, 2008; Brady *et al.*, 2011a).

Apraxia of speech

Around 10% of stroke survivors have acquired apraxia of speech (AOS) (Atkinson and McHanwell, 2018). AOS is 'usually caused by damage to the left frontal lobe, especially when the damage occurs near Broca's area' (Freed, 2023, p.302).

AOS is an inability to facilitate the motor plan in the primary motor cortex to direct movements for normal speech production (Duffy, 2020; Manasco, 2021). It is a bit like having a computer coding problem.

Characteristics of acquired AOS

- A slow rate of speech.
- Sounds will be longer than expected, and/or there will be pauses between syllables, or words.
- Vowels and consonants in words are distorted, changing how the word sounds.
- Sounds are substituted with other sounds.
- Prosody does not sound normal, for example, stress patterns in words can be different to expected and can therefore change meaning. Sometimes people with apraxia can sound like they have a different accent for parts of their speech (Wambaugh *et al.*, 2006).

Impact of AOS

For people with AOS, producing speech is usually very effortful, with struggle and multiple attempts to produce the words they want, even though orofacial muscle movement and tone remain normal. People with apraxia are only too aware of their difficulties and will often try repeatedly to correct their own speech, attempting to 'self-repair' the word (Manasco, 2021). One theory is that this effort comes about because the stroke survivor cannot access stored, learnt movement patterns (e.g., 'how are you?' is stored as one movement pattern). As a result, they have to put this together each time they say it sound by sound and syllable by syllable, which takes time (Varley and Whiteside, 2001).

AOS usually presents alongside some level of aphasia. This mixed presentation and continued theoretical debate amongst AOS experts may mean that the wider healthcare team are less aware of this speech disability (Molloy and Jagoe, 2019).

What do people with communication disability need from healthcare professionals?

Put incredibly succinctly, people with communication disabilities need healthcare staff to be good communication partners for them. Jo explains how a good communication partner can make you feel empowered.

> I found that the people that were kind enough to give me time, ask what I wanted and how I wanted to communicate in that instant and then checked that what they have done is correct always made me feel quite empowered and part of the processes rather than, you know, kind of rushed and not involved.
>
> *(Jo, 46, embolic stroke as a result of endocarditis, 20 years post stroke)*

If communication support needs are not attended to, there are risks to good healthcare practice. For example:

- Capacity may be questioned.
- Adverse events may occur.
- Reduced autonomy for the survivor.
- Unsuccessful communication.
- Dissatisfaction and disengagement (Zingelman *et al.*, 2024).

Time please!

The number one request from the EbyEs involved in writing this chapter is for healthcare professionals to allow people the time needed to (1) communicate effectively, (2) process information and (3) access appropriate quality of services (Parr *et al.*, 2003).

> They would make chit chat with me but because I couldn't speak, didn't ever give me the time to respond or answer and the conversation would move on too quickly and I never felt I was able to keep up... When you are having treatment, diagnosis or planning to go home discussions it is really important to give the person time.
>
> *(Jo, 47, ischaemic stroke, 20 years post stroke)*

The temporal norms in interaction mean people with communication disabilities experience discrimination (Parr *et al.*, 2003). Allowing time, being clear that as a partner in the interaction you will wait and not jumping in to guess what someone is trying to say is not just important – it is a reasonable and expected adjustment to communication disability (Equality Act, 2010, s20). The individual can often be derailed if the healthcare professional tries to guess where the conversation is going; they then must explain it was not what they wanted to say and by that time they have lost track of what they were saying in the first place!

People with aphasia or CCD may also need time to process and make sense of things they have heard before they can reply, so they may not reply immediately – waiting a couple of seconds extra may make an enormous difference. By observing the individual closely, there may be clues indicating they are still processing information.

Needing time to think about what they want to say (Dalemans *et al.*, 2010) and rehearse it is a common need for all people with post-stroke communication difficulties. It means the pace of conversation must be slower.

Listen!

It is important to listen to what is really being said. Healthcare professionals are taught active listening, but this is not always demonstrated. Take this example:

Student (sitting facing the patient): 'So why have you come to see us today?'
Stroke Survivor: 'um... I had a stroke 2 years ago....'
Student: 'Ok, great (nods head; maintains eye contact)'

The student is carrying out the instructions often given to demonstrate active listening (sitting, nodding and maintaining eye contact), but not really hearing what the stroke survivor has said – nothing about having a stroke is likely to be great. The 'great' is a response to the student's own internal narrative or an acknowledgement that an answer has been received, but the response has not fitted the prior turn in the conversation. A better response would be silence, an 'uh huh' or a nod of the head, known as a minimal/passing turn (Schegloff, 1982), which places the next turn in the conversation back with the stroke survivor to add more. This technique is especially helpful to provide the extra time needed by people with aphasia.

Listening well is also key to understanding when someone has reduced speech intelligibility. The listener may need to use everything the person is doing to understand, for example, observing facial expression, gestures such as air writing or holding fingers up to show a number, hearing the way something has been said or noting part words/phrases – a bit like piecing together a jigsaw – the sum of the parts is more than each individual piece.

It also means *not pretending to understand*. EbyEs are very clear that they know if healthcare professionals have not understood them! People with speech difficulties are usually more than happy to keep repeating themselves until they are understood, but sharing the burden for this really helps make it easier. This can be done by saying something such as 'I'm sorry I didn't quite get that', then ask 'tell me again'. Sometimes for people with aphasia, you also need to say 'can you show me?' or 'Can you tell me another way?' This might enable the individual to use different ways to communicate such as using gestures, drawing or writing, or pulling out resources and simple techniques (which are suggested later on in this chapter) to help.

Listening to understand allows the healthcare professional to fully absorb what the person has said (Mannix, 2021). Without realising it, health professionals are often keen to be helpful and jump into conversations, offering solutions or talking about next steps before the full story has been heard and understood. Several stories have been shared with the author where stroke survivors and family members do not feel listened to. For example, a survivor's husband explained that the problem she had with her leg was repeatedly put down to her stroke, despite her husband explaining this was not the case. It was only when he insisted on showing a video of her walking after her post stroke to compare it with her current walking that the professional reconsidered the diagnosis. This delayed treatment for the condition, and the stroke survivor lived with considerable pain, all because they were not *listening to understand*.

Try questions such as:

- Is this normal for you since your stroke?
- Can you tell me how this differs from your usual?
- Can you show me a picture or a video?

Use simple techniques that support conversation

Use a technique known as supported conversation for adults with aphasia (SCA™) (Kagan, 1998). This approach aims to acknowledge and reveal the person with aphasia's competence. The communication partner shares the responsibility for the conversation. It uses simple techniques that support understanding (getting information in), expression (getting information out) and checking (known as verifying) that the communication partner has understood.

> Often the nurses can be the person that advocates what mode of communication you are using; they must make sure other people are aware of your mode of communication whether that be a notepad and pen or nowadays more likely to be apps. If your pad or paper has been moved to the other side of your body that you can't move, or moved away from you where you can't reach it in the middle of the night … and the doctor comes to see you, it's really important that actually, especially on call doctors, that a nurse speaks up and tells them your mode of communication and then gives it to you. Many times, I heard people say, 'oh yeah, she communicates through pen and paper', and then I wasn't given my pen and paper to communicate. So, it kind of seems like, obvious, but these are the things that happen all the time.
>
> *(Jo, 47, embolic stroke as a result of endocarditis, 20 years post stroke)*

In the same way that physical access to buildings is provided by installing ramps, access to communication/conversation is also needed. Conceptually, the idea of communication ramps is based in the social model of disability – the way in which the world is organised means people with communication difficulties cannot access communication in the way society expects, but providing ramps removes some of the barriers to participation.

There are lots of everyday items that can act as brilliant conversation ramps, helping to get to know stroke survivors and to engage those with communication disabilities in meaningful conversations. These are particularly helpful for people with aphasia or sometimes CCD but can also be used to understand what people with speech difficulties are saying too. Visual support benefits everyone – just think how emojis add context to texts/emails.

- *Calendars:* Handy if you are talking about the next appointment, plans for future treatment or sharing a conversation about an upcoming wedding anniversary.
- *Maps:* For if you are talking about a holiday or where they or family live.
- *Menus:* Helpful to choose food options, show the kinds of food they enjoy or make plans for future social events.
- Photos of family/friends/places/pets that are important.
- Newspapers, magazines or online news sites are great for conversations about current affairs.
- Leaflets (for places visited or for services).
- Free published communication support resources (e.g., the communication picture book published by the Stroke Association – see box 1).

- Searches using Google, image searches or Wikipedia.
- *Alphabet chart:* These are especially useful for people with preserved writing skills, such as those with dysarthria or AOS.
- Apps or accessibility options to make devices more useful and enable some reading or writing (e.g., increasing font size, using predictive text and using text-to-speech options).

Make these resources something to look at together collaboratively, and layers of conversation and understanding can be built up – they may also take the conversation in a different and more important direction.

What communication resources do you already have in your setting and what could you add? How should these be managed so resources are available to you and your service? so resources are available for you and your service users when they are needed?

Write keywords down as you talk

This method of keyword documenting is incredibly helpful to support getting information in. It has multiple other benefits:

- It naturally slows down the pace of interaction.
- It gives the stroke survivor methods to use to express themselves. Later in conversation, the person might come back to words that have already been written to use to support a new point.
- It can make the healthcare professional sit with the stroke survivor.
- It can make the stroke survivor feel listened to and valued.

Imagine a conversation: The healthcare professional would say something like 'we need to talk about going home'.

In this method, the healthcare professional would write down the keyword 'home' for the person to see *at the same time as it is spoken* (see Figure 3.3). The

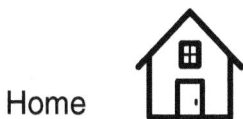

Home

FIGURE 3.3   An example of keyword documenting.

Washing?

Dressing?

Cooking?

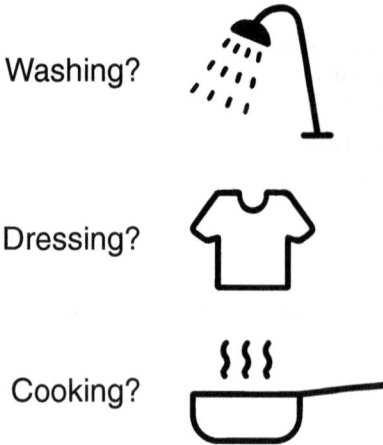

FIGURE 3.4 An example of keyword documenting with pictures to support discussion.

healthcare professional could also draw a simple outline of a house too to add extra support for understanding.

This can also be used to give people choices (see Figure 3.4) – for example, talking about what help someone might need to go home.

Drawings need to be simple and do not have to be great works of art as you can see in the examples given.

Give information

In small chunks

When healthcare professionals are explaining things, it should be done in simple steps, with one idea presented at a time. This helps people understand and process the information.

> If you tell me too much it is like you are a Spanish person talking to me – I have no idea what you are talking about.
>
> *(Kelly, 55, ischaemic stroke, 7 years post stroke)*

It can help to break information into manageable stages. Some people with CCD or Aphasia find it useful to have a plan laid out at the beginning of the conversation. This can be written at the time as a shared, agreed document. It can also help to agree or send this information ahead explaining 'this is what I would like to cover in your appointment' (see Figure 3.5).

Today:

① Things at home?

② Scan results

③ Exercises

④ Next steps

⑤ Anything else?

FIGURE 3.5 An example agenda for an appointment.

About the health condition

Many EbyEs describe not having enough information/not knowing what was wrong with their talking at the time they had their stroke.

> Nobody told me I had aphasia. My daughter found it on Dr Google. Of course we didn't know anything about aphasia.
>
> *(Kelly, 55, ischaemic stroke, 7 years post stroke)*

Kelly now spends a lot of time talking to healthcare students about aphasia and is heavily involved in awareness-raising campaigns to improve the general public's knowledge of aphasia.

Many describe those early days after a stroke as like a fog, so they are not sure that they would remember information clearly if they had been given it. The EbyEs, therefore, recommend that healthcare professionals give information about a stroke survivor's diagnosis such as the type of stroke and communication disability in a written, accessible format that can be left with them.

> They need something so that you can receive that information…even if you can't read it properly in one go, you've got that information. You can study it later and come back to it and go over it and over it.
>
> You can have too much information that isn't relevant. What you're really looking for as that person, is what's wrong with **me**.
>
> *(Jan, 80, ischaemic stroke, 14 years post stroke)*

The information also needs to be current. A number of the EbyEs report stories of being told about recovery, plateau and time limits that do not fit with current knowledge of stroke recovery and rehabilitation. For example, stroke survivors should be considered to have the potential to benefit from rehabilitation at any point after their stroke as recommended by section 4, National Clinical Guideline for Stroke in the United Kingdom and Ireland (National Clinical Guideline for Stroke for the UK and Ireland, 2023).

Keep vocabulary simple

Try to do this whilst also keeping it adult and respectful. It can be helpful to avoid metaphors, especially for people with comprehension difficulties. Technical terms become everyday words for healthcare professionals, but they are not always understood by others, and people do not always ask for explanations. It is important to make sure the language used is accessible, for example, instead of talking about a haemorrhagic stroke, talk about a 'bleed in the brain'.

Use phrases like 'I know you know'

This is also based on the theoretical approach of Supported Conversation for Adults with Aphasia (SCA™) (Kagan, 1998). This simple phrase shows that you respect the individual, and you know they are a competent, intelligent individual, but that they are struggling to share their ideas. It takes some of the anxiety out of the situation, often enabling the words to come or frustration to be reduced. It is ok to pause a conversation and come back to it later if things are particularly difficult.

Check if you have understood

It is important for the communication partner to confirm whether they have understood correctly, especially for people with aphasia and people with CCD where they may have swapped words for ones with similar meaning. This verification (Kagan, 1998) reduces assumptions, avoids conversations being derailed and increases satisfaction. For example: 'Let me just check I have understood; you want me to call your daughter? You want her to bring toothpaste?'

> I think that the best advocacy is asking 'is that ok? Is that what you meant?' Not only saying or reading out what you've written, but checking that's what you meant or what you want(ed) to say.
>
> *(Jo, 47, embolic stroke as a result of endocarditis, 20 years post stroke)*

Using written keyword documenting can really help here too, for example, circling confirmed ideas and crossing out things that do not apply, as illustrated in Figure 3.6.

Show your face

It can help some people with aphasia and people with hearing loss if they can see your face and mouth as you speak. Mask wearing in healthcare settings may be

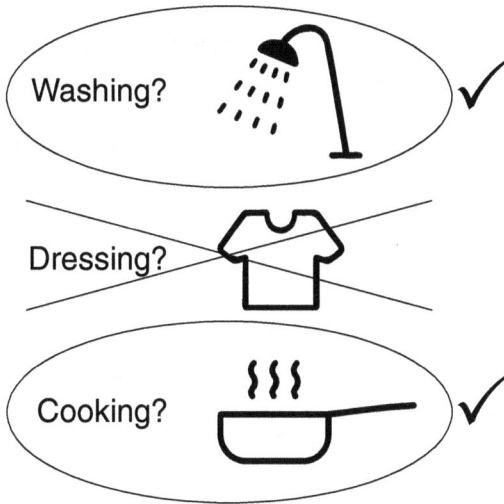

FIGURE 3.6 Clarifying what support someone needs when they go home.

necessary, but exploring clear masks can help. It can also help if the environment is maximised:

- Turn off devices/radio/television.
- Use a quiet place, if possible.
- Sit facing each other.
- Make sure lights are on.
- If working online, it can sometimes help to put a background on to lighten the screen.

Ultimately, the key message in this section is that the healthcare professional shares responsibility for the success of the communication, recognising the reasonable adjustments they can make in their practice to enhance communication as much as possible.

Risks when you have a communication disability

Stroke and its resulting communication difficulties have a 'ripple effect' impacting everyone around the stroke survivor as well as the individual themselves. Anecdotally, it is clear that the long-term effects of communication disabilities are not always considered.

When I was (a year after) finally signed off by the specialist, physically can you do this (points to eyes); can you stand up, can you walk round the corner, that's it, (mimes signing pieces of paper). There is no suggestion can you speak alright? They were purely interested in my physical ability and that's all that was signed off.

(Jan, 80, ischaemic stroke, 14 years post stroke)

Assumptions about capacity and competence

In the United Kingdom, the Mental Capacity Act (2005) states that a person has capacity unless proven otherwise. Experiences of people with communication difficulties show that this assumption is not always made in everyday practice, and many report being treated as if they are not competent adults:

They used to talk over her, they wouldn't talk to her... they would say 'we're doing this' but not to her, to each other. They seemed to be talking between themselves, to each other, and not to her, which if you are doing personal care it needs to be personal. And my mum had got everything about her up here, she couldn't say things and she struggled, but she knew exactly what they were talking about. She felt very, very uncomfortable at times.

(Steph, daughter and carer)

Low mood, anxiety and depression

These are frequent consequences of communication difficulties, although this is not well studied for AOS.

Me, me, I can't do it [crying] Why, why me? Why me, Why ME? (Michelle, 61, ischaemic stroke, 4 years post stroke), when talking about being depressed/ low mood.

You've changed. I spent several months thinking why me, why me? I'm a good man, I've helped hundreds, thousands of young people ... so why me? But eventually I realised, it isn't why me, but adding up victories, little victories throughout my troubles and eventually I needn't ask myself why me? Here, it happened, I can do things. Those victories show us the way.

(Les, 78, ischaemic stroke, 2 years post-stroke)

Accessing behavioural therapy or psychological interventions, both recommended by NICE (2023), for post-stroke aphasia, may be challenging with communication disability, but the need for more appropriate therapies is recognised in SLT research. This is recommended before antidepressant medication (NICE, 2023). Northcott *et al.* (2021) have been using solution-focused brief therapy effectively for this group.

Loss of identity and big feelings

Living with communication disability can be very challenging. The EbyE community describes feelings of anger, frustration, loss, grief and, at times, despair.

> The loss was gigantic.
>
> *(Jo, 47, embolic stroke as a result of endocarditis, 20 years post-stroke)*
>
> In that four, five months, I got very angry, shouting, I used to be frustrated cos I couldn't say the word. I didn't want to go anywhere because friends had left me. One day I had a falling out with my son. I had a little breakdown, spoke to the doctor, and had a mental health doctor who spoke with me, not just me but the family, but gave me some understanding because the behaviour, wasn't me. It helped everyone. I'm this ripple in this sea.
>
> *(Kelly, 55, ischaemic stroke, 7 years post-stroke)*

Isolation, exclusion and loss of social connectedness

For people with communication disabilities, there are negative effects on social participation and social connectedness that are shown to be more significant than for those stroke survivors without communication disability (Hewetson *et al.*, 2018). Where people manage to maintain social participation, it is associated with greater wellbeing (Haslam *et al.*, 2008). Brady *et al.* (2011a) found that, for people with dysarthria, other people's reactions to their speech resulted in experiences of social exclusion, citing examples of healthcare staff speaking to carers instead of the people with dysarthria.

Ensuring that people have opportunities for social connectedness is a key aspect of healthcare management for this population. The EbyE community involved in this book feels strongly that this should be with people experiencing communication disability rather than a general stroke support group. For some, it can feel like home – they have found their tribe. Hersh *et al.* (2024) found that for people living alone experiencing aphasia, attending aphasia and stroke support groups helped many keep busy and connect socially, though it did not suit everyone.

EbyE, Les sums this up beautifully, saying to his fellow aphasia group members:

You, in this group, are a godsend I really wish I had me in the ward 7 years ago – speech and language therapists, doctors, nurses, they are fantastic (but) they don't get it either. I really wish I'd met somebody on the other side. That community we have here – that's a lifeline. (Les, 78, ischaemic stroke, 3 years post stroke)

I've met some wonderful friends. Because its isolating…it's very isolating.
(Kelly, 55, ischaemic stroke, 7 years post-stroke)

Healthcare staff can help by finding out what opportunities there might be locally. These could be:

- Peer befriending services (such as those described by Moss *et al.*, 2022).
- Remote or face-to-face conversation/support groups.
- *Social media:* There are several stroke survivors with communication difficulties sharing their experiences, providing positive role models and hope.
- *Forums:* Some EbyE communities operate WhatsApp groups using photos, emojis, voice/video notes as well as text.
- *An aphasia choir:* Preserved/more fluent singing abilities experienced by some stroke survivors mean choirs can be a source of joy, improved wellbeing and peer support (Fekete and Eckhardt, 2022).

Useful resources: support/communication support

Stroke Association: www.stroke.org.uk/aphasia

- *Learn more about aphasia*: It contains helpful videos on what happens to communication after a stroke and a video guide on good communication strategies showing examples of techniques mentioned above in use.
- *Order a free communication support pack*: It contains a communication picture book, which is useful to have on wards or in clinics and an aphasia-friendly guide to stroke and communication problems. This has been produced with people who have communication problems themselves (Stroke Association, 2023).
- *Accessible information guidelines:* www.stroke.org.uk/sites/default/files/aig_low_res.pdf
- *Aphasia etiquette:* www.youtube.com/watch?v=hTh86NoQh7Q

Say Aphasia: www.sayaphasia.org

- Order a free 'I have Aphasia' support card.
- Order a free 'Say Aphasia' information booklet.
- Find real-life stories of people with aphasia who can be great role models.

Aphasia Institute: www.aphasia.ca/health-care-providers/education-training/self-directed-elearning/

There is an excellent free training resource in SCA™ (Kagan *et al.*, 2025), an evidence-based practical module. This explores the ideas mentioned earlier.

Useful people to know

There are many fantastic role models of people living well with communication disability after their stroke. Share these examples with patients and families. As a healthcare professional, it really helps to know what the positive potential outcomes can be. Not everyone has access to support groups but simply knowing there are other people out there 'like me' can really help.

Meet Carly and Jan: www.youtube.com/@alifeafterstroke-aphasiaaw3396/featured
Meet Sarah Scott: www.facebook.com/SarahScottAphasia/

Self-evaluation

Take a moment to complete the following activity to support your self-evaluation.

- Reflect on the first activity: What new knowledge do you have about communication disability following a stroke?
- What one change can you implement to be a good communication partner for your stroke survivors?
- What one action will you take to reduce the risks for people with communication disability?

Conclusion

In this chapter, there has, rightly, been a focus on the challenges that people with communication disability face when living their lives – this has been necessary to draw attention to how all healthcare professionals can better support this population of stroke survivors. It is, however, important to note how people with communication disability manage to return to life after stroke with incredible success and resilience. The author has had the privilege to meet and work with amazing communities who have come together because of their communication difficulties and achieved something that seemed unimaginable. The resilience of people with communication disability, their family and friends and the mountains that they climb is incredible. It is possible to live well with communication disability after stroke.

References

Atkinson, M., and McHanwell, S. (2018). *Basic Medical Science for Speech and Language Therapy Students*. 2nd edn. Albury, Guildford: J&R Press Ltd.

Blake, M. L. (2021). Communication deficits associated with right hemisphere brain damage. In: Damico, J., Muller, N., and Ball, M. J. (Eds.). *The Handbook of Language and Speech Disorders*. 2nd edn. Hoboken, NJ: Wiley-Blackwell.

Blake, M. L. (2022). Communication disorders associated with right-hemisphere brain damage. In: Papathanasiou, I., and Coppens, P. (Eds.). *Aphasia and Related Neurogenic Communication Disorders*. 3rd edn. Chicago: Jones & Bartlett Learning, pp. 405–434.

Brady, M. C., Clark, A. M., Dickson, S., Paton, G., and Barbour, R. S. (2011a). The impact of stroke-related dysarthria on social participation and implications for rehabilitation. *Disability and Rehabilitation*, 33(3), pp. 178–186.

Brady, M. C., Clark, A. M., Dickson, S., Paton, G., and Barbour, R. S. (2011b). Dysarthria following stroke – the patient's perspective on management and rehabilitation. *Clinical Rehabilitation*, 25(10), pp. 935–952.

Copland, D. A., McNeil, M. R., and Meinzer, M. (2018). Aphasia theory, models, and classification. In: LaPointe, L. L., and Stierwalt, J. A. G. (Eds.). *Aphasia and Related Neurogenic Language Disorders*. 5th edn. New York: Thieme, pp. 23–34.

Côté, H., Payer, M., Giroux, F., and Joanette, Y. (2007). Towards a description of clinical communication impairment profiles following right-hemisphere damage. *Aphasiology*, 21(6–8), pp. 739–749.

Dalemans, R. J. P., de Witte, L., Wade, D., and van den Heuvel, W. (2010). Social participation through the eyes of people with aphasia. *International Journal of Language & Communication Disorders*, 45(5), pp. 537–550.

Dhufaigh, N. N., Haughey, M., and Gillen, C. (2019). 170 admissions to a stroke unit in an Irish rehabilitation hospital: A review from speech and language therapy. *Age and Ageing*, 48(Supplement 3), pp. iii1–iii16.

Dickson, S., Barbour, R. S., Brady, M., Clark, A. M., and Paton, G. (2008). Patients' experiences of disruptions associated with post-stroke dysarthria. *International Journal of Language & Communication Disorders*, 43(2), pp. 135–153.

Duffy, J. R. (2020). *Motor Speech Disorders: Substrates, Differential Diagnosis, and Management*. 4th edn. Edinburgh: Elsevier.

Duffy, J. R., Fossett, T. R. D., Thomas, J. E., and Stierwalt, J. A. G. (2018). Care for people with aphasia and related neurogenic communication disorders in acute hospital settings. In: LaPointe, L. L., and Stierwalt, J. A. G. (Eds.). *Aphasia and Related Neurogenic Language Disorders*. 5th edn. New York: Thieme, pp. 44–54.

Equality Act (2010). *Equality Act 2010*. Available at: www.legislation.gov.uk/ukpga/2010/15/part/2

Fekete, Z., and Eckhardt, F. (2022). Hungarian aphasia choir coping online during the COVID-19 pandemic. *Voices: A World Forum for Music Therapy*, 22(1), pp. 1–9.

Ferré, P., and Joanette, Y. (2016). Communication abilities following right hemisphere damage: Prevalence, evaluation, and profiles. *Perspectives of the ASHA Special Interest Groups*, 1(2), pp. 106–115.

Freed, D. B. (2023). *Motor Speech Disorders : Diagnosis and Treatment* (4th edition). San Diego: Plural Publishing.

Hallowell, B. (2017). Cited in Johnson, L. W. (2020). Factors influencing assessment for bilingual adults. In: Scott, D. M. (Ed.). *Cases on Communication Disorders in Culturally Diverse Populations*. San Diego, CA: Plural Publishing, pp. 196–216.

Haslam, C., Holme, A., Haslam, S. A., Iyer, A., Jetten, J., and Williams, W. H. (2008). Maintaining group memberships: Social identity continuity predicts well-being after stroke. *Neuropsychological Rehabilitation*, 18(5–6), pp. 671–691.

Hersh, D., Williamson, C., Brogan, E., and Stanley, M. (2024). 'It's day to day problems': Experiences of people with aphasia who live alone. *International Journal of Speech-Language Pathology*, 26(3), pp. 367–379.

Hewetson, R., Cornwell, P., and Shum, D. (2018). Social participation following right hemisphere stroke: Influence of a cognitive-communication disorder. *Aphasiology*, 32(2), pp. 164–182.

Hilari, K. (2011). The impact of stroke: Are people with aphasia different to those without? *Disability and Rehabilitation*, 33(3), pp. 211–218.

Kagan, A. (1998). Supported conversation for adults with aphasia: Methods and resources for training conversation partners. *Aphasiology*, 12(9), pp. 816–830.

Kagan, A., Shumway, E., Thesenvitz, J., Brookman, C., Han., S., Gierman, N., Draimin, R., Kant, L., and Chan., M. T. (2025). Aphasia Institute Community Hub: Introduction to SCA™ eLearning (Second Edition). Aphasia Institute. Available at: www.aphasia.ca/hea lth-care-providers/education-training/self-directed-elearning/

Kauhanen, M. L., Korpelainen, J. T., Hiltunen, P., Määttä, R., Mononen, H., Brusin, E., Sotaniemi, K. A., and Myllylä, V. V. (2000). Aphasia, depression, and non-verbal cognitive impairment in ischaemic stroke. *Cerebrovascular Diseases*, 10(6), pp. 455–461.

LaPointe, L. L., and Stierwalt, J. A. G. (Eds.). (2018). *Aphasia and Related Neurogenic Language Disorders*. 5th edn. New York: Thieme.

Lingraphica (2024). *What Is Paraphasia?* Available at www.aphasia.com/aphasia-library/ symptoms-of-aphasia/paraphasia/

Manasco, H. (2021). *Introduction to Neurogenic Communication Disorders*. 3rd edn. Burlington, MA: Jones & Bartlett Learning.

Mannix, K. (2021). *Listen: How to Find the Words for Tender Conversations*. London: William Collins.

Mental Capacity Act (2005). *Mental Capacity Act 2005*. Available at www.legislation.gov. uk/ukpga/2005/9/contents (accessed 19 August 2024).

Mitchell, C., Gittins, M., Tyson, S., Vail, A., Conroy, P., Paley, L., and Bowen, A. (2021). Prevalence of aphasia and dysarthria among inpatient stroke survivors: Describing the population, therapy provision and outcomes on discharge. *Aphasiology*, 35(7), pp. 950–960.

Molloy, J., and Jagoe, C. (2019). Use of diverse diagnostic criteria for acquired apraxia of speech: A scoping review. *International Journal of Language & Communication Disorders*, 54(6), pp. 875–893.

Morris, R., Eccles, A., Ryan, B., and Kneebone, I. (2017). Prevalence of anxiety in people with aphasia after stroke. *Aphasiology*, 31(12), pp. 1410–1415.

Moss, B., Behn, N., Northcott, S., Monnelly, K., Marshall, J., Simpson, A., Thomas, S., McVicker, S., Goldsmith, K., Flood, C., and Hilari, K. (2022). 'Loneliness can also kill:' A qualitative exploration of outcomes and experiences of the SUPERB peer-befriending scheme for people with aphasia and their significant others. *Disability and Rehabilitation*, 44(18), pp. 5015–5024.

Nasios, G., Messinis, L., Dardiotis, E., Pisani, A., and Pisani, A. (2019). From Broca and Wernicke to the neuromodulation era: Insights of brain language networks for neurorehabilitation. *Behavioural Neurology*, 2019 (July), pp. 1–10.

National Clinical Guideline for Stroke for the UK and Ireland (2023). *National Clinical Guideline for Stroke for the UK and Ireland*. London: Intercollegiate Stroke Working Party; May 4. Available at: www.strokeguideline.org.

National Institute for Health and Care Excellence (NICE) (2023). *Stroke Rehabilitation in Adults* (NICE guideline 236). Available at: www.nice.org.uk/guidance/ng236

Northcott, S., and Hilari, K. (2011). Why do people lose their friends after a stroke? *International Journal of Language and Communication Disorders*, 46(5), pp. 524–534.

Northcott, S., Simpson, A., Thomas, S., Barnard, R., Burns, K., Hirani, S. P., and Hilari, K. (2021). 'Now I Am Myself': Exploring how people with poststroke aphasia experienced solution-focused brief therapy within the SOFIA trial. *Qualitative Health Research*, 31(11), pp. 2041–2055.

Norvik, M., and Goral, M. (2020) in Lanza, Elizabeth. *Multilingualism across the Lifespan*. Blackwood, R. J., and Røyneland, U. (Eds.). New York: Routledge.

Parr, S., Paterson, K., and Pound, C. (2003). Time please! Temporal barriers in aphasia. In: Parr, S., Duchan, J., and Pound, C. (Eds.). *Aphasia Inside Out*. Berkshire: McGraw-Hill Education, pp. 127–144.

Purdy, M. (2018). Communication and cognition. In: LaPointe, L. L., and Stierwalt, J. A. G. (Eds.). *Aphasia and Related Neurogenic Language Disorders*. 5th edn. New York: Thieme, pp. 240–249.

Rouse, M. H. (2016). *Neuroanatomy for Speech Language Pathology and Audiology*. Burlington, MA: Jones and Bartlett Learning.

Say Aphasia (2023). *What Is Aphasia*. Available at: www.sayaphasia.org/what-is-aphasia

Schegloff, E. (1982). Discourse as an interactional achievement: Some uses of uh huh and other things that come between sentences. In: Tannen, D. (Ed.). *Analyzing Discourse: Text and Talk*. Washington, DC: Georgetown University Press, pp. 71–93.

Sheppard, S. M., Stockbridge, M. D., Keator, L. M., Murray, L. L., and Blake, M. L. (2022). The company prosodic deficits keep following right hemisphere stroke: A systematic review. *Journal of the International Neuropsychological Society*, 28(10), pp. 1075–1090.

Stroke Association (2021). *Communication Problems after a Stroke: Guide. Version 5*. www.stroke.org.uk/communication_problems_after_stroke_guide.pdf

Stroke Association (2023). *Communication Support Pack*. www.stroke.org.uk/webform/order-your-communication-support-pack (accessed 10 November 24).

Swaydon, K. J., Anderson, K. K., Connelly, L. M., Moran, J. S., McMahon, J. K., and Arnold, P. M. (2012). Effect of sitting vs. standing on perception of provider time at bedside: A pilot study. *Patient Education and Counseling*, 86(2), pp. 166–171.

Varley, R., and Whiteside, S. P. (2001). What is the underlying impairment in acquired apraxia of speech? *Aphasiology*, 15(1), pp. 39–84.

Walshe, M. (2011). The psychosocial impact of acquired motor speech disorders. In: Lowit, A., and Kent, R. D. (Eds.). *Assessment of Motor Speech Disorders*. San Diego: Plural Publishing, pp. 97–122.

Wambaugh, J. L., Duffy, J. R., McNeil, M. R., Robin, D. A., and Rogers, M. A. (2006). Treatment guidelines for acquired apraxia of speech: A synthesis and evaluation of the evidence. *Journal of Medical Speech-Language Pathology*, 14(2), pp. xv–xxxiii.

Worrall, L., Simmons-Mackie, N., Wallace, S. J., Rose, T., Brady, M. C., Kong, A. P. H., Murray, L., and Hallowell, B. (2016). Let's call it 'aphasia': Rationales for eliminating the term 'dysphasia'. *International Journal of Stroke*, 11(8), pp. 848–851.

Zingelman, S., Wallace, S. J., Kim, J., Mosalski, S., Faux, S. G., Cadilhac, D. A., Alexander, T., Lannin, N. A., Olaiya, M. T., Clifton, R., Shiner, C. T., Starr, S., and Kilkenny, M. F. (2024). Is communication key in stroke rehabilitation and recovery? National linked stroke data study. *Topics in Stroke Rehabilitation*, 31(4), pp. 325–335.

4

KEEPING COMFORTABLE AND KEEPING GOING

Supporting and promoting wellbeing post-stroke

Rachel Hayden and Gill Hoad

Learning objectives

- To understand the ongoing challenges faced by stroke survivors and how they can impact their wellbeing.
- To appreciate the importance of listening to the stroke survivor and building rapport.
- To understand the potential impact of post-stroke pain.
- To have an increased awareness of low mood and anxiety post stroke and how to support stroke survivors to manage the ongoing psychological impact of stroke.
- To have an awareness of the range of strategies that are available to support stroke survivors with pain management and wellbeing.

Background

Stroke is a traumatic event which often results in a loss of identity, changed reality and threat to self (Large *et al.*, 2019). Stroke recovery and life post-stroke are rarely a smooth path, and instead are likely to involve setbacks and challenges, both during the initial recovery process and in the longer term. Examples of these challenges may be pain, fatigue, reduction in cognitive abilities, physical impairment, adjustment struggles, new health concerns, anxiety and depression. Many patients undergo a period of rehabilitation following stroke, but their journey continues once this formal rehabilitation period ends. They are often left navigating this long-term journey with little support from healthcare professionals, which can be daunting and frightening for stroke survivors and their loved ones. In addition, new problems can develop even once stroke survivors have found some stability, possibly even years after the stroke, and this can lead to disappointment, frustration and anxiety.

DOI: 10.4324/9781003426196-5

> ... everything you've built and everything you think you can do starts to fade away again, and that's really upsetting and frustrating.
>
> *(Jo, 47, embolic stroke as a result of endocarditis, 20 years post stroke)*

Acceptance of the long-term nature of ongoing issues may take some time, and this process itself may include ups and downs, bringing with it new emotions.

> It was a couple of years in, when you start to realise actually I'm not going to get fully better, I'm not going to get back to who I was. I have lost a great deal of my independence and abilities, and I'm always tired. And all of that came with a hell of a lot of emotion – anger, sadness, disappointment, fear for the future and what's going to happen to me.
>
> *(Jo, 47, embolic stroke as a result of endocarditis, 20 years post stroke)*

Healthcare professionals can help support stroke survivors throughout the long-term challenges, by listening to their concerns and then exploring options with them to help them to overcome or manage their issues. Each stroke survivor is unique and what works for one person may not necessarily work for another, so it is key to listen to their experiences and work collaboratively to find the best combination of solutions or strategies to optimise the individual's wellbeing.

It is also important to consider that most stroke survivors will have had a lot of interactions with healthcare professionals during their journey, not all of which will have been positive. As a result, they may come into healthcare appointments in a negative headspace and anticipate that they will need to fight to be listened to. Healthcare professionals need to be empathetic and remember that the patient is the expert on their condition. Staff who take the time to listen to and support patients to get their point across are appreciated by stroke survivors. In conversation about their experiences in both inpatient and outpatient settings, stroke survivors will often recall those staff who stood out for them because they supported them and advocated for them in situations where they felt anxious, frustrated or vulnerable.

> I know that the nurses had to fight my case .... They had clearly listened to all my worries and concerns and taken them and pleaded my case well (with the Consultant) ... and I know that it would have taken me a really long time to get an appointment with the Consultant to discuss this, whereas the nurse practitioners were able to do that really swiftly .... And I was very grateful for that.
>
> *(Jo, 47, embolic stroke as a result of endocarditis, 20 years post stroke)*

Taking the time to really listen to and understand the individual is invaluable in supporting stroke survivors and will improve both outcomes and the experience for stroke survivors. Access to psychology and mental health support can be limited, which reinforces the need for *all* healthcare professionals to allow stroke survivors to be heard and supported, regardless of their individual discipline.

Pain post-stroke

Pain is common following stroke, with up to half of patients reporting it, although pain levels vary widely in the literature (Harrison and Field, 2015; Westerlind *et al.*, 2020). However, pain is not universal, and every person will have their own unique experience of pain, and different responses to pain management strategies. As such, it is crucial that assessment and management of pain following stroke take a truly individualised approach. This is underlined in the National Institute for Health and Care Excellence (NICE) guideline on the assessment and management of chronic pain (NICE, 2021) which recommends a person-centred assessment to identify factors contributing to pain, and how the pain affects the person's life.

Although pain may occur after any stroke, certain risk factors are associated with developing pain, including increased severity of stroke, lower levels of functional independence, anxiety, increased muscle tone, reduced upper limb movement and sensory deficits (Harrison and Field, 2015; Ali *et al.*, 2023; Westerlind *et al.*, 2020). Problematic pain is also more common following thalamic and brainstem strokes (Klit *et al.*, 2011). Additionally, many stroke survivors have co-morbidities that may also result in pain, such as osteoarthritis or diabetic neuropathy. Even if the pain is not a direct result of the stroke it will still impact on the lived experience of the stroke survivor, so it is important to take a holistic view. There is also a link between pain and depression, with each being a significant risk factor for the other (Docking and Tarrant, 2018), so this should be considered when working with stroke survivors.

The most common types of pain following stroke are central post-stroke pain (CPSP), pain secondary to spasticity, shoulder pain, complex regional pain syndrome (CRPS) and headache (O'Donnell *et al.*, 2013; Hansen *et al.*, 2012). Pain experienced by stroke survivors may be either nociceptive or neuropathic, or a combination of both. Nociceptive pain is that which arises from actual or potential tissue damage, whereas neuropathic pain is initiated or caused by a primary lesion or dysfunction in the peripheral or central nervous system (Schofield, 2018). The two may have distinct characteristics and require different management both in terms of pharmacology and holistic management. Pain may occur at varying time points post-stroke, for example, CPSP often has a gradual onset, but once present, is severe and unrelenting. Interestingly, reports of extreme pain have been found to be highest beyond 2 years post-stroke (Ali *et al.*, 2023).

Pain is a subjective and multifaceted experience that is influenced by many factors and requires a biopsychosocial lens. The exact mechanisms of pain are not yet clearly understood, but according to the neuromatrix theory of pain (Melzack, 2001), pain involves networks that are related to cognition (mental processes such as knowledge, thought, memory, perception and attention) sensory and motivational brain networks. Therefore, pain can be influenced by, and also impact, psychological states. Evidence from traumatic brain injury research suggests that injured brain tissue can cause pain interference and maladaptive processing of pain (Kuner and Flor, 2017). This can make pain management more challenging and have a deleterious effect on wellbeing, with pain intensity being associated with poorer psychological states including post-traumatic stress disorder, depression and anxiety (Cherup *et al.*, 2023).

Advances in imaging studies have helped our understanding of the multiple different areas of the brain involved in this 'pain matrix', although our knowledge remains incomplete, particularly in relation to chronic and neuropathic pain (Moisset and Bouhassira, 2007). The key areas thought to be involved in the pain matrix are the primary and secondary somatosensory cortices, the insular cortex, the anterior cingulate cortex, the thalamus and the prefrontal cortex, although other more diffuse areas are also thought to be involved (see Figure 4.1). These multiple areas create a fluid system of several interacting networks which produce the pain that we experience and remember (Garcia-Larrea and Peyron, 2013). The first network within the pain matrix relates to the nociceptive elements of pain, including identifying where in the body the stimulus is coming from. The second-order network is where the nociceptive stimulus becomes conscious pain, and the final layer involves the affective-emotional and cognitive aspects of pain (Garcia-Larrea and Peyron, 2013). There can be a large top-down influence on nociceptive areas dependent on contextual factors, and the pain experience can be modified through beliefs, emotions and expectations. Pain perception is an active process, and as such, it is constantly restructuring. This allows for potential change in the pain experience, which is the focus of the non-pharmacological approaches to pain management. In Figure 4.1 illustrates the multiple and complex connections between the different brain areas involved with pain perception.

The impact of pain on stroke survivors

Pain can have an enormous impact on stroke survivors' lives and on their wellbeing. More frequent pain has been shown to be associated with poorer health-related quality of life and self-perceived recovery following stroke (Westerlind *et al.*, 2020), and there is a strong link between pain and depressed mood (Docking and Tarrant, 2018).

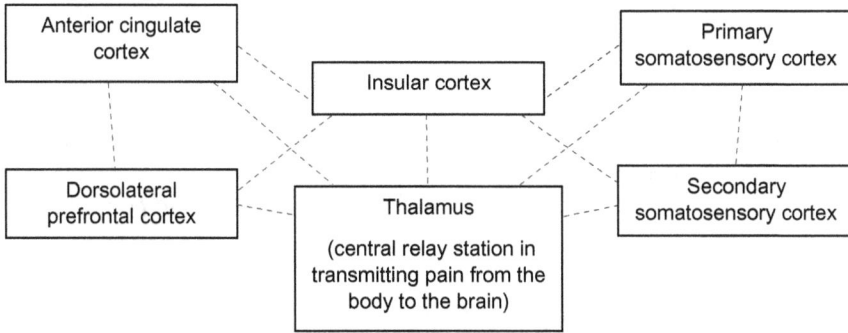

FIGURE 4.1   Basic structures of the pain matrix. (The arrows illustrate the multiple and complex connections between the different brain areas involved with pain perception.) Key: ACC, anterior cingulate cortex; dlPFC, dorsolateral prefrontal cortex; INS, insular cortex; SII, secondary somatosensory cortex; SI, primary somatosensory cortex.

Source: Monroe *et al.* (2015).

For some stroke survivors, pain can dominate their lives.

> My mind won't remember a day when I wasn't in pain. I can't imagine a day without pain. Which is my biggest thing. That's every single day, 24 hours a day. It's there constantly …. Sitting here now I am in pain, but I know as soon as I stand up it's like someone is driving knives into my leg.
>
> *(Phil, 59, embolic stroke, 2 years post stroke)*

The pain experience post-stroke can be difficult for patients to describe, particularly neuropathic pain, as this may be unlike any other pain that they have experienced before. Patients may also suffer from allodynia, where pain occurs in response to a stimulus that would not usually provoke pain, such as heat or light touch. This can make everyday activities excruciating:

> Because of the hot/cold thing, the water splashing off the base of the shower hitting my right leg feels like a bunch of needles driving into me.
>
> *(Phil, 59, embolic stroke, 2 years post stroke)*

Living with pain may also have a negative impact on sleep, which may exacerbate the fatigue that many stroke survivors suffer from. The combination of pain and fatigue may adversely affect mood, potentially leading to a vicious circle as the relationship between depression and pain is complex, with each potentially impacting on each other (Docking and Tarrant, 2018).

> When you get more tired, you have a worse day. And if you're really tired, which happens very easily, you get very negative.
> *(Phil, 59, embolic stroke, 2 years post stroke)*

The importance of listening to patients

Identification of pain is important as it can have an enormous impact on wellbeing and quality of life. It is recommended that healthcare professionals should enquire directly regarding pain, as otherwise this may not be disclosed by patients, particularly the elderly (Langhorne *et al.*, 2000). Language may be key when discussing pain, for example, older people may deny 'pain', but when asked about 'soreness' or 'aching' they may respond differently (Cox and Cannons, 2018).

The most reliable and accurate evidence regarding the existence of pain and its intensity is self-report from the individual themselves (Cox and Cannons, 2018). Assessment is not just about completing a pain scale but must involve an opportunity for the individual to talk about their pain experience (Schofield, 2018). Evaluation of pain should consider its multidimensional nature, so in addition to the sensory elements (e.g. intensity, location) assessment should explore the emotional component and the impact on the person. Stroke survivors may need encouragement and support to talk about pain or other issues such as depression, but getting their story across is a key part in helping them to manage their issues:

> Since I had my stroke, I've had to learn to talk to people more. I've never been one to express my feelings or anything like that, but since this, I've learnt I have to. Because if I want any help with what I'm going through, I've got to be honest with people, tell them what I am feeling.
> *(Phil, 59, embolic stroke, 2 years post stroke)*

Time spent listening to the person and establishing trust is invaluable in supporting the individual suffering from pain to have a positive outcome. A key component of effective interaction is that the person feels believed and has their experience validated (NICE, 2021). A trusting, supportive and collaborative relationship with the healthcare professional is more likely to result in good adherence to self-management suggestions, as well as improved resilience and confidence in their ability to self-manage (NICE, 2021). This evidence reiterates that effective listening and collaborating with stroke survivors struggling with pain improves not only the patient experience but also outcomes.

It is important to consider that many stroke survivors have barriers to communication, such as aphasia or cognitive impairment, which will affect how they can express their pain, potentially resulting in unmet needs and ongoing distress. Many stroke survivors are older adults, who may have additional co-morbidities that make assessment more challenging, for example, dementia or reduced hearing. In these situations, it is important to work with stroke survivors, their carers and family to try and explore their pain as thoroughly as possible. Even in patients with impaired cognition or communication, self-reporting may be the best and most reliable method of gaining information about the pain, but language and communication methods may need to be adapted, for example, using pictorial prompts. For stroke survivors where the barriers to communication are too significant, healthcare professionals may need to use observational pain scores such as the Pain Assessment in Advanced Dementia (PAINAD) Scale (Warden *et al.*, 2003) or Abbey Pain Score (Abbey *et al.*, 2004), and advocate for those patients who are unable to communicate their own needs.

- Think about the different words that can be used to describe pain.
- How many words can you list?
- Circle the words that you have heard your patients use most frequently when describing pain.
- Think about how you could change your questions when asking people about their pain.

Pain management

Pain management should take an individualised holistic approach, including the use of a range of elements such as education, pharmacological management, exercise, relaxation, activity management/pacing and more cognitive-based interventions such as acceptance commitment therapy (ACT) or cognitive–behavioural therapy (CBT) where appropriate. There are a wide range of pharmacological options available, which are a vital part of pain management. Although medications are the principal approach to pain control, this topic is not within the scope of this chapter, which instead focuses on the non-pharmacological elements which are often used alongside these.

Management of post-stroke pain can be difficult and may involve a trial-and-error approach (Harrison and Field, 2015). It is important to stress that pain management is *management*, not a cure. It can be thought of as providing the stroke survivor with a full toolbox of resources to help them minimise the impact of the pain on their lives. Support may be required intermittently on a long-term basis, including helping patients to access a wide range of resources to help them find the combination of pain management approaches that work for them.

> You have to find the pain management that works for you. There is no pain management that works 100% for you 100% of the time. But if you can find the pain management that works for you and helps you to have most of your time, not pain-free, but pain-managed, that makes your well-being and your mental health much easier. I have tried every single pain management option, and I have found that the combination of different things work, it's never one thing on its own.
>
> *(Jo, 47, embolic stroke as a result of endocarditis, 20 years post stroke)*
>
> Don't give up, keep trying. Have a positive attitude. You've got to keep trying. Try everything that's offered to you, and fight for stuff that isn't offered to you, if you think it might help.
>
> *(Phil, 59, embolic stroke, 2 years post stroke)*

Providing information and education to patients suffering from pain is good clinical practice (NICE, 2021). It helps empower the stroke survivor to manage their own pain and provides family and carers with knowledge and skills to support those stroke survivors who are less able to manage independently. Having the pain explained may also help individuals to feel listened to, rather than having their pain dismissed, particularly in cases of neuropathic pain, as this may not link to a particular stimulus and so is harder to understand. However, it must be remembered that just because information has been given to an individual, this does not mean that the information has been received and understood. It is important to check understanding level, and information giving may need to be re-visited and repeated at different points during the stroke survivor's journey.

Exercise may be one part of pain management, and it can be a simple, cost-effective approach. The evidence review for the NICE (2021) guidelines on chronic pain found convincing evidence from many studies that showed exercise reduced pain (23 studies) and improved quality of life (22 studies). There are several potential mechanisms through which exercise may reduce pain sensitivity and increase pain threshold; these may include immediate effects such as modulation of endogenous opioids and endocannabinoids, and reduced inflammation through inhibition of microglia activation, as well as longer-term effects including regulation of synaptic plasticity within the pain matrix, creating changes in some of the brain pathways that process pain (Ma *et al.*, 2022). In addition, exercise may also provide many other physiological benefits, for example, improving physical function, reducing cardiovascular risk factors and improving mood.

However, it is important to note that much of the research into the pain response following exercise has been done in healthy populations, and in individuals with chronic pain the pain response appears to be more variable, possibly even causing an increase in pain sensitivity following exercise in some people, particularly in the early stages of starting an exercise regime (Rice *et al.*, 2019). This may cause poor adherence to exercise and limit the longer-term benefits, so it is important to work together with the individual stroke survivor to grade the exercise to a level appropriate for them and set achievable exercise goals, as well as only increasing exercises as the stroke survivor feels confident to do so, rather than to a pre-determined schedule. A greater feeling of perceived control may improve compliance, optimising the chance of individuals achieving multiple physiological and psychological benefits that exercise can potentially deliver.

Stroke survivors may have additional barriers to exercise other than pain, so these should be explored with appropriate healthcare professionals. Cardiovascular risk factors must be considered, particularly in the more acute stages post-stroke, and exercise may need to be adapted accordingly. Stroke survivors may have a wide range of deficits, and this may result in a need to think more creatively about how to exercise. Exercise can encompass a wide range of activities, for example aerobic exercise, strength training, yoga, walking and seated cycling, and stroke survivors should be supported to try a variety of activities to help them find forms of exercise that are beneficial and that they can sustain either independently or with support from those around them. For those more physically able, activities such as Parkrun, www.parkrun.org.uk/, which has the option of walking, can be a great way to engage in exercise in a supportive community.

Exercise may feel daunting for someone who is suffering from pain, but explaining the potential benefits to the stroke survivor and supporting them may give them the courage to try.

> The idea of doing exercise worries me as I think it will make my pain worse, but when reframed as physio to help my pain it's strangely less threatening and I am more willing to try it.
>
> *(Jacqueline, 42, ischaemic stroke whilst pregnant, 12 years post stroke)*

Other forms of pain management may include Mindfulness and Acceptance Commitment Therapy, which are explored in more detail later in this chapter. Anxiety is associated with increased pain perception and reduced pain tolerance (Clancy and McVicar, 2009) and so approaches to manage this can have a significant impact on pain as well as wellbeing.

Psychological wellbeing after stroke

Following a stroke there is a natural grief cycle and a period of time needed for a person to adjust and process how to live with their new self (see Figure 4.2). Stroke survivors often find this overwhelming and despair that they will not be able to live a fulfilling and meaningful life and that they may be a burden on their family and friends (Stroke Association, 2018). A vital part of the recovery process needs to focus on establishing psychological strategies to support long-term rehabilitation and psychological wellbeing, including coming to terms with what has happened and devising strategies to move on.

Anxiety after stroke is a very common emotion and is a physical, biological and psychological response to the sudden, life changing and potentially lifelong effects of stroke on a stroke survivors' life. Knapp *et al.* (2020) reported 25% of all stroke survivors suffer post stroke anxiety and highlighted the importance of understanding the anxiety triggers and recognising the symptoms to be able to develop coping strategies and target treatments to the individual.

What is anxiety?

Anxiety is triggered when the amygdala (part of the limbic system and found deep within the temporal part of the brain between the hippocampus and the

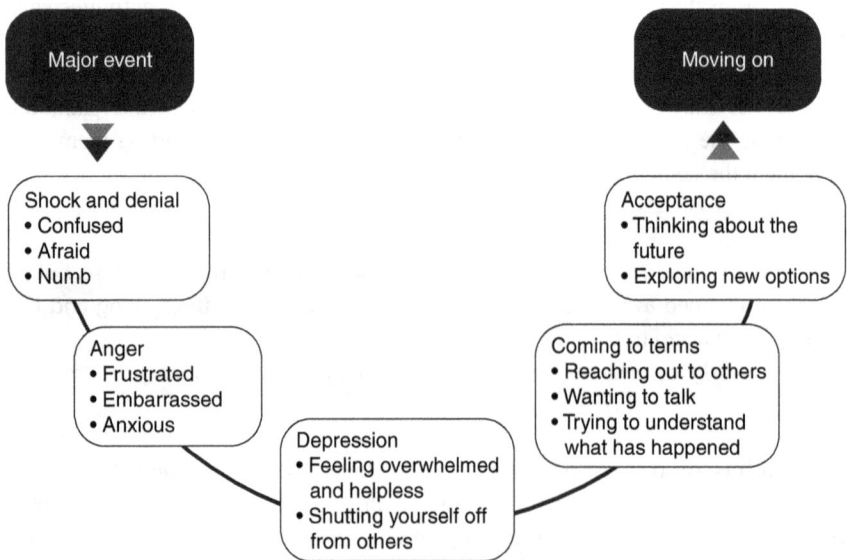

FIGURE 4.2 Grief cycle: a complete guide to emotional changes after Stroke 2018 v2.
Source: Küber-Ross (1969), adapted by Stroke Association.

hypothalamus) interprets stimuli as a threat. It sends a distress signal to the hypothalamus, which in turn relays the signal to the rest of the body by initiating the sympathetic nervous system. Adrenaline is released from the adrenal glands which sends the brain into a state of alertness. Signals are then transmitted to the hippocampus where the threat is assessed, and a decision made based on previous experience and memory, as to whether to respond to it or not (Guy-Evans, 2025; Mtui, Gruener and Dockery, 2015).

When the amygdala is activated and in a heightened state of readiness, the prefrontal cortex attempts to use aspects of our executive functioning, for example working memory, decision-making and emotional control to reduce the negative emotional response. However, the inhibitory response of the prefrontal cortex is reduced when glutamate, an excitatory neurotransmitter, is released by the amygdala; therefore the individual continues to experience feeling of heightened stress and anxiety (Guy-Evans, 2025) (see Figure 4.3).

Anxiety can be felt by anyone, for example the nerves felt just before an exam, when someone cannot eat and their heart begins to race. These are normal feelings and can be managed by an individual distracting themselves from the situation or seeking reassurance that everything will be ok. Anxiety after stroke however can develop into intense and overwhelming fear and nervousness preventing people from being able to enjoy their lives. Other symptoms may include irritability, difficulty sleeping and concentrating, rapid heart rate and feeling restless (Stroke Association, 2018). Some examples of anxiety triggers are shown in Figure 4.4.

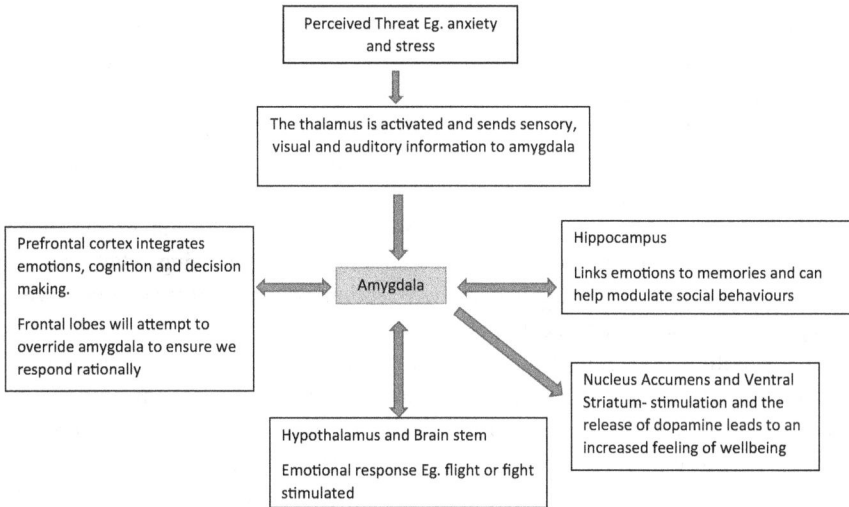

FIGURE 4.3 How perceived threat is interpreted by the brain.

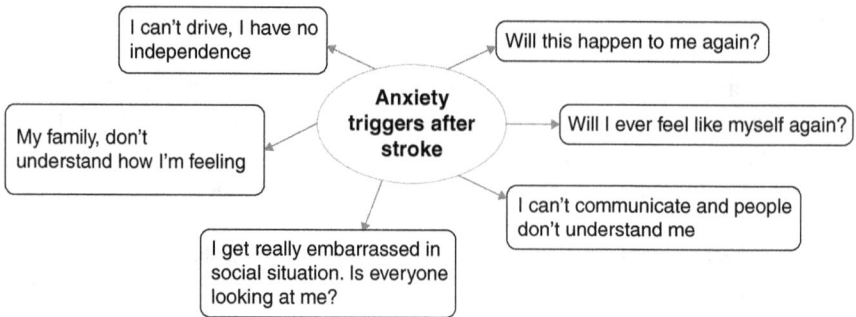

FIGURE 4.4 Some examples of anxiety triggers following a stroke.

Strategies for well-being

Mindfulness

Research has shown that there are a variety of ways to manage and address the psychological aspects of post-stroke recovery. Kabat-Zinn (2003) found that mindfulness could be highly effective for patients suffering from long-term physical health conditions that were affecting their quality of life. There are two main forms of mindfulness endorsed by the NICE National Clinical Guidelines for Depression in Adults: Treatment and Management (2022) – mindfulness-based stress reduction (MBSR) and mindfulness-based cognitive therapy (MBCT).

Mindfulness is rooted in Buddhism and Yoga which was synthesised with the physiology of stress and stress perception into a more secular Western context by Kabat-Zinn (2003). It is a method used to help people understand how they are feeling and to be aware of what triggers feelings of negativity and how to bring themselves out of this cycle. Enabling a person to develop an open, non-judgemental and non-reactive relationship with their internal thoughts, emotions and sensations may mean physical symptoms can be reduced and positive behaviour change is promoted (Luberto *et al.*, 2020).

Mindfulness creates a link between the mind and body with the aim of improving balance. It works at the level of metacognition, that is knowing what you are thinking when you are thinking it, and interoception, which involves knowing what is happening in the body at a certain point in time.

Whilst both MBSR and MBCT focus on self-regulating attention to the current moment and experience as the main feature of mindfulness, MBSR tends to be used more generally for a range of physical and emotional conditions. It teaches how to recognise habitual and unhelpful reactions to difficult thoughts, feelings and experiences and how to accept them and find a way to manage them. MBCT focuses more specifically on low mood, depression and recurring depressive episodes, enabling people to recognise the cyclic nature of their depression, what triggers these episodes and how to respond to them intentionally and purposefully (Hofmann and Gomez, 2017).

An MBSR course may involve up to eight 2-3 hour sessions involving individual and group sessions where the focus is on experiencing how the individual is feeling in that moment. An MBCT course may involve up to 20 sessions lasting 30-60 minutes. These sessions are aimed at identifying unhelpful thoughts, feelings and activities and finding ways to change them. Adaptations to this delivery structure can be made to accommodate the different needs of stroke survivors.

Mindfulness practice:
- Focus on your breath
- Close your eyes
- Inhale slowly and then exhale slowly
- What do you feel?
- What do you hear?
- How do your feet feel on the floor?
- What emotions do you feel?

Tip: Set an intention and if your mind wanders bring it back to focus.

How can mindfulness help recovery after stroke?

Neurobiological research has shown that mindfulness can help reduce the impact of the sympathetic nervous system and the hypothalamic–pituitary–adrenal response to acute stress; this improved immune response acts to lower the production of proinflammatory cytokines and reduce physiological stress (Willekens *et al.*, 2018). Marchand (2014) showed through neuroimaging that practising mindfulness techniques can lead to changes in brain function, which corresponded to areas associated with managing and regulating the body's emotional response.

Studies have shown that mindfulness can decrease mental fatigue, defined as an extreme reaction to mental and cognitive tasks and a reduced ability to deal with daytime fatigue in stroke survivors (Han, 2021). However, many of the studies focus on stroke survivors with mild to moderate deficits and those with minimal cognitive impairments who were able to follow an 8-week MBSR programme. In contrast to this, Wrapson *et al.* (2021) found that stoke survivors with more severe functional impairments who followed an individualised one to one approach to mindfulness could also benefit. Saban *et al.* (2022) highlighted that by shortening the sessions, allowing rest breaks, and modifying physical movements alongside sensory and memory support, mindfulness could be more accessible to a range of stroke survivors.

Mindfulness interventions that include caregivers and families have been shown to reduce the potential negative outcomes caused by emotional distress in the acute period after stroke (Bannon *et al.*, 2020). Louise's story given below highlights this.

Following my stroke, I was very anxious, and I found being on the stroke unit very stressful. It was noisy and I was spending my day worrying about everything from my recovery to how my husband and son were coping. I used noise cancelling headphones to try and block out the distractions on the ward to allow me to concentrate on being mindful and being in the moment, using mindfulness videos on the internet. These helped me to get to sleep and tapped into my unconscious. Since returning home I have continued using mindfulness techniques and I feel hopeful, and my son even joins me on occasions. Mindfulness techniques have helped us as a family to cope with my stroke and find a new way to live.

(Louise, 46, left thalamic intracranial haemorrhage, 18 months post stroke)

You may like to access the NHS Mindfulness website or signpost family for further information and practical advice Mindfulness – NHS (https://www.nhs.uk/mental-health/self-help/tips-and-support/mindfulness/).

Nature

Having a healthy lifestyle, enjoying time in the outdoors and exercising are all invaluable for reducing the risk of illness and improving a person's wellbeing. This is especially important following a life-changing event such as a stroke. In the clinicians' experience stroke patients in hospital often feel disconnected from the outside world and want to go outside to experience fresh air and regain a feeling of normality.

Anecdotally many patients report how important their gardens are to them and relate their rehabilitation goals to being able to return to their own gardens once they are discharged. Evidence suggests that increasing time spent doing activities in an environment that is relevant and meaningful can significantly improve mood, participation, engagement and help patients connect with past experiences which can lead to better stroke rehabilitation outcomes (Barello *et al.*, 2016). Spending time in the garden or outdoor spaces can also lead to improved immersive sensory experiences which link to improved memory, and cognitive abilities.

Spending time within nature can be beneficial in promoting both physical and emotional wellbeing (McMahan and Estes, 2015). There are several suggested mechanisms for the benefits of nature: the physical activity, the social factors of spending time with others and the air quality (Anderson *et al.*, 2021). For example, it has been suggested that antimicrobial compounds released by plants can boost immune functioning, and the sights and sounds of nature encourage relaxation, which can decrease blood pressure and increase parasympathetic activity (Kuo, 2015). The benefits of exposure to sunlight also contribute to increasing vitamin D, whilst working in a garden can lead to improved aerobic capacity and increased strength and dexterity (Sowah *et al.*, 2017). It can also boost sleep and result in improved immune functioning (Anderson *et al.*, 2021). Some stroke patients may have mobility issues or have reduced access to outside space which may prohibit getting outside into nature. In these cases, listening to sounds of nature through headphones could be beneficial, as it has been shown to moderate the stress response by decreasing sympathetic activity (Alvarsson *et al.*, 2010). Even observing nature by looking at pictures of nature can improve mood and reduce depression, stress, fear and pain (Jo *et al.*, 2019). Exposure to outdoor spaces can reduce the effects of health inequalities such as low socioeconomic status and deprivation, and the interaction of people with different functional and cognitive abilities can offer ongoing support and friendship in a safe environment (Fuller *et al.*, 2007).

There is a possible interaction between nature and the capacity for being mindful (Djernis *et al.*, 2019). Being in nature can be helpful in the process of attending to thoughts, feelings and sensations, encouraging the individual to focus on the moment.

Clinical experience suggests that many health professionals are realising that the physical and emotional impacts of gardening and being in the outdoors post stroke are huge, and that social prescribing and referring stroke survivors to ongoing community projects have significant long-term health benefits.

> The change of environment with different sensory inputs e.g. trees rustling, bird song and the warmth was uplifting for me.
>
> *(Stroke patient)*
>
> Lovely to get some fresh air and personal space.
>
> *(Stroke patient)*

Groups

Group sessions may have a valuable role in helping people to recover and adjust following stroke. In the acute setting, finding ways to increase the time that stroke patients spend in meaningful and task-specific activities is an important part of rehabilitation, as highlighted in the National Clinical Guidelines for Stroke (National Clinical Guideline for Stroke for the UK and Ireland, 2023). Clinical experience and patient feedback suggests that group work allows an opportunity for increased activity, and has a vital functional, social and emotional role to play.

Following discharge from hospital, continuing to address stroke survivors' abilities to come to terms with what has happened to them and giving them back a level of control promotes improved outcomes. However, many stroke survivors report that they feel lost and alone once they are discharged from hospital, and that community rehabilitation services do not always bridge that gap (ISWP, 2023). Community stroke support groups, tailored exercise groups and charity groups such as the Stroke Association therefore have a vital role in the long-term support of stroke survivors.

The National Clinical Guidelines for Stroke (National Clinical Guideline for Stroke for the UK and Ireland, 2023) recommend group work that is relevant to the person's needs, which will enhance recovery and allow them and their families to better understand their difficulties. It is important to acknowledge that stroke survivors need to be at the right stage of their rehabilitation to fully access and utilise this support. Furthermore, although groups can provide great benefits, it is important to carefully consider the mix of people within each group. Some stroke survivors report negative experiences where they have attended groups where they feel that they are with the 'wrong' people, and this can make them feel worse.

I felt too young to be attending a stroke group, they were all so much older than me. It made me feel depressed and I didn't find it a positive experience. I needed to work out where I fitted in, in my new world and find a way back to myself. I have since found an exercise group for people with neurological difficulties and I love it. I have help to adapt the exercises and I know I won't be judged if I rest and then carry on. I feel more like myself again.

(Louise, 46, left thalamic intracranial haemorrhage, 18 months post stroke)

I was looking at all these other people around me who'd had brain injuries and hadn't got better, really really poorly people .... It had a massive impact on me and how I felt.

(Jacqueline, 42, ischaemic stroke whilst pregnant, 12 years post stroke)

It is not only the age of the attendees that should be considered, but also other factors such as the severity of their impairments and the stage they are at in the post-stroke journey. Although it may never be possible to create a group of perfectly suited individuals, it is important to be cognisant of the impact the participants may have on each other and offer support as appropriate, particularly for new members joining an established group.

Acceptance Commitment Therapy (ACT)

Around a third of stroke patients will experience depression within the first year following stroke (Stroke Association, 2018), which may be due to struggles in adjustment, post-traumatic stress and pain, all of which can hamper rehabilitation and affect quality of life. There is already a body of evidence that acceptance commitment therapy (ACT) is successful in improving pain experiences and psychological outcomes for chronic pain; see Lai *et al.* (2023) for a meta-analysis. Whilst there is currently little evidence for other psychological therapies post stroke, ACT has demonstrated success in decreasing depression and increasing hopefulness in a small randomised controlled trial of a low-intensity group intervention (Majumdar and Morris, 2019). The key aim of ACT is to shift the focus away from avoiding sensations, thoughts and feelings that are unpleasant and move towards mindful observation of them (Hayes *et al.*, 2006). In doing this, a wellbeing approach of acceptance of a changed reality is adopted, individuals are mindful and present, develop goals and experience self-acceptance (Large *et al.*, 2019).

Music

Music is an easily accessible adjuvant therapy that can be beneficial for wellbeing (Viola *et al.*, 2023). There is a growing body of literature that reports on the benefits of listening to sounds and music in decreasing pain and increasing positive affect (Arnold, Bagg and Harvey, 2024; Chen, Yuan, Wang *et al.*, 2025; van der Valk Bouman *et al.*, 2025). There are individual differences when it comes to type of music, but there is evidence that preferred music is linked with reduced pain intensity (Timmerman, van Dijk and van den Bosch, 2023). Music can act as a distraction but is also associated with reduced stress and cortisol levels through modulation of stress (de Witte *et al.*, 2020). There is also some evidence to suggest that music listening during stroke rehabilitation may enhance cognitive recovery and reduce low mood (Särkämö *et al.*, 2008).

Motivation and goal attainment

Clinical experience has shown that low mood, anxiety and pain may all lead to feelings of frustration and undermine motivation to engage in therapy. A study looking into the views and beliefs of patients found that those determined to have high motivation understood what was expected of them, took an active role in their rehabilitation and were able to understand information given to them. However, those perceived to have low motivation did not understand the steps required to achieve a goal, made comparisons to other patients and relied on healthcare professionals to make decisions for them (Maclean *et al.*, 2000). Therefore, addressing these misconceptions and understanding what is important to a stroke survivor is key to understanding what motivates them and how to maximise their potential to achieve their rehabilitation goals. Self-efficacy, an individual's belief in their ability to achieve a goal, is the cornerstone of motivation and perseverance to succeed and to overcome setbacks (Bandura, 1997; Jones *et al.*, 2009). When a person is feeling in control, they are more likely to have higher self-esteem, less anxiety and more likely to engage in different activities (National Clinical Guideline for Stroke for the UK and Ireland, 2023; Pagnini, Bercovitz and Langer 2016).

By building confidence, improving skills through practice and knowledge through communication and information, stroke survivors and healthcare professionals can build a meaningful therapeutic relationship. Stroke survivors should have the opportunity to set their own goals whether these are huge or small, and work through steps to achieve these, reflecting on their progress and celebrating their successes however small.

Toolbox to support stroke survivors with longer-term issues and promote wellbeing	
Listen to their experience	Nature-based therapy
Support from family and friends	Music
Mindfulness	Attending groups
Acceptance Commitment Therapy	Setting goals
Exercise	Signposting to specialist onward support if required

> The impact of stroke is so varied affecting every inch of life, so having a varied approach and toolbox of strategies is vital to managing pain, well-being and living a fulfilled life after stroke.
>
> *(Jo, 47, embolic stroke as a result of endocarditis, 20 years post stroke)*

Conclusion

Stroke survivors may face ongoing challenges, and recovery is rarely a smooth path. Supporting the stroke survivor to have a toolbox of resources to use when challenges arise empowers them to be able to self-manage and reduce the impact of these difficulties on their day-to-day lives.

References

Abbey, J., Piller, N., De Bellis, A., Esterman, A., Parker, D., Giles, L., Lowcay, B. (2004). The Abbey pain scale: a 1-minute numerical indicator for people with end-stage dementia. *International Journal of Palliative Nursing*, 10(1), 6–13. Available at: https://doi.org/10.12968/ijpn.2004.10.1.12013

Ali, M., Tibble, H., Brady, M. C., Quinn, T. J., Sunnerhagen, K. S., Venketasubramanian, N., Shuaib, A., Pandyan, A., Mead, G., VISTA Collaboration (2023). Prevalence, trajectory, and predictors of poststroke pain: retrospective analysis of pooled clinical trial data set. *Stroke*, 54(12), 3107–3116. Available at: https://doi.org/10.1161/STROKEAHA.123.043355

Alvarsson, J. J., Wiens, S., Nilsson, M. E. (2010). Stress recovery during exposure to nature sound and environmental noise. *International Journal of Environmental Research and Public Health*, 7(3), 1036–1046. https://doi.org/10.3390/ijerph7031036

Arnold, C.A., Bagg, M.K., and Harvey, A.R. (2024). The psychophysiology of music-based interventions and the experience of pain. *Frontiers in Psychology*, 15, [online] Available at: https://doi.org/10.3389/fpsyg.2024.1361857

Andersen, L., Corazon, S., Stigsdotter, U.K. (2021) Nature Exposure and Its Effects on Immune System Functioning: A Systematic Review. *Int. J. Environ. Res. Public Health* 2021, 18, 1416. Available at: https://doi.org/10.3390/ijerph18041416

Bannon, S., Lester, E. G., Gates, M. V, McCurley, J., Lin A., Rosand, J., Vranceanu, A. M. (2020). Recovering together: Building resiliency in dyads of stroke patients and their caregivers at risk for chronic emotional distress; a feasibility study. *Pilot Feasibility Study*, 6, 75. Available at: https://doi.org/10.1186/s40814-020-00615-z

Bandura, A. (1997). *Self-efficacy: The exercise of control*. New York: Freeman.

Barello, S., Graffigna, G., Menichetti, J., Sozzi, M., Savarese, M., Albino Claudio, B., Corbo, M. (2016). The value of a therapeutic gardening intervention for post-stroke patients' engagement during rehabilitation: an exploratory qualitative study. *Journal of Participatory Medicine*, e9.

Chen, S., Yuan, Q., Wang, C., Ye, J. and Yang, L.. (2025). The effect of music therapy for patients with chronic pain: systematic review and meta-analysis. *BMC Psychology*, 13, 455. [online] Available at: https://doi.org/10.1186/s40359-025-02643-x

Cherup, N. P., Robayo, L. E., Vastano, R., Fleming, L., Levin, B. E., Widerström-Noga, E. (2023). Neuropsychological function in traumatic brain injury and the influence of chronic pain. *Perceptual and Motor Skills*, 130(4), 1495–1523. Available at: https://doi.org/10.1177/00315125231174082

Clancy, J., McVicar, A. (2009). *Physiology and Anatomy for Nurses and Healthcare Practitioners: A Homeostatic Approach*, 3rd ed. Routledge. Available at: https://doi.org/10.1201/b13385

Cox, F., Cannons, K. (2018). Self-report measures of pain assessment, in Schofield, A. (ed.). *The Assessment of Pain in Older People: UK National Guidelines. Age and Ageing*, 47, i1–i22. Available at: https://doi.org/10.1093/ageing/afx192

de Witte, M., Spruit, A., van Hooren, S., Moonen, X. and Stams, G.J.J.M (2020). Effects of music interventions on stress-related outcomes: a systematic review and two meta-analyses. *Health Psychology Review*, 14(2), 294–324. [online] Available at: https://doi.org/10.1080/17437199.2019.162789

Djernis, D., Lerstrup, I., Poulsen, D., Stigsdotter, U., Dahlgaard, J., O'Toole, M. (2019). A systematic review and meta-analysis of nature-based mindfulness: effects of moving mindfulness training into an outdoor natural setting. *International Journal of Environmental Research and Public Health*, 16(17), 3202. Available at: https://doi.org/10.3390/ijerph16173202

Docking, R., Tarrant, L. (2018). Pain assessment of older adults with mental health and psychological problems, in Schofield, A (ed). *The Assessment of Pain in Older People: UK National Guidelines. Age and Ageing*, 47, i1–i22. Available at: https://doi.org/10.1093/ageing/afx192

Fuller, R. A., Irvine, K. N., Devine-Wright, P., Warren, P. H., Gaston, K. J. (2007). Psychological benefits of greenspace increase with biodiversity. *Biol Letters*, 3, 390–394.

Garcia-Larrea, L., Peyron, R. (2013). Pain matrices and neuropathic pain matrices: a review. *Pain*, 154 (Suppl 1), S29–S43. Available at: https://doi.org/10.1016/j.pain.2013.09.001

Guy-Evans, O. (2025). Reviewed by Mcleod, S. Amygdala: What is it & it's functions. www.simplypsychology.org/amygdala.html

Han, A. (2021). Mindfulness- and acceptance-based interventions for stroke survivors: a systematic review and meta-analysis. *Rehabilitation Counseling Bulletin*, 66(2). Available at: doi:10.1177/00343552211043257

Hansen, A. P., Marcussen, N. S., Klit, H., Andersen, G., Finnerup, N. B., Jensen, T. S. (2012). Pain following stroke: a prospective study. *European Journal of Pain (London, England)*, 16(8), 1128–1136. Available at: https://doi.org/10.1002/j.1532-2149.2012.00123.x

Harrison, R., Field, T. (2015). Post stroke pain: identification, assessment, and therapy. *Cerebrovascular Diseases*, 39(3–4), 190–201. Available at: doi:10.1159/000375397. Epub 2015 Mar 5. PMID: 25766121.

Hayes, S. C., Luoma, J. B., Bond, F. W., Masuda, A., Lillis, J. (2006). Acceptance and commitment therapy: model, processes and outcomes. *Behaviour Research and Therapy*, 44(1), 1–25. https://doi.org/10.1016/j.brat.2005.06.006

Hofmann, S. G., Gomez, A. F. (2017). Mindfulness-based interventions for anxiety and depression. *Psychiatry Clinical North America*, 40(4), 739–749.

Intercollegiate Stroke Working Party (2023) *National Clinical Guideline for Stroke for the UK and Ireland*. London. Available at: www.strokeguideline.org

Jimenez, M.P., DeVille, N.V., Elliott, E.G., Schiff, J.E. Wilt, G.E. Hart, J.E., James, P. (2021). Associations between Nature Exposure and Health: A Review of the Evidence. *Int. J. Environ. Res. Public Health, 18*, 4790. Available at: https://doi.org/10.3390/ijerph18094790

Jo, H., Song, C., Miyazaki, Y. (2019). Physiological benefits of viewing nature: a systematic review of indoor experiments. *International Journal of Environmental Research and Public Health*, 16(23), 4739. https://doi.org/10.3390/ijerph16234739

Jones, F., Mandy, A., and Partridge C. (2009). Changing self efficacy in individuals following first time stroke: preliminary study of novel self management interventions. *Clinical rehabilitation*, 2, 522–533.

Kabat-Zinn, J. (2003). Mindfulness-based interventions in context: past, present and future. *Clinical Psychology: Science and Practice*, 10, 144–156.

Klit, H., Finnerup, N. B., Overvad, K., Andersen, G., Jensen, T. S. (2011). Pain following stroke: a population-based follow-up study. *PLoS One*, 6(11), e27607. Available at: https://doi.org/10.1371/journal.pone.0027607

Knapp, P., Dunn-Roberts, A., Thomas, S. A. (2020). Frequency of anxiety after stroke: an updated systematic review and meta-analysis of observational studies. *International Journal of Stroke*, 15(3), 244–255.

Kuner, R., Flor, H. (2017). Structural plasticity and reorganisation in chronic pain. *Nature Reviews Neuroscience*, 18, 20–30. https://doi.org/10.1038/nrn.2016.162

Kuber-Ross, E. (1969). *On Death and Dying: What the Dying Have To Teach Doctors, Nurses, Clergy & Their Own Families*. Scribner Book Company, New York.

Kuo, M. (2015). How might contact with nature promote human health? Promising mechanisms and a possible central pathway. *Frontiers in Psychology*, 6, 1093. Available at: https://doi.org/10.3389/fpsyg.2015.01093

Lai, L., Liu, Y., McCracken, L. M., Li, Y., Ren, Z. (2023). The efficacy of acceptance and commitment therapy for chronic pain: a three-level meta-analysis and a trial sequential analysis of randomized controlled trials. *Behaviour Research and Therapy*, 165, 104308. https://doi.org/10.1016/j.brat.2023.104308

Langhorne, P., Stott, D. J., Robertson, L., MacDonald, J., Jones, L., McAlpine, C., Dick, F., Taylor, G. S., Murray, G. (2000). Medical complications after stroke: a multicenter study. *Stroke*, 31(6), 1223–1229. Available at: https://doi.org/10.1161/01.str.31.6.1223

Large, R., Samuel, V., Morris, R. (2019). A changed reality; experience of an acceptance and commitment therapy (ACT) group after stroke. *Neuropsychological Rehabilitation*, 30(8), 1477–1496. Available at: https://doi.org/10.1080/09602011.2019.1589531

Luberto, C. M., Hall, D. L., Park, E. R., Haramati, A., Cotton, S. (2020). A perspective on the similarities and differences between mindfulness and relaxation. *Global Advances in Health and Medicine*, 9, 1–13.

Ma, Y., Luo, J., Wang, X. Q. (2022). The effect and mechanism of exercise for post-stroke pain. *Frontiers in Molecular Neuroscience*, 15, 1074205. Available at: https://doi.org/10.3389/fnmol.2022.1074205

Majumdar, S., Morris, R. (2019). Brief group-based acceptance and commitment therapy for stroke survivors. *The British Journal of Clinical Psychology*, 58(1), 70–90. Available at: https://doi.org/10.1111/bjc.12198

Marchand, W. R. (2014). Neural mechanisms of mindfulness and meditation: evidence from neuroimaging studies. *World Journal of Radiology*, 6, 471–479. Available at: doi:10.4329/wjr.v6.i7.471

Maclean, N., Pound, P., Wolfe, C., Rudd, A. (2000). Qualitative analysis of stroke patients' motivation for rehabilitation. *BMJ*, 321, 1051–1054.

McMahan, E., Estes, D. (2015). The effect of contact with natural environments on positive and negative affect: a meta-analysis. *The Journal of Positive Psychology*. 10. Available at: doi:10.1080/17439760.2014.994224

Melzack, R. (2001). Pain and the neuromatrix in the brain. *Journal of Dental Education*, 65, 1378–1382. Available at: https://doi.org/10.1002/j.0022-0337.2001.65.12.tb03497.x

Moisset, X., Bouhassira, D. (2007). Brain imaging of neuropathic pain. *NeuroImage*, 37(Suppl 1), S80–S88. Available at: https://doi.org/10.1016/j.neuroimage.2007.03.054

Mtui, E., Gruener G., and Dockery, P. (2015) Fitzgeralds Clinical Neuroanatomy and Neuroscience (E Book). Elsevier 7th Ed.

National Clinical Guidelines for Depression in Adults: Treatment and Management (2022, June 29). Available at Overview | Depression in adults: treatment and management | Guidance | NICE

National Institute for Health and Care Excellence (NICE) (2021). Chronic pain (primary and secondary) in over 16s: assessment of all chronic pain and management of chronic primary pain [NICE guideline 193]. Available at: www.nice.org.uk/guidance/ng193

O'Donnell, M. J., Diener, H. C., Sacco, R. L., Panju, A. A., Vinisko, R., Yusuf, S., PRoFESS Investigators (2013). Chronic pain syndromes after ischemic stroke: PRoFESS trial. *Stroke*, 44(5), 1238–1243. Available at: https://doi.org/10.1161/STROKE AHA.111.671008

Pagnini, F., Bercovitz K., and Langer, E. (2016). Perceived control and Mindfulness: Implications for Clinical Practice. *Journal of Psychotherapy Integration*, 26, 2, 91–102.

Rice, D., Nijs, J., Kosek, E., Wideman, T., Hasenbring, M. I., Koltyn, K., Graven-Nielsen, T., Polli, A. (2019). Exercise-induced hypoalgesia in pain-free and chronic pain populations: state of the art and future directions. *The Journal of Pain*, 20(11), 1249–1266. Available at: https://doi.org/10.1016/j.jpain.2019.03.005

Saban, K. L., Dina, T., De La Pena, P. (2022). Nursing implications of mindfulness-informed interventions for stroke survivors and their families. *Stroke*, 53, 3485–3493.

Särkämö, T., Tervaniemi, M., Laitinen, S., Forsblom, A., Soinila, S., Mikkonen, M., Autti, T., Silvennoinen, H. M., Erkkilä, J., Laine, M., Peretz, I., Hietanen, M. (2008). Music listening enhances cognitive recovery and mood after middle cerebral artery stroke. *Brain: A Journal of Neurology*, 131(Pt 3), 866–876. Available at: https://doi.org/10.1093/brain/awn013

Schofield, A. (2018). The assessment of pain in older people: UK national guidelines. *Age and Ageing*, 47, i1–i22. Available at: doi:10.1093/ageing/afx192

Sowah, D., Fan, X., Dennett, L., Hagtvedt, R., Straube, S. (2017). Vitamin D levels and deficiency with different occupations: a systematic review. *BMC Public Health*, 17, 519.

Stroke Association (2018). A complete guide to the emotional changes after stroke. Available at a_complete_guide_to_emotional_changes_after_stroke.pdf

van der Valk Bouman, E.S., Becker, A.S., Schaap, J., Cats, R., Berghman, M., and Klimek, M. (2025). Perceptions of music listening for pain management: a multi-method study. *BMJ Open*, 15, 3, e097233. [online] Available at: https://doi.org/10.1136/bmjopen-2024-097233

Viola, E., Martorana, M., Airoldi, C., Meini, C., Ceriotti, D., De Vito, M., De Ambrosi, D. and Faggiano, F. (2023). The role of music in promoting health and wellbeing: a systematic review and meta-analysis. *European Journal of Public Health*, 33,4, 738–745. Available at: https://doi.org/10.1093/eurpub/ckad063

Warden, V., Hurley, A. C., Volicer, L. (2003). Development and psychometric evaluation of the Pain Assessment in Advanced Dementia (PAINAD) scale. *Journal of the American Medical Directors Association*, 4(1), 9–15. Available at: https://doi.org/10.1097/01.JAM.0000043422.31640.F7

Westerlind, E., Singh, R., Persson, H. C., Sunnerhagen, K. S. (2020). Experienced pain after stroke: a cross-sectional 5-year follow-up study. *BMC Neurology*, 20(1), 4. Available at: https://doi.org/10.1186/s12883-019-1584-z

Willekens, B., Perotta, G., Cras, P., Cool, N. (2018). Into the moment: does mindfulness affect biological pathways in multiple sclerosis. *Frontiers in Behavioural Neuroscience*, 12, 1–9.

Wrapson, W., Dorrestein, M., Wrapson, J., Theadom, A., Kayes, N. M., Snell, D. L., Rutherford, S., Roche, M., Babbage, D. R., Taylor, S., *et al.* (2021). A feasibility study of a one-to-one mindfulness-based intervention for improving mood in stroke survivors. *Mindfulness*, 12:1148–1158. Available at: doi:0.1007/s12671-020-01583-4

5

ENJOYING FOOD AND DRINK

Sarah Davies, Konstantinos Eleftheriadis and Ruth Trout

Learning outcomes

- To understand the challenges of eating and drinking after a stroke and how these can be addressed.
- To raise awareness of malnutrition in stroke and long-term implications for nutrition and hydration.
- To apply principles related to shared decision-making, empowerment and choice.
- To analyse ethical considerations related to eating and drinking, including care of patients receiving palliative care.

Background

The British Association for Parenteral and Enteral Nutrition (BAPEN, 2023) estimates that around 30–40% of people admitted to hospitals or care homes in the UK are found to be actually or at risk of malnourishment or under-nutrition. Studies indicate that hospital nutrition and hydration need improvement, with poor food quality and limited patient support reported (Francis, 2013). Stroke can cause additional challenges with eating and drinking due to dysphagia, drowsiness, cognitive impairment, aphasia and weakness (Burgos *et al.*, 2018). These changes in health status can make meeting nutritional requirements complex and stressful for stroke survivors and their families. The National Institute for Health and Care

DOI: 10.4324/9781003426196-6

Excellence (NICE, 2023) and the UK National Clinical Guideline for Stroke (ISWP, 2023) recommend individuals should:

- Receive a swallow screen
- Be screened for malnutrition
- Be referred to a dietitian and receive dietary advice if at risk of malnutrition or if they have dysphagia
- Be considered for enteral nutrition if they are unable to meet their requirements via oral food/drinks
- Receive individualised dietary advice and monitoring.

It is therefore important that all parties are equipped to deal with the specific challenges related to eating and drinking following a stroke.

Malnutrition

Malnutrition affects about 50% of stroke survivors by the time of hospital discharge (Burgos *et al.*, 2018; Figure 5.1). Malnourishment results in lower survival rates, requires more intensive treatment, causes reduced quality of life (QoL) and makes people prone to illness. Causes include eating and drinking difficulties, poor diet quality, co-morbidities, unmet metabolic requirements and nutrient absorption issues (NICE, 2017). Wider issues, such as stroke side effects and survivors' priorities, also impact nutrition. For instance, aphasia and cognitive impairment may indirectly affect eating and drinking. These stroke effects further impair clinical outcomes and the enjoyment of food.

Table 5.1 outlines some of the signs and symptoms of malnutrition to be aware of (BAPEN, 2024).

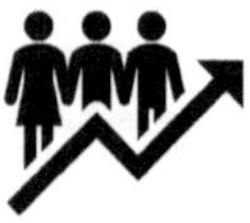	Three million people in the UK are malnourished or at risk. Danone report that 62% of the UK population cannot define malnourishment. Although it can happen to anyone, those most at risk are vulnerable people or those with existing health issues.
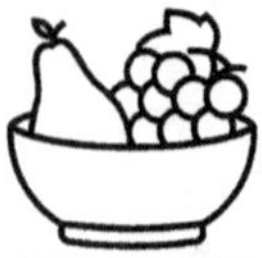	Malnutrition occurs when the body isn't receiving the right nutrients. This may be due to medical or societal factors.
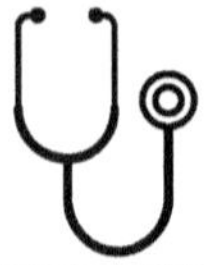	Malnutrition costs society approximately £3.5 billion and can cause long-term health effects if not detected early.

FIGURE 5.1   Malnutrition in the UK.

Strokes' impact on eating and drinking can significantly affect QoL (Burgos *et al.*, 2018). A study on QoL and perceptions regarding tube-feeding for long-term tube-fed stroke patients showed that QoL and nutritional support are considered the most important aspects of tube-feeding in adults living in the community following stroke (Eleftheriadis and Madden, 2024). Effective communication between healthcare professionals, adequate training to be able to self-care or provision of trained carers are important aspects to allow individuals to cope with changes after stroke and maintain QoL whilst receiving tube-feeding.

Everyone who is admitted to hospital must be screened for malnutrition within 24 hours of admission (ISWP, 2023). Someone may be well nourished upon admission, and sometimes, this may change after discharge from hospital. Anecdotal evidence suggests that some patients who are eating and drinking well in hospital may decline upon discharge due to new living arrangements or new care needs. Therefore, ongoing dietetic support post discharge from hospital is important for long-term health.

For individuals affected by stroke who want to assess their potential risk of malnutrition. This is a fast and free screening tool: https://www.malnutritionself screening.org/self-screening.html.

Nutritional support

Stroke survivors who are identified as at risk of malnutrition will require nutritional support (NICE, 2017). They will be assessed by ward-specific dietitians in UK hospitals, with specialised dietitians in stroke units. Not all patients receive input from dietitians, but their importance is well recognised. Care should be evidence based according to individual need, so it is clinically valuable (British Dietetic Association (BDA, 2020).

Nutritional support aims to maintain or improve nutritional status, support recovery and prevent or treat malnutrition. The options for nutrition support are (a) oral nutrition support, (b) enteral nutrition support and (c) parenteral nutrition support.

Oral nutrition support: Diet is supplemented with fortified meals and/or high-energy snacks/foods and/or oral nutritional supplements (otherwise known as sip feeds) (NICE, 2017).

TABLE 5.1 Signs and symptoms of malnutrition

Muscle weakness (sarcopenia)	*Cognitive impairment, Poor concentration*
Weight loss/reduced appetite	Dysphagia
Tiredness/feeling weak	Dry skin/lips (dehydration)
Low mood, sadness, depression	Dark urine (dehydration)
Impaired immunity and increased infections	Wounds healing slowly, pressure injuries

Enteral nutrition: This involves delivering nutrients directly to the gastrointestinal tract via a feeding tube. This method is normally used when a person has a functioning digestive system but cannot eat or drink enough by mouth. Forms of enteral nutrition include:

- Nasogastric (NG) tube: Inserted through the nose into the stomach.
- Nasojejunal (NJ) tube: Inserted through the nose and into the jejunum. These tubes also have a gastric port where medication can be administered.
- Percutaneous endoscopic gastrostomy (PEG) tube: Inserted directly into the stomach through an abdominal incision under endoscopic procedure.
- Radiologically inserted gastrostomy (RIG) tube: Inserted directly into the stomach through an abdominal incision guided under X-ray equipment
- Jejunostomy (JEJ) tube: Inserted directly into the small intestine.

Parenteral nutrition: Nutrients are delivered directly into the bloodstream intravenously. This approach is used when the digestive system is not functioning or accessible. It is rarely needed long-term for stroke patients.

While many stroke patients experience eating and drinking difficulties, not all need long-term nutrition support.

Diets for stroke prevention

Professional standards recognise the importance of promoting, protecting and maintaining health as well as preventing ill health (Nursing and Midwifery Council (NMC), 2018b, 2018c; Health and Care Professionals Council (HCPC), 2013a, 2013b). Educating and empowering patients effectively to improve their dietary habits or maintain them will improve QoL and have a beneficial effect in terms of reducing the risk of subsequent strokes. Managing stroke risk factors, such as diet and physical activity, can help prevent another stroke. A healthy diet controls hypertension, diabetes, obesity and high cholesterol.

Dietary changes may be difficult to adopt over the long term. A registered dietitian can help identify nutrients of concern and provide tailored dietary advice to minimise risk of further stroke.

The focus must be on foods that can be eaten rather than those that cannot so that good dietary habits can be reinforced.

Diets rich in fruits, vegetables, fibre, wholegrains, nuts, seeds and healthy fats, particularly olive oil, have been shown to be beneficial in reducing cholesterol levels and have an overall beneficial impact on secondary stroke prevention (NICE, 2023). The Mediterranean diet (ISWP, 2023) and Dietary Approaches to Stop Hypertension (National Heart, Lung and Blood Institute, 2021) have positive effects in terms of reducing cholesterol, blood pressure and risk of coronary heart disease. Principles to reduce stroke risk include:

- Follow the Eat-Well guide: eat five plus portions of fruits/vegetables daily and two portions of oily fish weekly.
- Reduce saturated fats, replacing them with monounsaturated fats like olive or rapeseed oil and olive-based spreads.
- Keep salt intake low by avoiding added salt and minimising processed foods.
- Maintain tight control of blood pressure and blood sugar levels.
- Limit alcohol intake to 14 units per week, spread over at least 3 days.
- Aim for a healthy body mass index (BMI) (NICE, 2023).

The NICE website contains a 'secondary prevention of stroke' page which contains further information on diet to aid stroke prevention. https://cks.nice.org.uk/topics/stroke-tia/management/secondary-prevention-following-stroke-tia

Stroke affects each patient differently. Malnutrition can impact rehabilitation and QoL and may require artificial nutrition support via one of the methods discussed above.

Dysphagia

Dysphagia is a reduced ability or difficulty with swallowing (Royal College of Speech and Language Therapists, 2023). Acute strokes often cause oesophageal dysmotility and gastroesophageal reflux, leading to aspiration and pneumonia. Gastroparesis, a slowing in gastric emptying, may result from intracranial haemorrhage (Tenny and Thorell, 2023), causing prolonged satiety, nausea, vomiting, poor appetite, pain and heartburn (National Institute of Diabetes and Digestive Kidney Diseases, 2023). Dysphagia strongly predicts mortality and other adverse clinical outcomes in stroke patients. Swallowing disorders are linked to a higher risk of aspiration (foreign objects being inhaled), chest infections and pneumonia. It often persists after discharge and is an independent predictor of QoL (Dziewas *et al.*, 2016).

It is important for professionals to have knowledge of the process of swallowing and successful eating and drinking. A 'normal' swallow requires the coordinated function of the respiratory, oral, pharyngeal, laryngeal and oesophageal anatomical structures, which depends on an intact motor and sensory nervous system. It involves several stages: (a) oral preparatory, (b) oral, (c) pharyngeal and (d) oesophageal.

The initial three phases collectively are known as the oropharyngeal phase (Royal College of Speech and Language Therapists, 2014).

In the pre-oral phase of swallowing, the presentation of food leads to salivation, which helps to moisten and break down the food. This is accompanied by cephalic anticipatory behavioural responses which prepare the body to digest, absorb and metabolise nutrients. The individual recalls sensory aspects of food and anticipates the enjoyment they will receive from ingesting it.

Once a bolus is ingested, laryngeal closure occurs to allow the airway to be protected and for food to be swallowed. Then swallowing is dependent on the upper oesophageal sphincter being open. This relaxation means that food can pass to the upper oesophagus as part of the successful swallow. If physiological changes occur following a stroke, then the function and ability of these muscles may be affected, meaning that swallowing is ineffective and unsafe. Furthermore, aspiration may occur, which will result in food entering the lungs. A primary protective action is the cough reflex, but this is dependent on the strength of the diaphragm and intercostal muscles, which may also be affected by stroke.

Cranial nerves are essential for an effective swallow (Florie *et al.*, 2021). Nervous system control of swallowing is automatic, with the functions of swallowing situated in the brain stem and midbrain. The cranial nerves responsible for mastication and swallowing include the trigeminal (V), facial (VII), glossopharyngeal (IX), vagus (X) and hypoglossal (XII) nerves. The cranial nerve components work in conjunction to achieve different aspects of swallowing, such as the control of movement and sensations in the face and tongue, the prevention of oral residue and the ability to achieve lip closure (V, VII, XII).

Impairment can compromise the preparatory and oral stages of swallowing; hence, food is not appropriately chewed or swallowed (V, IX). Additionally, impairments within the glossopharyngeal nerve can result in reduced perception of taste. The glossopharyngeal nerve, combined with branches of the vagus nerve, is responsible for the opening of the upper oesophageal sphincter; dysfunction can result in reduced transport of the pharyngeal bolus; hence food which should have been swallowed is still present.

Following a stroke, cranial nerve palsy may occur, resulting in decreased function or loss of cranial nerve actions. This can be bilateral or asymmetrical, and the ability to regain function will at least in part depend on the size of the lesion. Cranial nerve stimulation, where electrical signals are used to aid the nerve to regain function, may be used in clinical practice; however, its contribution to achieving a safe and effective swallow is unclear (Florie *et al.*, 2021).

Managing the safe swallow of patients is a key element of the role of speech and language therapists (SLT) (HCPC, 2013a). The National Institute for Health and Care Excellence (NICE) (2022)National Stroke Programme (2017) states that a swallow screen should be undertaken within 4 hours of arrival at hospital. However, recent data suggests that the proportion of cases when this occurs is falling, although the figure remains above 70% (Bhalla *et al.*, 2022). It is therefore important that nurses are also adequately trained to complete swallow screens to reduce the occurrence of aspiration pneumonia and promote sufficient nutrition and hydration (Sentinel Stroke National Audit Programme, 2022). Although formal guidance and various training courses related to dysphagia and swallowing are available (NHS England, 2023; NICE, 2013; Royal College of Speech and Language Therapy, n.d.), there is a paucity of evidence related to the extent to which they are accessed and utilised effectively. If the swallow is deemed to be unsafe, the use of nutritional supplements is essential and should be instigated as soon as possible. Patients who are unable to meet their nutritional requirements due to dysphagia via food and drinks will require tube-feeding.

What are the key considerations for enteral feeding?

Maintaining nutritional status after a stroke is crucial. Enteral feeding should be considered when patients have an inadequate or unsafe oral intake and are at risk of malnutrition, e.g. have a BMI of below 18.5 kg/m, have unintended weight loss, have eaten very little over several days, have poor nutritional absorption or high nutrient losses (NICE, 2017).

When an NGT is required, correct placement is essential; therefore, sufficient expertise and competence are necessary (National Patient Safety Agency, 2011). Misplaced NGTs can have serious consequences for patient safety (NHS Improvement, 2016a). The benefits of NGT feeding include adequate nutritional support and reducing pressure ulcers. However, associated difficulties can involve unpleasant experiences, risk of dislodgement and the long-term swallowing process being compromised.

Available research estimates that unplanned removal of NGT occurs in approximately one-third of cases, thus increasing the risk of aspiration. This is often due to neurological conditions such as dementia, but can also occur due to patient intent, resulting from discomfort or dissatisfaction with the intervention. Completing chest X-rays to ensure correct positioning creates a financial cost and means delays in feeding. Checking the pH of an aspirate obtained from the NGT establishes correct placement by identifying gastric secretions rather than aspirate from the respiratory tract (NHS Improvement, 2016b). The NICE (2017) advises that the pH should be obtained within the acceptable range of 5.5 or below, prior to the feed being commenced. However, obtaining an aspirate can be challenging in a large percentage of patients, with results not always accurately interpreted, hence increased risk. When patients have been dependent on NG feeding, an improved swallowing ability can lead to tube removal, and this often results in improved QoL and enjoyment.

Exercises to develop the swallow

Although enteral feeding has significant advantages, it can cause swallow rehabilitation to be limited. Swallow rehabilitation should be promoted alongside modification of food for management of dysphagia (Sentinel Stroke National Audit Programme, 2022). Using the Effective Swallow Protocol involving neuromuscular electrical stimulation has demonstrated improved swallow ability and clinical outcomes (NICE, 2018).

Swallowing exercises are also important. They are designed to develop and achieve a safe swallow. They aim to improve strength and range of movement to improve the reduced ability associated with dysphagia (ISWP, 2023). By consistently practising swallowing exercises, stroke patients can encourage recovery by promoting neuroplastic adaptive changes in the brain. In addition to stimulating brain recovery, practising swallowing exercises can improve oral–motor coordination and help strengthen the muscles associated with swallowing. These exercises include:

- Tongue strengthening exercises: Stick the tongue out as far as it can reach, stretch the tongue to the left, holding for a few seconds, stretch the tongue to the right, holding for a few seconds. Return to midline. Push the tongue towards the top of the mouth, behind the front teeth. Press and hold for a few seconds, and release. Repeat 10 times.
- Effortful swallow: This exercise practises the mechanics of swallowing and can increase the strength of muscles involved. To complete an effortful swallow, swallow hard while pushing the tongue against the top of the mouth. Repeat 10 times.
- Laryngeal elevation: Focuses on raising the larynx (voice box), which is an essential component of swallowing. Take a deep breath, then say the sound 'eeee' in a low pitch. Gradually slide the voice into a high-pitched 'eeee' and hold for a few seconds. Repeat 10 times Flint Rehab (2024).

More comprehensive exercises can be found at: www.flintrehab.com/swallowing-exercises-for-stroke-patients/#benefits

Oral intake

So what are the challenges?

Any person who has recently had a stroke should be monitored closely when they are eating and drinking, even if an abnormal swallow has not been detected. For those with confirmed dysphagia, monitoring is even more important and positioning to maximise a safe swallow is vital.

Patients should be:

- Sat upright in an erect position
- Sat with their chin forward, head slightly down
- Supported on their weak side

- Sat at the same level as (or slightly above) the person who is helping them to eat
- Fed into the stronger side of their mouth
- Facilitated to eat by ensuring food is not put into any 'blind spots' secondary to visual field deficit and food is placed within the reach of the unaffected side of the body Nutricia (2023)

Dehydration – thickened fluids and considerations for care

Dehydration is commonly observed among stroke survivors, with dysphagia being a key risk factor (Buoite Stella *et al.*, 2019). The use of thickened fluids is common practice when a patient's swallowing ability is significantly affected. Increased viscosity is thought to negate swallowing deficits by reducing the rate at which fluid travels from the mouth to the oropharynx (the back of the oral cavity). This gives additional time for closure of the epiglottis (a structure that covers the trachea); hence food is prevented from entering the respiratory tract, reducing the risk of aspiration.

The effectiveness of thickened fluids among those experiencing dysphagia following a stroke is frequently debated (Steele, 2021). Fluid intake is often suboptimal for individuals prescribed thickened fluids; one explanation for this is that unmodified fluids are often associated with improved enjoyment and QoL. Patients often report choosing not to adhere to prescribed thickened fluid regimes due to dissatisfaction, reduced palatability and because they do not effectively reduce the physiological sensation of thirst. Research suggests patients are not only aware of but are also willing to accept consequences of avoiding thickened fluids, including an expected reduction in life span.

Whilst medical intervention can be used to address fluid intake insufficiency, ideally, the focus should be shifted to rehabilitation and enablement. Ensuring correct positioning (>45 degrees at mealtimes) is an important element of care, and patients are often more accepting of postural adaptation in place of adherence to thickened fluid regimes.

Achieving the correct consistency of fluids can be difficult. The International Dysphagia Diet Standardisation Initiative (2019a) provides detailed guidance on the preparation of thickened fluids and texture-modified food along with testing methods (International Dysphasia Diet Standardisation Initiative, 2019b). Whilst it is important that thickening agents are available for use if needed, appropriate storage, protocols and documentation are also needed to ensure patient safety (NHS England, 2015) as accidental ingestion can result in serious harm. However, some people find thickened fluids helpful – their value may be at least partly dependent on the degree to which swallowing is affected.

Free water protocols, in which people with dysphagia drink un-thickened fluids, may be considered. Whilst there is a risk of aspiration and potentially adverse consequences, these are managed by strict guidelines. Lower rates of dehydration and chest infections have been shown to occur when free water protocols are used. Safety is an important factor, but research findings suggest that choice, control and QoL for patients can sometimes override safety considerations. In light of the issues previously identified, it is important that shared decision-making between clinicians and stroke survivors (and, if appropriate, carers/family members) occurs with the various advantages and disadvantages of treatment options being discussed, allowing individuals to make an informed choice. This supports personalised care and increases choice and control (NHS England and NHS Improvement, 2019). It also means care can be empowering and based on individual need (NICE, 2023). However, stroke survivors are often not involved in the decision to use thickened fluids and receive little explanation for their use.

> Following my second stroke I experienced a lack of saliva control, often dribbling and needing suction. I had a raging thirst which was unquenched by intravenous or enteral fluids. The mouth swabs and sponges offered to give me feelings of hydration and moisten my mouth were really ineffective and unpleasant. I felt I was able to swallow despite knowing it wasn't effective. I received little education from clinicians related to the importance of a safe and effective swallow and the dangers of aspiration which I would have found helpful. This led to me and my family to make what in hindsight I know were considered as 'unwise decisions' by taking on water using syringes and consequently experiencing aspiration; however, I was also grateful for family support. I requested frequent swallow assessments because of the desire to drink.
>
> *(Jo, 47, embolic stroke as a result of endocarditis, 20 years post stroke)*

The Stroke Association has a web page which may be useful for individuals experiencing dysphagia/swallowing difficulties www.stroke.org.uk/stroke/effects/physical/swallowing-problems

For practice areas, information leaflets can be ordered by the Stroke Association in a standard or accessible format for communication adaptations.

Comprehensive, individualised care

Family members and sometimes stroke survivors feel disempowered by a lack of education and involvement, which then leads to a variation of food and fluid intake that is not in line with the care plan or professional recommendations. This may also occur due to relatives feeling helpless whilst at the same time believing they are the most appropriate person to have insight into the preferences and best interests of their loved one. Preferred food and drinks may be brought into a clinical setting by friends and relatives, reducing the patient's intake of the food provided. This can create various dilemmas in relation to safety, meeting nutritional requirements and food storage. However, in the case of individuals with capacity, they should be allowed to make informed decisions about their intake.

In the event of stroke, survivors or their families who want to deviate from the prescribed nutrition and hydration plan must be encouraged to work together with healthcare professionals to find solutions and compromises rather than working against each other. This could avoid harm.

Is it all about food?

The social and emotional impact of dysphagia and other concerns related to eating and drinking can be significant for the individual and their family members, especially when needs are unmet. High-quality individualised assessment is an essential element of care. Humiliation and frustration are commonly reported emotions when patients are unable to control or manipulate food or open packets due to weakness on one side or when requiring practical support. Pureed food is considered almost universally unappealing, which leads to reduced enjoyment and nutritional intake. Some individuals may want to eat alone as they are embarrassed about dropping food or dribbling. Part of the healthcare professionals' role is to encourage and empower the individual to engage with others within the limits of their comfort.

Consider how you can facilitate social eating within our workplace. Could a lunch club be organised which allows stroke survivors to eat together without fear of judgement?

What needs to be considered during assessment?

Some practitioners caring for patients with dysphagia feel confident in making appropriate adaptations to diets and ensuring appropriate positioning for meals, whereas others are acutely aware of their lack of skills, knowledge and competence in this area. Limitations in the ability to engage with patient education may result in a reluctance to improve swallow and engage in rehabilitation. A lack of clear goals and attaining achievable targets is often highlighted as an area of difficulty in regaining control of eating.

When caring for my husband Malcom professionals incorrectly assumed an impaired swallow, hence he was given a soft diet. I don't recall Malcom ever receiving swallow assessments or having his eating and drinking skills/abilities recorded. I was also asked by staff to assist Malcom with meals. I took Malcom carrot cake which he was able to eat without any difficulties. Inaccurate assumptions were made by professionals about Malcom's rehabilitation potential in terms of independence and I was advised he would require significant support with all aspects of daily living including assistance with feeding, it was suggested that residential care would be required. However, Malcom was able to return home and used a knife and fork to complete meals.

(Gill, 71, wife of Malcom, 80, bilateral thalamic infarct, 14 years post stroke)

High-quality assessment and communication are essential to prevent assumptions being made by professionals. Furthermore, it is always beneficial to focus on the strengths and abilities of patients in terms of what they can do instead of what they cannot.

Hydration and nutrition needs are considered essential for health and wellbeing and are imperative to physical comfort (Royal Collage of Nursing (RCN), 2015), and this is something that is strongly voiced by patients. The NMC (2018a) Code states that ensuring adequate access to nutrition and hydration, as well as providing assistance, should be a priority. The RCN (2015) suggest referring to the seven 'Ps' when supporting patients with hydration and nutrition, considering preference, palatability, presentation, portions, position, patience and provision of oral care. Awareness of these different elements of oral intake will promote a patient's ability and desire to eat at various stages of their care and treatment (Care Inspectorate, 2020).

Your nutritional needs and preferences

Reflect upon and consider your daily eating and drinking. Think about whether you eat habitually or spontaneously.

How aware are you of hunger?

What foods or meals do you enjoy or dislike?

What about portion sizes or preference of texture, temperature, taste and utensils or plates and dishes?

Do you prefer hot or cold drinks?

Do you like these a certain way? How do your individual needs differ from others?

Now, imagine you are completely dependent on professional staff for all eating and drinking needs including physical assistance. They are unaware of your personal preferences, you are being rushed during assistance with meals, mouthfuls are too big, you do not have enough time to chew and swallow, so you are scared of choking. Portions are too large or too small, you find some foods difficult to chew and are given meals you do not enjoy. You are thirsty most of the time, and you are given tea, but only like coffee.

How would this impact your physical/emotional wellbeing, risk of malnutrition and QoL?

Hopefully, this activity has reinforced how essential communication is to understand personal preferences and needs, but it is also important to recognise that pre-existing preferences may have changed following a stroke. Utilising personalised information is paramount to provide high-quality care to ensure patients feel valued, respected and important.

Oral care – why it is more than brushing teeth

Effective oral care has positive implications not only for clinical outcomes but also for cost effectiveness. Oral care for patients is essential as this can help avoid pain and discomfort secondary to oral caries or gum disease, thereby improving QoL. In patients who have swallowing issues, it is important that the oral burden of bacteria is minimised as effectively as possible, for in the event of aspiration, the bacteria-loaded fluid can reach the lungs and cause significant infection.

Those with cognitive or learning difficulties or individuals cared for in residential settings may be at increased risk of poor care due to reduced cognition, perceptual and physical ability. This means they can be heavily reliant on others, whilst some may be unwilling or unable to seek assistance. Extensive guidance for oral care is provided by the British Society of Geroontology (2016). It discusses the impact of facial paralysis resulting in food debris accumulation; hence, dietary modification and effective oral care are imperative. Despite its importance, oral hygiene is often considered a low priority, with barriers existing to efficacy. Practitioners may lack training in oral assessment and effective hygiene techniques and have poor confidence, often being concerned about the occurrence of aspiration during oral care.

Increased assistance, guidance, training and resources for both patients and carers, along with teaching related to assessment and management of oral hygiene for professionals, are likely to be beneficial.

Think about your preferences/routine for oral hygiene; this might include time, frequency, duration and occurrence before or after meals. Also consider your choice of toothbrush (hard/soft, electric/manual), preferred toothpaste, mouthwash or dental floss. Think about the sensory elements, e.g. pressure, feeling and taste.

How would it feel if someone else assisted you? How would you feel if they were not aware of your preferences? Imagine you were unable to meet your oral hygiene needs and sometimes received no support, so you were left with unpleasant tastes, pain and discomfort.

Reflect, making notes about the importance of oral hygiene to you. How would you feel if your needs were unmet or if routine and preferences were not maintained? Would it have emotional impacts, affect your QoL, enjoyment of other activities or motivation to eat and drink? Consider trying to brush your teeth with your non-dominant hand or asking someone else to clean your teeth, and see if it is equivalent to brushing your own teeth.

Ethical considerations for the multiprofessional team

Professionals need to consider four ethical principles of autonomy, beneficence, non-maleficence and justice in relation to nutrition (Beauchamp and Childress, 2019). These principles are particularly pertinent when decisions relate to withdrawal of hydration and nutrition or commencing enteral feeding. Hydration and nutrition are regarded in law as a basic human right (United Nations, 2010a, 2010b); however, enteral feeding and intravenous administration of fluids are medical interventions, so may be withheld after carefully considering the ethical implications.

The ethical implications of enteral feeding for stroke patients involve several key considerations (Druml *et al.*, 2016).

Autonomy

- **Informed consent:** Patients must be fully informed about the risks, benefits and alternatives to enteral feeding, ensuring they understand the procedure and its impact on their QoL.
- **Decision-making capacity:** Assessing the patient's ability to make informed decisions is crucial. If they lack capacity, decisions should be guided by surrogate decision-makers or advance directives, reflecting the patient's prior wishes.

Beneficence and non-maleficence

- **Balancing benefits and risks:** Enteral feeding can provide essential nutrition and support recovery but also carries risks like infection and discomfort. Healthcare providers must ensure that the benefits outweigh the risks.
- **Quality of life:** The potential health benefits must be weighed against the possible reduction in QoL due to the physical and psychological burden of tube-feeding.

Justice

- **Resource allocation:** Enteral feeding requires specialised equipment and trained staff, raising ethical issues about the fair distribution of healthcare resources.
- **Equity of access:** Ensuring equal access to enteral feeding for all patients, regardless of socio-economic status, is essential.

Cultural and individual preferences

- **Respect for cultural values:** Healthcare providers must respect and incorporate cultural perspectives on artificial feeding.
- **Personal preferences:** Individual values and preferences should guide the decision to use or withdraw enteral feeding.

Palliative and end-of-life care

- **Palliative care focus:** For patients with poor prognoses, the decision to use enteral feeding should consider the goals of palliative care, prioritising comfort and QoL.
- **Ethical withdrawal:** Decisions to withdraw enteral feeding must be made sensitively, respecting the patient's wishes and the overall goals of care.

Navigating the ethical implications of enteral feeding requires a compassionate, patient-centred approach that balances medical benefits with respect for autonomy, QoL and equitable resource distribution.

Loss of hunger is commonly experienced post stroke (Stroke Association, 2023). Individuals motivated to eat may be more aware of how it promotes health and energy to participate in daily activities. Sharing meals with others and eating at social occasions may have been previously valuable but often become more challenging leading to avoidance, withdrawal and isolation. Some may eat out of duty or to acknowledge the support and efforts of healthcare professionals or family members. For patients receiving palliative care, nutrition may be reduced as hunger is not experienced or it is not regarded as pleasurable. Motivation can be determined by an individual's feelings in terms of being 'ready to die'.

Ensuring professional responsibility and accountability

Healthcare professionals have a clear duty and responsibility to enable and empower patients to meet their hydration and nutritional needs to promote health and recovery; this can be achieved through effective multiprofessional team working.

Why it is the role of the professional to promote choice, increase control and signpost effectively

Stroke survivors should be empowered with informed decision-making (HCPC, 2016). Professional bodies highlight the importance of recognising choice (NMC, 2018a) empowering informed choices (BDA, 2020) as well as allowing individuals to take control of their own health, behaviours and care (NMC, 2018b). Patients often strive for control which is perceived as being able to eat safely and properly. Frustration occurs when assistance is needed and eating pace is dictated. Negative feelings and emotions may result when being reminded or prompted by others regarding safe eating behaviour. Limited control can lead to avoidance of social situations due to fear of embarrassment.

Effective signposting to services and appropriate information promote access, reducing health inequalities (Health and Social Care Alliance Scotland, n.d.) and promoting choice (NHS England, n.d.). This increases awareness of practical solutions for meals, healthy recipes, restoring weight and eating well to reduce the risk of further strokes.

Patients may find uncovering or handling food challenging due to the complex and multifaceted nature of eating. It is therefore important that professionals and caregivers provide practical support when appropriate, but also use a person-centred approach to empower rehabilitation. Participation in decision-making and recognition of ability can support a sense of personal identity. Hence, awareness of personal preferences will help individuals feel valued and achieve a sense of control.

Stroke survivors consider dignity as paramount when eating with others; therefore, food avoidance or restrictions often occur due to reduced ability. Concerns often relate to appearance, leading to napkins being used frequently. The use of napkins rather than protective clothing covering is considered to promote dignity (Ageing and Dementia Research Centre, 2019). Security may be found within the home, with individuals feeling permitted to eat at their own pace, receive assistance and without feeling exhausted by the company of others, but this increases the risk of isolation.

Social support is key to rehabilitation and eating. Individuals may be entitled to concessions designed to support them with this aspect of their life (SCOPE, 2022; Disability Grants, 2023); however, patients can be reluctant to utilise these even when considered beneficial because of fears related to dignity.

Conclusion

Determination, persistence and patience to cope with change are needed by individuals who experience dysphagia. Alteration in taste and food preference is often experienced with meals taking longer to complete and difficulties with saliva management. Adapting to physical, cognitive and emotional changes after stroke is a challenge in relation to eating and drinking. Individualised advice from speech therapists and dietitians is essential to overcome these challenges. Safety should remain a key consideration, particularly when enteral feeding and thickened fluids are used.

Eating and drinking can present significant challenges for patient's following a stroke. Whilst it is important that professionals provide effective assessment, guidance and support to avoid dehydration and malnutrition, this should be done in a person-centred way to ensure individual needs are met. The social and emotional aspects of eating should not be underestimated, particularly in relation to choice, control, isolation and dignity. Research highlights the need for ongoing support and rehabilitation to maintain safety and improve QoL.

References

Ageing and Dementia Research Centre (2019) *Eating and Drinking Well with Dementia* . Available at: www.ageuk.org.uk/bp-assets/contentassets/2d42698f64294f3993e75b378 eb3292a/eating-and-drinking-well-carers-guide.pdf

BAPEN (2024) *About Malnutrition.* https://malnutritionselfscreening.org

Beauchamp, T. L., and Childress, J. F. (2019) *Principles of Biomedical Ethics*. 8th edition. New York: Oxford University Press.

Bhalla, A., McMullen, E., and Afsar, A. (2022) *The Road to Recovery: The Ninth SSNAP Annual Report*. Available at: www.strokeaudit.org/Documents/National/Clinical/Apr 2021Mar2022/Apr2021Mar2022-AnnualReport.aspx

British Dietetic Association (BDA) (2020) *Code of Professional Conduct*. Available at: www.bda.uk.com/uploads/assets/ef8656c5-320e-4d8d-b5c7ff7c82519d47/Code-of-Conduct.pdf

British Society of Gerodontology (2016) *Guidelines for the Oral Healthcare of Stroke Survivors [PDF]*. Available at: www.gerodontology.com/content/uploads/2014/10/stroke_guidelines.pdf

Buoite Stella, A., Gaio, M., Furlanis, G., Douglas, P., Naccarato, M., and Manganotti, P. (2019) Fluid and energy intake in stroke patients during acute hospitalization in a stroke unit. *Journal of Clinical Neuroscience*, 62, pp. 27–32. Available at: www.sciencedirect. com/science/article/pii/S0967586818320861

Burgos, R., Breton, I., Cereda, E., Desport, J. C., Dziewas, R., Genton, L., Gomes, F., Jesus, P., Leischker, A., Muscaritoli, M., Poulia, K. A., Preiser, J. C., Van der Marck, M., Wirth, R., Singer, P., and Bischoff, S. C. (2018) ESPEN guideline clinical nutrition in neurology. *Clinical Nutrition*, 37, pp. 354–396.

Care Inspectorate (2020) *Eating and Drinking Well in Care: Good Practice Guidance for Older People*. Available at: https://hub.careinspectorate.com/how-we-support-improvem ent/care-inspectorate-programmes-and-publications/eating-and-drinking-well-in-care-good-practice-guidance-for-older-people/

Danone (2023) *Hidden Epidemic of Malnutrition Impacts 3 Million and Starves the NHS of Funds [Online]*. Available at: www.danone.co.uk/media/articles-list/Hidden-Epidemic-Of-Malnutrition-Impacts-3-Million.html

Disability Grants (2023) *Disability Discounts*. Available at: www.disability-grants.org/dis ability-discounts.html

Druml, C., Ballmer, P. E., Druml, W., Oehmichen, F., Shenkin, A., Singer, P., Soeters, P., Weimann, A., and Bischoff, S. C. (2016) ESPEN guideline on ethical aspects of artificial nutrition and hydration. *Clinical Nutrition [Online]*. Available at: http://dx.doi.org/10.1016/j.clnu.2016.02.006

Dziewas, R., Michou, E., Trapl-Grundschober, M., Lal, A., Arsava, E. M., Bath, P. M., Clavé, P., Glahn, J., Hamdy, S., Pownall, S., Schindler, A., Walshe, M., Wirth, R., Wright, D., and Verin, E. (2016) European Stroke Organisation and European Society for Swallowing Disorders guideline for the diagnosis and treatment of post-stroke dysphagia. *European Stroke Journal*, 6 (3), pp. LXXXIX–CXV. https://doi.org/10.1177/23969873211039721

Eleftheriadis, K., and Madden, A. M. (2024) An exploration of the experiences and attitudes of healthcare professionals towards enteral tube feeding for adults living in the community following stroke. *Journal of Human Nutrition and Dietetics*, 37, pp. 1050–1060. Available at: https://onlinelibrary.wiley.com/doi/epdf/10.1111/jhn.13320

Flint Rehab (2024) *10 Swallowing Exercises for Stroke Patients to Recover from Dysphagia.* Available at: www.flintrehab.com/swallowing-exercises-for-stroke-patients/#benefits

Florie, M. G. M. H., Pilz, W., Dijkman, R. H., Kremer, B., Wiersma, A., Winkens, B., and Baijens, L. W. J. (2021) The effect of cranial nerve stimulation on swallowing: A systematic review. *Dysphagia*, 36 (2), pp. 216–230. Available at: https://link.springer.com/content/pdf/10.1007/s00455-020-10126-x

Francis (2013) *Report of the Mid Staffordshire NHS Foundation Trust Public Inquiry Volume 1: Analysis of Evidence and Lessons Learned (Part 1) [PDF]*. The Stationery Office. Available at: https://assets.publishing.service.gov.uk/government/uploads/system/uploads/attachment_data/file/279115/0898_i.pdf

Health and Care Professionals Council (HCPC) (2013a) *Standards of Proficiency: Speech and Language Therapists*. Available at: www.hcpc-uk.org/globalassets/resources/standards/standards-of-proficiency---speech-and-language-therapists.pdf

Health and Care Professionals Council (HCPC) (2013b) *Standards of Proficiency: Dietitians*. Available at: www.hcpc-uk.org/globalassets/resources/standards/standards-of-proficiency---dietitians.pdf?v=637018068040000000

Health and Care Professionals Council (HCPC) (2016) *Standards of Conduct, Performance and Ethics*. Available at: www.hcpc-uk.org/globalassets/resources/standards/standards-of-conduct-performance-and-ethics.pdf

Health and Social Care Alliance Scotland (n.d.) *Developing a Culture of Health [PDF]*. Available at: www.alliance-scotland.org.uk/wp-content/uploads/2017/10/ALLIANCE-Developing-a-Culture-of-Health.pdf

Intercollegiate Stroke Working Party (ISWP) (2023) *National Clinical Guideline for Stroke for the United Kingdom and Ireland*. Available at: www.strokeguideline.org/app/uploads/2023/04/National-Clinical-Guideline-for-Stroke-2023.pdf

International Dysphasia Diet Standardisation Initiative (2019a) *Complete IDDSI Framework Detailed Definitions [PDF]*. Available at: https://iddsi.org/IDDSI/media/images/Complete_IDDSI_Framework_Final_31July2019.pdf

International Dysphasia Diet Standardisation Initiative (2019b) *IDDSI Framework Testing Methods [PDF]*. Available at: www.iddsi.org/images/Publications-Resources/DetailedDefnTestMethods/English/V2DetailedDefnEnglish31july2019.pdf

NHS England (2015) *Patient Safety Alert Stage One: Warning Risk of death from asphyxiation by accidental ingestion of fluid/food thickening powder [PDF]*. Available at: https://www.england.nhs.uk/wp-content/uploads/2015/02/psa-thickening-agents.pdf

NHS England (n.d.) *Active Signposting [PDF]*. Available at: www.england.nhs.uk/wp-cont
ent/uploads/2017/10/west-wakefield-general-practice-case-study.pdf

NHS England (2015) *Patient Safety Alert: Stage One: Warning Risk of Death from
Asphyxiation by Accidental Ingestion of Fluid/Food Thickening Powder*. Available
at: www.england.nhs.uk/wp-content/uploads/2015/02/psa-thickening-agents.pdf

NHS England (2023) *Dysphasia Guide*. Available at: www.e-lfh.org.uk/programmes/dys
phagiaguide/

NHS England and NHS Improvement (2019) *Shared Decision Making: Summary Guide
[PDF]*. Available at: www.england.nhs.uk/wp-content/uploads/2019/01/shared-decis
ion-making-summary-guide-v1.pdf

NHS Improvement (2016a) *Patient Safety Alert: Nasogastric Tube Misplacement:
Continuing Risk of Death and Severe Harm*. Available at: www.england.nhs.uk/wp-cont
ent/uploads/2019/12/Patient_Safety_Alert_Stage_2_-_NG_tube_resource_set.pdf

NHS Improvement (2016b) *Resource Set Initial Placement Checks for Nasogastric and
Orogastric Tubes*. Available at: www.england.nhs.uk/wp-content/uploads/2016/07/
Resource_set_-_Initial_placement_checks_for_NG_tubes_1.pdf

National Heart, Lung and Blood Institute (2021) *The Science Behind the DASH Eating Plan*.
Available at: www.nhlbi.nih.gov/education/dash/research (accessed 12 December 2023).

National Institute for Health and Care Excellence (NICE) (2013) *Stroke Rehabilitation in
Adults*. Available at: www.nice.org.uk/guidance/cg162/resources/stroke-rehabilitation-
in-adults-pdf-35109688408261

National Institute for Health and Care Excellence (NICE) (2017) *Nutrition Support for
Adults: Oral Nutrition Support, Enteral Tube Feeding and Parenteral Nutrition. Clinical
Guideline*. Available at: www.nice.org.uk/guidance/cg32/resources/nutrition-support-
for-adults-oral-nutrition-support-enteral-tube-feeding-and-parenteral-nutrition-pdf-
975383198917

National Institute for Health and Care Excellence (NICE) (2018) *Transcutaneous
Neuromuscular Electrical Stimulation for Oropharyngeal Dysphagia in Adults [PDF]*.
Available at: www.nice.org.uk/guidance/ipg634/resources/transcutaneous-neurom
uscular-electrical-stimulation-for-oropharyngeal-dysphagia-in-adults-pdf-189987404
3109061

National Institute for Health and Care Excellence (NICE) (2022) Stroke and Transient
Ischaemic Attack in Over 16s: Diagnosis and Initial Management. NICE Guideline
[NG128] [PDF]. Available at: www.nice.org.uk/guidance/ng128/resources/stroke-and-
transient-ischaemic-attack-in-over-16s-diagnosis-and-initial-management-pdf-6614166
5603269

National Institute for Health and Care Excellence (NICE) (2023) *National Clinical
Guideline for Stroke*. Available at: www.strokeguideline.org/app/uploads/2023/04/Natio
nal-Clinical-Guideline-for-Stroke-2023.pdf?_gl=1*1b91rlz*_up*MQ..*_ga*MTc4M
zUwODIyNy4xNzAyNDcyNTkx*_ga_EE3BZMVLRT*MTcwMjQ3MjU5MC4xLjE
uMTcwMjQ3MjU5NS4wLjAuMA

National Institute for Health Research (2017) *Nutrition Support for Adults: Oral Nutrition
Support, Enteral Tube Feeding and Parenteral Nutrition. Clinical Guideline [CG32]*.
London: NICE.

National Institute of Diabetes and Digestive Kidney Diseases (2023) *Gastroparesis*.
Available at: www.niddk.nih.gov/health-information/digestive-diseases/gastroparesis

National Patient Safety Agency (2011) *Patient Safety Alert NPSA/2011/PSA002: Reducing
the Harm Caused by Misplaced Nasogastric Feeding Tubes in Adults, Children and*

Infants. Available at: hwww.cas.mhra.gov.uk/ViewandAcknowledgment/ViewAttachm ent.aspx?Attachment_id=101342

National Stroke Programme: Working Group – Swallow Screen Sub-Group (2017) *National Guideline for Swallow Screening in Stroke 2017 [PDF].* Available at: www.hse.ie/eng/ about/who/cspd/ncps/stroke/resources/national-clinical-guideline-for-stroke.pdf

Nursing and Midwifery Council (NMC) (2018a) *The Code.* Available at: www.nmc.org.uk/ globalassets/sitedocuments/nmc-publications/nmc-code.pdf

Nursing and Midwifery Council (NMC) (2018b) *Future Nurse: Standards of Proficiency for Registered Nurses.* www.nmc.org.uk/globalassets/sitedocuments/standards/2024/standa rds-of-proficiency-for-nurses.pdf

Nursing and Midwifery Council (NMC) (2018c) *Standards of Proficiency for Nursing Associates.* Available at: www.nmc.org.uk/standards/standards-for-nursing-associates/ standards-of-proficiency-for-nursing-associates/ (accessed 11 June 2023).

Nutricia (2023) *Top Tips – Mealtime Positioning for People with Swallowing Problems.* Available at: www.nutricia.co.uk/patients-carers/articles-stories/feeding-with-dyspha gia-swallowing-problems.html (accessed 06 August 2024).

Occupational Therapists Registration Board (n.d.) *Standards of Proficiency for Occupational Therapists.* Available at: www.coru.ie/files-education/otrb-standards-of-proficiency-for-occupational-therapists.pdf

Royal Collage of Nursing (RCN) (2015) *Getting It Right Every Time: Fundamentals of Nursing Care at the End of Life. Publication code*: 004 871.

Royal College of Speech and Language Therapists (2014) *RCSLT Resource Manual for Commissioning and Planning Services for SLCN. London. Available from* https://rcslt. org/wp-content/uploads/media/Project/RCSLT/slcn-resource-manual.pdf

Royal College of Speech and Language Therapists (2023) *Dysphagia and Eating, Drinking and Swallowing Needs Overview.* Available at: www.rcslt.org/speech-and-language-ther apy/clinical-information/dysphagia/

Royal College of Speech and Language Therapy (n.d.) *Guidance on the Management of Dysphagia in Care Homes [PDF].* Available at: www.rcslt.org/wp-content/uplo ads/media/Project/RCSLT/guidance-on-the-management-of-dysphagia-in-care-homes.pdf

SCOPE (2022) *Disability Discounts for Days Out and Travel.* Available at: www.scope.org. uk/advice-and-support/free-discount-event-pa

Sentinel Stroke National Audit Programme (2022) *Acute Organisational Audit 2021.* Available at: www.strokeaudit.org/Documents/National/AcuteOrg/2021/2021-AOANat ionalReport.aspx

Intercollegiate Stroke Working Party (2023) *National Clinical Guideline for Stroke for the UK and Ireland. London.* Available at: www.strokeguideline.org

Steele, S. J., Ennis, S. L., and Dobler, C. C. (2021) Treatment burden associated with the intake of thickened fluids. *Breathe,* 17 (1), p. 210003. Available at: www.ncbi.nlm.nih. gov/pmc/articles/PMC8291955/

Stroke Association (2023) *Changes to Taste and Smell.* Available at: www.stroke.org.uk/effe cts-of-stroke/physical-effects-of-stroke/taste-and-smell#The%20impact%20of%20ta ste%20and%20smell%20changes

Tenny, S., and Thorell, W. (2023) *Intracranial Haemorrhage.* Available at: www.ncbi.nlm. nih.gov/books/NBK470242/

The British Association for Parenteral and Enteral Nutrition (2023) *Enteral Nutrition.* Available at: www.bapen.org.uk/education/nutrition-support/enteral-nutrition/

United Nations (2010a) *The Human Right to Water and Sanitation.* Available at: https://dig itallibrary.un.org/record/686927?ln=en#record-files-collapse-header

United Nations (2010b) *The Right to Adequate Food.* Available at: www.ohchr.org/sites/defa ult/files/Documents/Publications/FactSheet34en.pdf

6

MANAGING AND MAINTAINING CONTINENCE

Ruth Trout, Fiona Chalk and Julia Williams

Learning objectives

- To understand the physiology of micturition and defaecation.
- To understand the physical, cognitive and emotional challenges relating to continence for a stroke survivor and their family/carer.
- To explore continence rehabilitation and recovery approaches.
- To explore the importance of therapeutic relationships to maximise continence.

Background

Stroke is frequently associated with continence difficulties, necessitating comprehensive physical and psychological support. Koike *et al.* (2015) highlight that together with bathing, continence is ranked among the most burdensome of consequences following stroke by survivors and their family/carers. Their paramount concern is maintaining independence, learning techniques to manage continence to reduce problems with urination and defaecation and to remain continent.

The effects of a stroke are complex and diverse. Any impairment following a stroke will depend on the type of stroke, the affected location and the severity of the damage, and will be unique for each survivor. Treating stroke survivors as individuals is vital for successful rehabilitation; therefore, developing person-centred care is imperative. Generic continence assessment tools are not necessarily going to be adequate to address the individuals' complex needs (Brady *et al.*, 2016).

Urinary incontinence affects an estimated 40–60% of people admitted to hospital following a stroke. According to a Cochrane Review, approximately 25%

DOI: 10.4324/9781003426196-7

of patients continue to experience incontinence at discharge, and around 15% remain incontinent one year post-stroke (Thomas *et al.*, 2019). About one in three people experience some loss of bowel control after a stroke (Bladder and Bowel Community, 2019). It's understandable that many stroke survivors worry about changes in their bladder and bowel habits. Urinary and bowel complications can lead to increased morbidity and mortality secondary to skin breakdown, pressure ulceration (Intercollegiate Stroke Working Party (ISWP), 2023) and catheterisation. However, there is evidence that bladder and bowel problems could be more proactively researched and managed by healthcare professionals (ISWP, 2023) and that stroke survivors are not always fully informed of the options available to them for regaining continence.

For many, the loss of bladder and/or bowel control is a very sensitive and personal issue, impacting on quality of life due to loss of dignity.

> Before this happened (the stroke) I used to go out most nights, drinking with the 'lads', watching the local football team at weekends, generally doing what I wanted, when I wanted. But not now you see, I've had to stop most of this 'cos of the tablets and injections I'm on, right now, only going places I feel safe enough to have an accident, if you know what I mean.
>
> *(Male, age 55, 2 years post stroke)*

Neurological links to micturition

The process of micturition, also known as urination, plays a crucial role in eliminating metabolic by-products and toxic wastes that have been filtered by the kidneys. This essential bodily function involves an intricate relationship of signals between the nervous system and the urinary tract, forming the micturition reflex. The effective storage and subsequent emptying of the bladder rely significantly on the functionality of these neurological pathways. Figure 6.1 illustrates the process of urination.

Micturition is controlled by two areas within the brain:

- The frontal lobe houses the cortico-inhibitory centre for micturition. It allows for voluntary control of elimination. Assisted by the pudendal nerve, voluntary inhibitory signals are transmitted, so that urine can be held in the bladder until such time that it is appropriate to urinate, supporting continence.
- The pontine micturition centre, located within the brainstem, plays a central role in coordinating both micturition and continence. Responding to impulses from the frontal lobe, the pontine micturition centre sends signals to the detrusor muscle of the bladder and internal sphincters to contract or relax to either initiate urination or maintain continence.

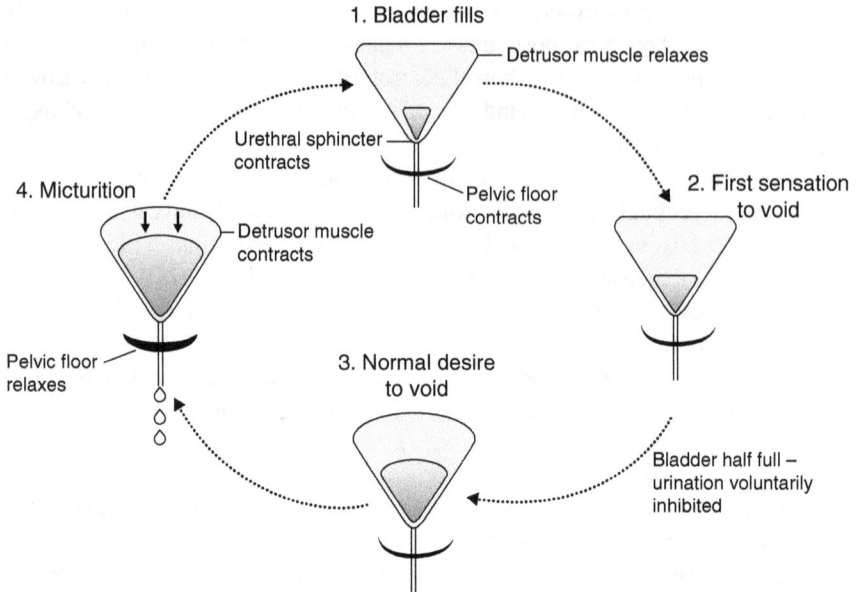

FIGURE 6.1   The bladder, pelvic floor, muscles and sphincters involved in urination.

After a stroke, if the damage has affected either of these areas within the brain, the stroke survivor will experience some degree of urinary problems (see Table 6.1), which ultimately changes the bladder patterns they have been used to.

Since my stroke, I dribble urine most of the time because I can't get up and out to the loo quickly enough. My doctor, he says it's all to do with how my stroke has affected my ability to have a wee. So, I wear a pad and change it often, but still worry that I smell. It's so embarrassing and definitely restricts me going out, unless I plan ahead. This does reduce the anxiety, but it's still on my mind, all the time. I try to work out where all the loos are, when I am out and about, that helps. It's OK if I'm with people who know me, but not so much if they don't. I really don't want to have to explain myself, it's just too embarrassing. I'm not old yet you know!

Reflect on the stroke survivor's experience and ask yourself:

- What type of urinary problem do you think she has?
- Which part of her brain has been affected by the stroke?
- Do you think she fully understands why she is having problems with continence?
- How could you support the lady in relation to her situation?

Neurological links to defaecation

The passage of faeces can vary in a healthy person from three times a day to three times a week (Royal College of Nursing (RCN), 2019b). Incontinence of

TABLE 6.1 Types of urinary problems following stroke

Bladder problem	Description
Frequency	Passing urine more often than is usual
Urgency incontinence	Involuntary, sudden, urgent and uncontrollable feeling of needing to pass urine, often with no time to get to the toilet
Nocturia	Waking from sleep with an urgent need to pass urine
Nocturnal enuresis	Wetting the bed while still asleep
Stress incontinence	Small dribbles of urine leakage during exertion, e.g., coughing or sneezing. Due to weak or damaged pelvic floor muscles (this is likely to have been present before a stroke)
Reflex incontinence	Unconsciously passing urine when bladder reaches capacity
Urinary retention +/− overflow incontinence	Hesitancy commencing urination, weak urine stream, straining to void. Likely to have significant postvoid residual urine measurement (>300 ml)
	May or may not have overflow incontinence – bladder leaks due to being too full
Functional incontinence	When the physical effects of the stroke make it difficult to reach the toilet or unfasten clothing in time

Source: Thomas *et al.* (2019).

faeces is generally associated with more severe strokes. Clinically, it is usually more difficult to manage than urinary incontinence. Additionally, constipation is common, occurring in 55% of people within the first month of stroke. This can compound urinary and faecal incontinence (ISWP, 2023).

Signals descending from the cerebral cortex and hypothalamus are responsible for the motor control of defaecation. This is another complex system.

- The *vagus nerve* has an effect on downward movement in the gut, including peristalsis.
- The *pudendal nerve* has vital input into the voluntary control of defaecation.
- The *anus has two sphincters* – internal and external – which are ring-like muscles controlling the release of stool.
- The *internal anal sphincter* is under involuntary nervous control.
- The *external anal sphincter* is under voluntary nervous control.

Any damage to these nerves can cause a change in the rhythm of intestinal activity or an inability to maintain faecal continence. Therefore, stroke survivors can suffer from a change to their bowel pattern and control.

The passage of faeces is facilitated by the relaxing and contracting of the associated structures. The rectum is part of the large bowel. It is involved in the storage of faeces and is usually empty before defaecation. Faeces are propelled into the rectum by peristalsis, which brings about the urge to evacuate the bowel or defaecate. Neurological control is facilitated by the enteric nervous system, sympathetic and parasympathetic nerves, which convey information between the

TABLE 6.2 Types of bowel problems

Bowel problem	Description
Faecal incontinence	Uncontrolled bowel movement. This can be caused by damage to the part of the brain controlling the bowel. It can also happen if the stroke survivor has reduced mobility and is unable to get to the toilet in time (functional incontinence)
Constipation with overflow	Large hard stools can get stuck and block the bowel. Liquid stools may flow around it, causing watery stools to leak
Faecal impaction/ constipation	Dry, hard stools collect in the bowel and can be difficult and painful to pass

brain and the lower bowel when the rectum is full. The internal anal sphincter relaxes involuntarily, while the external anal sphincter relaxes voluntarily, allowing the stool to be expelled when it is convenient to do so.

In stroke survivors, factors such as muscle tone, neural pathways, psychological wellbeing, hydration, consistency of stool, mobility, physical ability and communication can collectively affect the process of defaecation and overall bowel function (see Table 6.2).

Here, an expert by experience shares their experiences of how their bowel pattern has changed.

> I'm nowhere near as active as I was, so I get constipated. I manage with meds but you can't get away from it. If you've had a stroke, then you've had a stroke. It's always with you.

Reflect on this scenario and ask yourself:

- What are some of the reasons for this stroke survivor to be experiencing constipation?
- How might his issues with constipation affect him physically and psychologically?
- How could you support the patient in relation to his situation?

The RCN (2019a) states caring for a person experiencing a change in their bladder or bowel control is an important part of the nurse's role. Providing such care must be approached with the upmost sensitivity, compassion and competency to ensure the dignity and privacy of the individual are always respected. Urinary and bowel problems can lead to psychological effects, which include stress, depression, sexual dysfunction, shame and loss of self-respect and self-confidence (ISWP, 2023). Generally, continence is undertaken alone, within a specifically designated and purposefully designed space – heightening the importance of independence in toileting for stroke survivors. For many people, continence is a taboo subject that should not be raised in everyday conversation, which can lead to challenges when trying to support someone with continence issues (Thomas *et al.*, 2019).

- Imagine you need to discuss bladder or bowel issues or incontinence with a stroke survivor. How might you prepare yourself, the survivor (and carer/s) and the environment to facilitate this discussion?
- What are some of the enablers and barriers to an open and frank conversation – How might you use this knowledge to facilitate a productive discussion or interaction?

Promoting and regaining continence

Before any continence care management plan is instituted, it is important to recognise the difference between *containment and management of incontinence* and *promotion and rehabilitation of continence*. Many healthcare professionals focus primarily on the former, believing that they are doing the latter. However, it is important to recognise that incontinence following stroke can be improved and sometimes cured if appropriate rehabilitation techniques are implemented (Brady *et al.*, 2016; ISWP, 2023). For some, both approaches might be needed initially as the individual slowly recovers and regains continence. Most, but not all, continence problems following stroke will improve to some degree (ISWP, 2023); however, sometimes there will be little response to simple interventions, and more invasive treatment is needed. Many of these interventions will be discussed in the following pages.

Assessment

To effectively plan and deliver care for stroke survivors who are experiencing urinary and bowel problems, it is crucial to initiate an individual continence assessment. This will help those providing care to have a clear understanding of the issues, ensuring identification of the appropriate intervention(s) needed to support the stroke survivor.

Managing continence is often complex, requiring attention to a combination of physical, cognitive and emotional challenges. Premorbid issues can include both physical conditions (including pre-existing continence issues) and cognitive problems, for example, such as those caused by dementia, frailty, diabetes or arthritis. Following a stroke the individual may have new mobility or cognitive issues secondary to the stroke, or premorbid issues may be exacerbated. These all need to be considered as part of the assessment. Any of these conditions can make maintaining continence challenging (ISWP, 2023). Alongside this, each individual is unique with their own personal challenges and strengths, for example, one person may be very open to discussions about their incontinence and proactively address it with healthcare professionals, another may be very embarrassed and might try to hide the problem. Stroke unit staff, therefore, should be trained in the use of standardised assessment and management protocols for incontinence and constipation in people with stroke (ISWP, 2023).

> I was coming to grips with the fact that I was incontinent and that was taking up most of my thoughts [how to deal with it]. So somebody coming in and saying 'you'll do this or you won't do that' or 'what's this or that' didn't really mean much to me – because I was too worried about having to go the toilet.
>
> *(Male, age 71, 6 years post stroke)*

> So, my boys say 'dad come up here for a couple of weeks' but I can't travel [because of my incontinence]. If I'm on a train or in a car or something and I've got to go, I've got to go ... I miss my boys.
>
> *(Male, age 58, 1 year post stroke)*

Assessment needs to be individualised, but all initial assessments should include:

- history taking: recording past medical history (PMH), medication review and details of signs and symptoms;
- investigations including simple diagnostic tests (urinalysis, post void residual abdominal ultrasound, input/output recordings);
- general and neurological physical examination;
- exploration of the effects of the stroke on continence.

Later more detailed information may be gathered as per the ISWP (2023) guidelines which state people who have continued loss of bladder and/or bowel control after 2 weeks should be reassessed to identify the cause of incontinence. It should be noted that often these interventions begin sooner than 2 weeks after onset of stroke:

- Bladder/continence diary – used to gather baseline information for planning management and rehabilitation strategies
- Further invasive diagnostic tests (urodynamic investigations).

The assessment in Figure 6.2 offers a problem-solving approach to delivering personalised care.

History taking

A detailed medical history should be taken, documenting co-morbidities, previous surgery, usual bladder and bowel habits and current medication

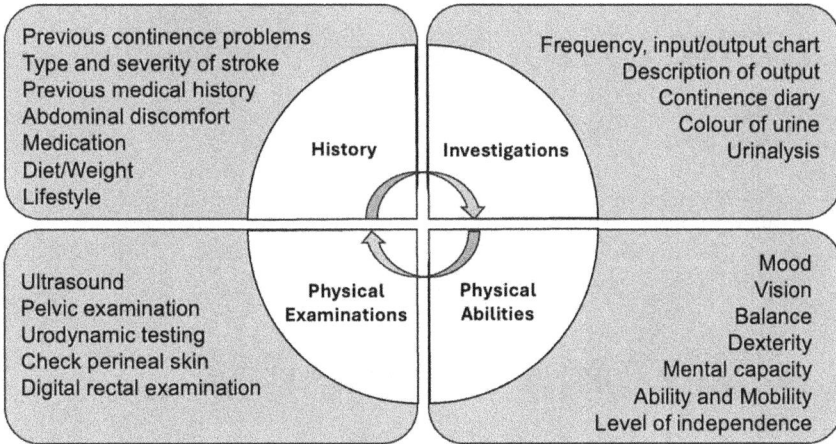

FIGURE 6.2   Continence assessment for stoke survivors.

(National Institute for Health and Care Excellence (NICE), 2023). For women, gynaecological surgery and previous pregnancies should be discussed, including how many times the woman has been pregnant, the delivery approach and whether there is any ongoing stress incontinence following pregnancies. This evaluation provides insight into the individual's health status before the stroke. Generally, older adults may be more likely to have long-standing bladder and bowel problems. Regular medication requires review as some medications, such as sedatives or analgesics, are known to affect continence. The type, location and severity of stroke should also be established to determine how continence is likely to be affected.

Asking the right questions, in the right manner and at the right time can improve outcomes, particularly when taking the history.

Consider the type of questions to meet this requirement. Think particularly about open-ended questions which discourage a yes/no answer, or including follow up questions. Such as: Do you ever feel an urgent need to rush to the toilet? If yes, do you make it in time? Do you have any discomfort or pain when passing urine? Can you describe the feeling to me. For more detailed advice about taking a history, consider reading Bickley *et al.* (2021).

Investigations

Several simple investigations should be completed. Fluid input and urinary and faecal output should be recorded, alongside the frequency of episodes of passing urine and incontinence (Nazarko, 2013). This is particularly useful, as this information may lead to the identification of the type of incontinence. Whilst monitoring input and output, the output should be noted for its colour and

 Type 1 Separate hard lumps, like nuts

 Type 2 Sausage-like but lumpy

 Type 3 Like a sausage but with cracks in the surface

 Type 4 Like a sausage or snake, smooth and soft

 Type 5 Soft blobs with clear-cut edges

 Type 6 Fluffy pieces with ragged edges, a mushy stool

 Type 7 Watery, no solid pieces

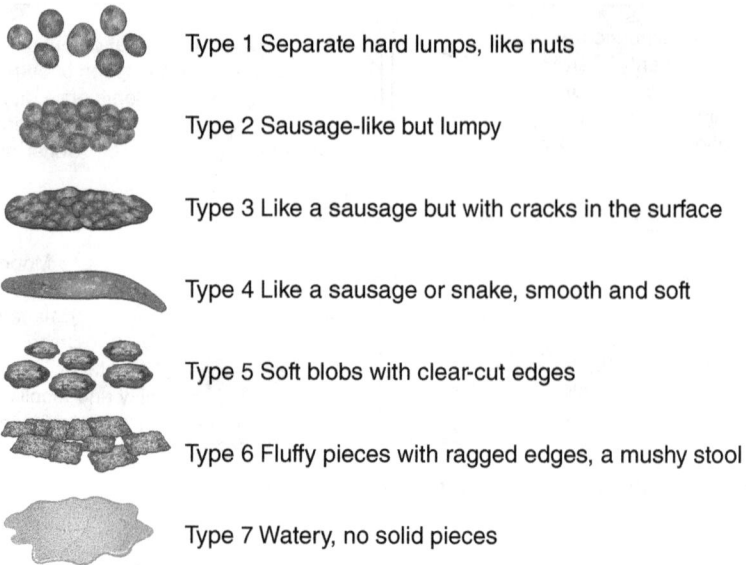

FIGURE 6.3 Bristol Stool Chart.
Source: (Lewis and Heaton, 1997).

consistency. Undertaking simple tests such as a urinalysis can help to exclude co-morbidities, such as urinary tract infection or dehydration, although guidelines may vary from country to country.

Monitoring bowel function should encompass gathering information about both dietary intake and the timing and appearance of bowel movements. Assessing both the frequency and consistency of stools is essential for identifying an individual's normal bowel pattern. The Bristol Stool Chart (Lewis and Heaton, 1997) is the most popular stool form chart (see Figure 6.3). Based on the transit of the gut, it classifies stools into seven different categories, with types 1 and 2 hard stool indicating constipation, types 3 to 5 'normal range' and types 6 and 7 loose stools, in keeping with diarrhoea. This can be useful in diagnosing constipation and overflow incontinence.

Physical examination

Physical examination is an important part of the assessment. This would include:

- A simple examination of the perineal skin to check for signs or soreness or infection. Reviewing skin changes can help identify the significance of the continence problem and prompt timely intervention to support skin integrity, comfort and hygiene (NICE, 2023).
- A vaginal examination to look for evidence of a vaginal prolapse (if history suggests this is needed) (NICE, 2023).

- An examination of the rectum may be necessary to determine the presence of faecal matter in the rectum, the amount and consistency. This examination is known as a digital rectal examination (DRE) and should only be undertaken by a healthcare professional who is deemed competent to do so (Nursing and Midwifery Council (NMC), 2018; RCN, 2019b).
- Assessment of anal tone (sometimes referred to as the 'anal wink') determines whether the anal sphincter is functioning (NICE, 2023).
- Abdominal palpation or use of bladder scan to assess whether the bladder is completely empty following micturition (NICE, 2023).

Physical ability

The assessment of physical ability evaluates the consequences of the type and severity of the stroke. Physical ability refers to the stroke survivors' ease of being able to manage the movements of toileting that include physical, cognitive and emotional limitations post stroke. For example, patients with stroke-related hemiplegia must use the non-paretic side to compensate for weaknesses of the paretic extremities to achieve independent toileting. This requires physical and cognitive coordination and may increase the time taken to reach the toilet.

Given the challenges that stroke survivors face in terms of walking, balance and coordination, the process of engaging in toileting can become a considerable task. As a result, physical challenges such as bathroom accessibility, walking (aided or unaided), being able to adjust lower garments whilst standing or sitting, balance, strength, muscle weakness to one side of the body, dexterity and sight will compound any acquired bladder and bowel problems following the stroke. For example, decreased mobility will result in additional physical exertion, making it more challenging to sustain bladder and bowel control and reduced mobility will increase the likelihood of constipation. The task of using the toilet involves a series of steps (see Table 6.3), with each step bringing about challenges.

The problems related to continence in stroke survivors may cause serious health concerns, and are associated with an increased frequency of falls, post-stroke depression and reduced quality of life (Kawanabe *et al.*, 2018). In addition, bathroom-related issues are associated with role loss, admission to institutional care, skin or urinary tract infection and mortality. Therefore, stroke survivors, as well as their families, seek to rebuild independent continence, and this should be addressed during rehabilitation.

A stroke survivor's ability to master their environment and to carry out daily activities efficiently and effectively has been shown to affect their mental health, wellbeing and overall quality of life profoundly (Brady *et al.*, 2016). Cognitive challenges, including memory loss, diminished attention span, difficulties in planning, scheduling and slower thinking, can adversely affect the individual's ability to independently manage continence and may worsen the issues. This may require the stroke survivor to re-learn essential daily living skills to maintain

TABLE 6.3 Steps to use the toilet and how stroke may affect this

1. Mobility to and from the toilet (cognitive issues, unilateral weakness, fatigue)
2. Transferring on and off the toilet (cognitive issues, unilateral weakness, loss of proprioception)
3. The re-arrangement of clothing – pulling down and pulling up of lower garments (cognitive issues, unilateral weakness, balance issues, loss of proprioception or somatosensory association area damage)
4. Control of continence (urine and/or faeces)
5. Tearing toilet paper away from roll (cognitive issues, unilateral weakness, balance issues, loss of proprioception or somatosensory association area damage)
6. Cleaning perineal skin (cognitive issues, unilateral weakness, balance issues, loss of proprioception or somatosensory association area damage)
7. Washing of hands (cognitive issues, unilateral weakness, balance issues)

Source: Adapted from Kawanabe *et al.* (2018).

independence. Communicating the need for the toilet may also be an issue as some stroke survivors may experience aphasia. However, Brady *et al.* (2016) found that patients in hospitals often feel that they are trying to communicate their concerns to healthcare professionals but feel ignored or that their concerns are misunderstood.

Any obstacles delaying the ability to get to the toilet may lower mood and increase feelings of frustration and anxiety potentially leading to less social interaction (Gillham and Clark, 2011). A full assessment allows for identification of the bladder and/or bowel problem as well as any other problems that make it difficult for the stroke survivor to remain continent.

The inability to maintain continence is regarded negatively by many stroke survivors as summed up by this male stroke survivor:

> ...it (being incontinent) was 'absolutely awful ... positively disgraceful ... a humiliating thing, simply degrading ... words aren't enough'.
> *(Male, age 71, 6 years post stroke)*

Practical care and management of bladder and bowel problems

Continence problems are debilitating, often cause embarrassment and are life-changing. Helping the individual maximise their continence and managing any problems is a fundamental skill. Identifying when incontinence has occurred, responding to care needs sensitively and supporting stroke survivors and their families and/or carers needs to involve the multidisciplinary team (Cheesley,

2017). However, a nurse-led approach is recommended (ISWP, 2023) and nurse education programmes have been shown to improve long-term continence (ISWP, 2023; Brady *et al.*, 2016). Nurses and other carers should cultivate strong communication skills, including active listening and considering appropriate timing of conversations, while consistently upholding dignity and respect. It is equally important to have a thorough understanding of how neurological damage can affect the practical aspects of continence care.

A focus on the somatosensory association area (parietal lobe). In the simplest terms, the somatosensory system is a network of neurons that helps us recognise objects and discriminate textures via touch.

Think about when you wake in the night and reach for your bedside table in the dark. You can touch and exclude your phone and your book before you find your drink – all without even opening your eyes! We use this shortcut constantly in our everyday lives. Think about how going to the toilet is affected if you have lost this function:

- You have to look down to find and undo your zip – a risk if your weakness causes balance issues.
- You might not receive feedback from your thighs and buttocks telling you when you are safely on the toilet.
- You have to turn around and visually find the toilet paper – risking toppling over or sliding from the toilet seat.
- You have to look down to see where the toilet paper is and where it needs to go to wipe yourself, you cannot do this by touch anymore as that sensation is lost – more risk, due to loss of balance.

Interventions to manage incontinence and promote rehabilitation

The multidisciplinary approach to managing urinary incontinence can encompass a range of interventions, including the use of absorbent pads, home environment modifications for easier bathroom access and, in more persistent cases, the consideration of long-term solutions such as intermittent self-catheterisation (ISC) or a suprapubic catheter or a stoma. There is, however, some basic advice that can be offered in the first instance (see Table 6.4) that may offer some resolution, before moving on to more structured management and rehabilitation methods.

Approaches to improve urinary incontinence

People who continue to have loss of bladder and/or bowel control 2 weeks after their stroke should be reassessed to identify the cause of incontinence. The individual and their family/carers should be involved in developing a treatment plan with the

TABLE 6.4 General advice for urinary/bowel problems

Advice	Rationale
Increase fluid intake	Strong concentrated urine irritates the bladder, increasing the urge to urinate
Reduce caffeine intake	Caffeine stimulates the production of urine
Weight loss	Improves bladder control in the longer term
Reduce or stop smoking	Coughing can increase urinary leakage
Increase fibre within the diet to prevent constipation	Straining on defaecation weakens pelvic floor muscles
Reduce alcohol intake	Alcohol is a diuretic so will increase urinary output
Environmental modifications: move the individual closer to the toilet	To reduce the time taken to reach the toilet
Clothing modification: Use pull-up trousers rather than trousers with buttons, zips and ties. Consider not wearing underwear	To reduce the time taken to pull trousers down

appropriate members of the multidisciplinary team (ISWP, 2023). The treatment plan should include:

- treatment of any identified cause of incontinence
- training for the person with stroke and their family or carers in the management of incontinence
- arrangements for an adequate continued supply of continence aids and access to services
- referral for specialist treatments and behavioural adaptations if the person is able to participate (ISWP, 2023).

Behavioural adaptations and interventions can be customised to the individual; to improve continence, help manage chronic symptoms and maximise chances of complete resolution of incontinence.

Table 6.5 summarises some of the techniques which can be used to maintain continence/manage incontinence.

Which continence approach or product is best will depend on the ability of the stroke survivor and what support they have. See Table 6.6.

Reviewing product use on a regular basis is important to ensure it is fit for purpose (Association of Continence Advice, 2017). Attention and care to the perianal skin are important, particularly when using the pads or pull-up pants and penile sheath.

TABLE 6.5 Techniques which can be used to maintain continence/manage incontinence

Adaption	Technique to avoid incontinence
Regular toileting	The individual is taken to the toilet regularly, perhaps every 2 or 3 hours, whether they need to go or not. This helps to retrain the bladder into a regular urination pattern.
Timed/prompted voiding	Toilet breaks are scheduled at specific times to avoid the sudden and uncontrollable need to pass urine. The timing is based on information from a bladder diary. The individual is encouraged to go to the toilet 15–20 minutes before their normal routine. The goal is to increase the length of time between scheduled bathroom breaks.
Urgency control	A combination of deep breathing and complex mental tasks (for example, counting backwards from 100) helps the individual to ignore the need to pass urine.
Ensuring continence aids are available at the bedside	Urinals and bedpans should be placed close to the individual so that they can access them easily. Carer support also needs to be available when needed for those less mobile.
Containment and absorption devices	This includes absorbent pads and pull-ups, tampons and washable bed pads. Some products are available on the NHS, however, depending on location, services vary. Penile sheaths may be used in men to allow urine to drain into a bag
Urinary catheterisation	Intermittent self-catheterisation/suprapubic catheterisation for long-term management. Allows urine to be drained directly into the toilet or a bag.
Medication: anti-muscarinics	Contraction of the bladder is stimulated by muscarinic receptors on the detrusor muscle, which respond to release of acetylcholine. Anti-muscarinic drugs (anti-cholinergics) are recommended for treatment of overactive bladder in neurological disorders. They block the muscarinic receptors on the detrusor, thereby reducing bladder contractions. They are also thought to reduce the sensation of urgency. They are non-selective so they can cause systemic side effects such as a very dry mouth
Botulinum toxin-A	This powerful neurotoxin blocks the release of acetylcholine and causes temporary muscle paralysis. Injected into the detrusor muscle regularly (approximately every 4–6 months) to treat overactive bladder

Sources: ISWP (2023), NICE (2023).

TABLE 6.6 Techniques to improve bladder storage/regain continence

Adaption	Techniques to improve bladder storage/regain continence
Bladder retraining	Involves scheduling toilet breaks at specific times to avoid the sudden and uncontrollable need to go, but the goal is to gradually increase the length of time between scheduled bathroom breaks by 15–30 minutes. This builds bladder storage capacity. Can take weeks or months to be effective. Demands a large degree of motivation from the patient and carer and requires planning, cognition and cooperation.
Urgency control.	A combination of deep breathing and complex mental tasks (for example counting backwards from 100) helps the individual to ignore the need to pass urine.
Transcutaneous electrical nerve	Electrical stimulation for the treatment of urinary incontinence. If used for over 6 months, it has been found to improve nocturia, urgency and frequency.
Pelvic floor exercises	Also known as Kegel exercises. Strengthens pelvic floor muscle tone, improving muscle and bladder control. Involves repetitive voluntary contraction and relaxation of the pelvic floor muscles to improve the strength and coordination of these muscles. There is evidence it is effective for stress incontinence for people with neurological disorders
Weighted vaginal cones	Used to help women to train their pelvic floor muscles. Cones are inserted into the vagina and the pelvic floor is contracted to prevent them from slipping out.

Sources: Evans (2015), NICE (2011, 2023), ISWP (2023).

Try passing urine into an incontinence pad.

- How easy is it to start the flow?
- What are your sensations and thoughts as you pass urine?
- How long are you prepared to wear the wet pad?

Now, consider these questions in the context of stroke survivors. Has this exercise changed the way you will practice, or influenced the advice you provide compared with your previous approach?

Long-term indwelling catheters should be used with caution due to recurrent infection, which can lead to further illness and subsequent hospital admission (John *et al.*, 2018). An indwelling catheter is an independent mortality risk factor following stroke. In the acute period (up to 2 weeks (Woodward, 2014)) after stroke, an indwelling (urethral) catheter should not be inserted unless indicated to relieve urinary retention or when fluid balance is critical (ISWP, 2023).

ISC is an intervention that can be discussed and taught by a continence specialist or experienced healthcare professional. ISC is when the stroke survivor inserts a catheter into their bladder via the urethra. This allows urine to flow into a container or the toilet, ensuring the bladder is empty. Careful patient selection is required, as success relies on dexterity, balance and strength. The procedure can be supported by a family member and/or carer.

Surgical procedures for urinary diversion, such as an ileal conduit, may be considered as a last resort.

Care for bowel problems

The most common bowel problems for stroke survivors are faecal incontinence, constipation with overflow and faecal impaction – the retention of a large, hardened mass of stool in the rectum or distal colon that cannot be evacuated voluntarily. It may result in partial or complete bowel obstruction, associated discomfort or pain, and can lead to complications such as overflow diarrhoea, rectal mucosal damage, or urinary retention. Stroke survivors can adopt several simple interventions to improve or maintain bowel function. The first step should involve a discussion about a healthy lifestyle, including weight management, smoking cessation, moderation of alcohol intake, dietary adjustments and regular physical activity.

Dietary and fluid intake are important. NICE (2007) recommend an individual's diet should promote an ideal stool consistency (see Figure 6.3). The nurse can advise the stroke survivor on their nutritional needs by looking at the presenting symptoms and consider whether to follow any interventions to improve bowel function. For example, when a stroke survivor has faecal incontinence a low-residue diet is recommended. Reducing the fibre intake can decrease the motility of the gut and make the stool firmer; likewise, increasing fibre will increase the motility of the gut, making the stool softer (see Table 6.7).

TABLE 6.7 Dietary and fluid intake advice

Bowel problem	Diet advice	Fluid advice	Result
Faecal incontinence	Low residue Bulking agents (whole grain) Fibre supplements	Reduce caffeine (coffee and diet drinks) Reduce alcohol	Firmer stool
Faecal overflow with constipation	Bulking agents (whole grain)	Reduce caffeine (coffee and diet drinks) Reduce alcohol	Softens hard stool/ firms loose stool
Constipation	High fibre Bulking agents (whole grain)	Herbal teas	Softens hard stools

Management of faecal incontinence will require some kind of containment product to help the stroke survivor maintain their dignity. There are a limited number of products available that are both reliable and specifically designed. The smell of faeces is difficult to contain or disguise. Some survivors use a deodoriser or perfume spray, but this is not always helpful. Current availability of products includes pads, pull-up pants, faecal collectors or bowel management systems. Their successful use all depends on the stroke survivor's dexterity, balance and strength.

Anal plugs and inserts are effective interventions for managing mild faecal leakage, supporting continence, reducing the risk of skin breakdown and promoting patient comfort, dignity and independence. Anal plugs are made of a soft slightly absorbent foam, that once in contact with bowel mucosa, open out into a cup shape that can collect a small amount of faecal matter. Anal inserts work in a similar way but are made of soft silicone so block the anus rather than collect faecal matter. When successful, both devices are useful and provide increased confidence and self-esteem. Faecal collectors and bowel management systems are only helpful to bed-ridden patients. Although slightly different, both systems adhere externally to the anus to collect the faecal matter; therefore, they are unsuitable for someone who is mobile.

A wide range of pads and pull-up pants are available but should be selected depending on the patient's degree of incontinence as seepage is common (Association of Continence Advice, 2017). Hygiene and skin care are of importance to prevent perianal soreness and excoriation, or incontinence-associated dermatitis. A healthcare professional should support and guide the stroke survivor on how to maintain good skin care (Gethin *et al.*, 2020). Enzymes in faecal matter possess alkaline properties. In the event of seepage, contamination occurs, leading the alkaline substances to impact the protein layer of the skin (keratin), resulting in redness and discomfort. If not addressed promptly, the affected area may deteriorate, becoming excoriated and posing a risk of infection. At this stage, there may be significant pain. Therefore, perianal skin protection is essential. This can be maintained by using moist toilet paper and a light barrier cream regularly. If perianal skin does deteriorate, thicker barrier creams or sprays are required to aid healing.

There are several bowel emptying techniques that can support the management of emptying the rectum effectively to avoid faecal leakage and aid constipation (see Table 6.8). Some of these techniques require a specialist nurse or doctor who has undergone advanced training. However, the fundamentals of proper defaecation should never be underestimated, and every nurse should be able to provide advice on them. Additional techniques include biofeedback, a non-invasive behavioural treatment that can serve as an alternative or adjunct for patients with functional bowel disorders. Biofeedback training helps individuals learn which muscles to

TABLE 6.8 Bowel emptying techniques relevant to stroke

Technique	Explanation
Digital Stimulation of the Rectum (DSR)	A lubricated gloved finger is inserted into the anus and slowly rotated in a circular movement. Maintaining contact with the rectal mucosa, the anal canal is gently stretched. This helps relax the sphincter and stimulates the rectum to contract and empty
Transanal Bowel Irrigation (TAI)	Warm water is passed into the rectum with the use of a rectal catheter. This softens the stool so ease evacuation.
Digital Removal of Faeces (DRF)	This should only be performed by an experienced practitioner and is not the first choice of management. A gloved finger that is lubricated passes gently into the rectum via the anus and gently removes any faecal matter in the immediate locality.

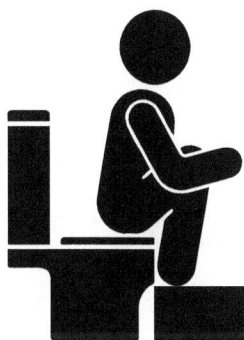

FIGURE 6.4   Recommended position to defaecate.

engage, the timing of their use, and the appropriate contraction strength to prevent leakage (Collins and Bradshaw, 2016).

The art of defaecation relies on positioning on the toilet or commode. Where possible, feet should be elevated on a stool to ensure the knees are above the hips (see Figure 6.4). The patient should then lean forward between their knees while keeping the back straight. By slowly rocking back and forth – a method known as the brace and pump technique – they can increase intra-abdominal pressure while simultaneously relaxing the external anal sphincter and puborectalis sling, thereby facilitating the expulsion of faeces.

Medication can support the management of faecal incontinence and constipation. This can be administered orally or rectally with an appropriate prescription. These include anti-diarrhoeal medications, bulk-forming agents, stimulants, laxatives and softeners. These can be combined with bowel emptying techniques to enhance the effectiveness.

While these products and interventions for bladder and bowel problems provide a sense of security and comfort for stroke survivors, facilitating a more normal way of life, it is crucial not to overlook their potential impact on dignity and self-esteem.

As a healthcare professional, you have a key role in safeguarding a person's dignity, particularly in relation to toileting and continence needs. This includes respecting their privacy, protecting their autonomy and providing care with sensitivity. Reflect on your own practice: how can you ensure individuals always have the privacy they require? What steps can you take to create a supportive, respectful environment that upholds dignity in these sensitive aspects of care?

It feels so overwhelmingly embarrassing to have to go to the toilet on a ward full of visitors with only a curtain to separate you.
(Jo, 47, embolic stroke as a result of endocarditis, 20 years post stroke)

When supporting inpatients, where possible, allow the individual to have the privacy of the bathroom over use of a commode behind a curtain on the ward. Even if this means pushing the patient from bedside to bathroom when there are mobility issues. This promotes privacy and dignity, and is especially important during visiting times.

Multidisciplinary approach

Effective continence care yields numerous advantages for both stroke patients and their caregivers. While complete restoration of continence may not always be achievable, implementing a variety of interventions can significantly enhance the patient's quality of life, subsequently fostering increased involvement in stroke rehabilitation. Enhanced continence management, encompassing both voiding and defaecation, may facilitate the transition from hospitalisation to home for older stroke patients and may improve quality of life for all. It is noteworthy that the improvement of continence issues post-stroke is feasible, contingent upon factors such as the type and extent of the stroke.

Continence care must have a multidisciplinary approach, including nursing and allied health professionals. Support services, including the occupational therapist, physiotherapist, dietitians and social services, all play an important role. The physiotherapist and occupational therapist will focus on rehabilitation to support recovery. Assessments will include adapting areas in the home to make getting to the bathroom easier, such as installing handrails, whilst also supplying walking aids, commodes, bedpans and handheld urinals to facilitate toilet use.

Dietitians offer valuable recommendations for a well-balanced diet and appropriate fluid intake, suggesting dietary changes that may continue to improve the stroke survivor's wellbeing. Community health services can organise support needed when the stroke survivor returns home, such as carers, and may introduce people to the local support network and like-minded people (see Table 6.9). There are many volunteer-run survivor groups, and stroke survivors should always explore what is available in their local area. Social services extend assistance to address any financial concerns, helping the stroke survivor to access benefits and secure grants, especially if adjustments to the bathroom become a large project.

Coping with continence challenges poses difficulties. Stroke survivors dealing with continence issues might experience discomfort or shame when broaching the topic with others. The reluctance to acknowledge the problem may prevent them from seeking the necessary support and advice that could enhance their quality of life. Living with incontinence instils a constant fear, especially in public settings, potentially triggering feelings of shame and embarrassment and fostering a sense of isolation. Healthcare professionals and carers play a crucial role by providing care and support through toilet training and ensuring the appropriate use of continence products tailored to their specific needs.

Analyse the assessment, planning and evaluation required to care for stroke survivors concerning alterations in urinary and bowel patterns. What are some of the enablers and barriers to effective continence care? Consider yourself, the stroke survivor and your work environment.

TABLE 6.9 Self-help

Tip	Contact
'Just Can't wait' card. Gains access to toilets anywhere	Bladder and Bowel community
RADAR key. Provides access to public disabled toilets	The National Key Scheme
Support groups	www.stroke.org.uk https://differentstrokes.co.uk https://abilitynet.org.uk/
getUbetter App – free physio support including pelvic floor exercises	Via the App store
The Stroke Association Helpline – offers support for the individual and carers. Advisors can also put individuals in contact with local carer support services	www.stroke.org.uk/stroke/support/helpline
Bladder Health UK	https://bladderhealthuk.org/continence-support
Bladder and Bowel community	www.bladderandbowel.org/

Bladder and Bowel UK
www.bbuk.org.uk (Offer free 'Just Can't Wait' Toilet Cards)

British Toilet Association
www.btaloos.co.uk

Disabled Living Foundation
www.dlf.org.uk

Disabled Living
www.disabledliving.co.uk

RCN Bladder and Bowel Forum
Royal College of Nursing
www.rcn.org.uk

RADAR Key Company
www.radarkey.org

Conclusion

Incontinence is a common and often persistent problem following stroke. It can affect the individual physically and psychologically and can have an impact on the ability to mobilise, return to work and enjoy social occasions. Incontinence can add an extra burden on carers and it is commonly recognised as one of the most burdensome sequelae following stroke.

It is important to recognise that there is a difference between managing incontinence and promoting continence. Both may need to be goals at times, but ultimately, strategies for regaining continence should be a key focus of rehabilitation.

References

Association of Continence Advice (2017) *Guidance for the provision of containment products for adult incontinence. A consensus document.* ACA. Available at: www.bladderandboweluk.co.uk/wpcontent/uploads/2017/07/Guidance_provision_of_product_adults_V8_May_2017_Final_ACA-2.pdf

Bickley, L. S., Szilagyi, P. G., Hoffman, R. M., and Soriano, R. P. (2021) *Bates' guide to physical examination and history taking, 13e.* Philadelphia: Lippincott Williams & Wilkins.

Bladder and Bowel Community (2019) *Bladder care (online).* Available at: www.bladderandbowel.org/bladder/

Brady, M. C., Jamieson, K., Bugge, C., Hagen, S., McClurg, D., Chalmers, C., and Langhorne, P. (2016) Caring for continence in stroke care settings: A qualitative study of patients' and staff perspectives on the implementation of a new continence care intervention. *Clinical Rehabilitation* 30(5), 481–494.

Cheesley, A. (2017) Why continence should be the seventh 'C' for all nurses. *Nursing Standard* 31(27), 29.

Collins, B., and Bradshaw, E. (2016) *Bowel dysfunction. A comprehensive guide for healthcare professionals*. Switzerland: Springer.

Evans, P. (2015) Validating the inter-rater reliability of an anorectal assessment tool. *Gastrointestinal Nursing* 13(5), 42–46.

Gethin, G., Probst, S., Weller, C., Kottner, J., and Beeckman, D. (2020) Nurses are research leaders in skin and wound care. *International Wound Journal* 17(6), 2005–2009. https://doi.org/10.1111/iwj.13492

Gillham, S., and Clark, L. (2011) *Psychological care after stroke – improving stroke services for those people with cognitive and mood disorders*. NHS Improvement. Available at: www.nice.org.uk/media/default/sharedlearning/531_strokepsychologicalsupportfinal.pdf (accessed 28 January 2024).

Intercollegiate Stroke Working Party (ISWP) (2023) *National Clinical Guideline for Stroke for the UK and Ireland*. London. Available at: www.strokeguideline.org (accessed 28 October 2024).

John, G., Primmaz, S., Crichton, S., and Wolfe, C. (2018) Urinary incontinence and indwelling urinary catheters as predictors of death after new-onset stroke: A report of the South London Stroke Register. *Journal of Stroke and Cerebrovascular Diseases* 27(1), 118–124. https://doi.org/10.1016/j.jstrokecerebrovasdis.2017.08.018

Kawanabe, E., Suzuki, M., Tanaka, S., Sasaki, S., and Hamaguchi, T. (2018) Impairment in toileting behaviour after a stroke. *Geriatrics & Gerontology International* 18, 1166–1172. https://doi.org/10.1111/ggi.13435

Koike, Y., Sumigawa, K., Koeda, S., Shiina, M., Fukushi, H., Tsuji, T., Hara, C., and Tsushima, H. (2015) Approaches for improving the toileting problems of hemiplegic stroke patients with poor standing balance. *Journal of Physical Therapy Science* 27(3), 877–881.

Lewis, S. J., and Heaton, K. W. (1997) Stool form scales a useful guide to intestinal transit time. *Scandinavian Journal of Gastroenterology* 32(9), 920–924.

National Institute for Health and Care Excellence (NICE) (2007) *Faecal incontinence in adults: Management (CG49)*. London: NICE. Available at: www.nice.org.uk/Guidance/CG49

National Institute for Health and Care Excellence (NICE) (2011) *Percutaneous tibial nerve stimulation for faecal incontinence (IPG395)*. London: NICE. Available at: www.nice.org.uk/guidance/ipg395

National Institute for Health and Care Excellence (NICE) (2023) *Urinary incontinence in neurological disease: Assessment and management (CG148)*. London: NICE. Available at: www.nice.org.uk/guidance/cg148

Nazarko, L. (2013) Continence series 4: The importance of assessment. *British Journal of Healthcare Assistants* 7(3), 118–124.

Nursing and Midwifery Council (NMC) (2018) *The code: Professional standards of practice and behaviour for nurses, midwives and nursing associates*. London: NMC.

Royal College of Nursing (RCN) (2019a) *Continence care (online)*. Available at: https://rcni.com/hosted-content/rcn/continence/home

Royal College of Nursing (RCN) (2019b) *Bowel care (online)*. Available at: www.rcn. org.uk/-/media/royal-college-of-nursing/documents/publications/2019/september/007-522.pdf

Thomas, L. H., Coupe, J., Cross, L. D., Tan, A. L., and Watkins, C. L. (2019) *Interventions for treating urinary incontinence after stroke in adults (Cochrane Review)*. Wiley. https://pmc.ncbi.nlm.nih.gov/articles/PMC6355973/

Woodward, S. (2014) Managing urinary incontinence after stroke. *British Journal of Neuroscience Nursing* 10(2). https://doi.org/10.12968/bjnn.2014.10.Sup2.25

7

WASHING AND DRESSING

Sarah Thirtle and Annette Palmer

Learning outcomes

- To discuss the impact of stroke on washing and dressing activities.
- To explore the importance of assessing washing and dressing as part of a holistic approach to recovery.
- To identify strategies for managing the impacts of stroke on washing and dressing in hospital and at home.

> When doing personal care, it needs to be personal.
>
> *(Steph, daughter and carer)*

Introduction

The Global Burden of Disease (GBD) 2019 Stroke Collaborators (2021) highlight that stroke is a leading cause of disability worldwide and that a third of stroke survivors are permanently disabled because of their stroke. For stroke survivors, the journey towards recovery is multifaceted, presenting both physical and emotional challenges for individuals and those in their support networks. Belagaie (2017) acknowledges that rehabilitation is a vital aspect of stroke care and regaining independence in daily activities like washing and dressing is a key goal in a stroke survivor's journey facilitating not only a return to self-care but also increased autonomy and dignity. This chapter explores the complexities surrounding washing and dressing for stroke survivors, offering insights, strategies and practical advice

DOI: 10.4324/9781003426196-8

for stroke survivors, and professional and informal caregivers regarding this critical aspect of ongoing rehabilitation.

Following a stroke, individuals may face a range of physical impairments, which can have varying significance on their daily lives. Motor deficits, sensory changes and cognitive impairments can impact stroke survivors' ability to perform activities of daily living independently. Washing and dressing, previously routine tasks, may present challenges post stroke and could require adaptation and support. Developing solutions to physical challenges is essential, but it is equally important to recognise and address the psychological impacts of having a stroke, given the need for individuals to navigate the long-term effects of stroke and any changes to their self-identity (van Dongen *et al.*, 2021).

The Care Quality Commission (CQC) (2011) highlights that life after stroke can include feelings of loss, confusion, frustration and anxiety, in addition to a sense of relief at having survived. Difficulties in performing self-care tasks independently can exacerbate these already complex emotional challenges. Supportive networks play a vital role in the journey to self-care. Support and empowerment are essential for recovery and rehabilitation and taking a person-centred approach which emphasises the empowerment and interpersonal connection between the individual and caregiver is essential (Kristensen *et al.*, 2016). Collaboration between stroke survivors, family and caregivers, and healthcare professionals can lead to significant progress and increased independence in washing and dressing.

The impact of stroke on washing and dressing

The ability to wash and dress contributes to a person's overall level of personal hygiene and while there may be varying opinions surrounding what constitutes good personal hygiene, the importance of maintaining basic washing and dressing practices should not be underestimated. Decreased function in this area can contribute to an increase in the risk of illness or disease, poor skin health, as well as having negative impacts on mental health, social interactions, self-esteem and over all wellbeing (Barclay, 2023).

The impact of stroke on washing and dressing activities can be linked to the underlying pathophysiology of the stroke, particularly in terms of how the location and severity of brain damage affect specific functions and abilities. Stroke affecting the left hemisphere can result in motor and sensory deficits, known as hemiparesis or hemiplegia on the right side of the body, whereas stroke impacting the right hemisphere may lead to similar difficulties on the left side (Sturgeon, 2018). This can lead to significant challenges in activities of daily living including washing and dressing, particularly if the person's previously dominant side is affected. Strokes affecting the frontal lobe can lead to changes in a person's ability to think or process and respond to information. This poses further challenges related to decision-making and function when washing and dressing, as well as presenting barriers to communication between stroke survivors and those assisting them. Following stroke, motor, sensory and cognitive impairments, spatial awareness and perceptual deficits and emotional and psychological factors can all impact a person's ability to wash and dress independently.

- Choose a pair of shoes with laces and a coat with buttons or a zip
- Sit down in a comfortable and safe environment
- Using only one hand (consider using your non-dominant hand), attempt to tie the shoelaces and fasten the coat.

Identify the main challenges you encountered during the activity and reflect on how the activity made you feel.

- Consider how the activity increased your awareness of the impact of physical limitations on your ability to dress yourself
- Explore potential solutions or adaptive strategies to mitigate the challenges encountered
- How might changes in cognitive function as the result of stroke further impact your ability to complete this activity?

Motor impairments

Stroke can result in hemiparesis or hemiplegia, affecting one side of the body (Sturgeon, 2018). Weakness or paralysis, particularly to the previously dominant side can lead to difficulties in undertaking the fine motor tasks required for washing and dressing, such as gripping objects, reaching overhead and manipulating buttons, zips and shoelaces. In addition to these fine motor challenges, gross motor skills can also be negatively impacted following stroke. Maintaining balance when walking and standing can present problems, increasing the risk of falls and injury. Post-stroke spasticity has a significant impact on those who develop it and can affect up to 40% of people suffering from severe weakness after their stroke (Intercollegiate Stroke Working Party (ISWP), 2023). Dressler *et al.* (2018) define spasticity as involuntary muscle overactivity in central paresis, caused by slow or rapid passive joint movement or sensory stimulation. Increased muscle stiffness and spasm can exacerbate mobility issues, resulting in painful movements which can have a significant impact on washing and dressing ability and can lead to severe disability in 15% of individuals post stroke (ISWP, 2023). Alan describes the difficulties he experienced with mobility following his stroke and their impact upon washing and dressing. Furthermore, Jo also highlights the importance of selecting appropriate clothing to mitigate motor impairment and to promote independence in dressing.

> I struggled putting clothes on and I couldn't get into a bath. No chance! So, I had to shower putting a hand against a wall and kneeling into the wall. I could step in to the bath, but I could not sit down as I would not be able to get back up again. I couldn't wear a zip-up coat or anything, I had to wear pullovers.
>
> *(Alan, 50, ischaemic stroke, 4 years post stroke)*

> While I was in hospital, my family chose clothes that I could put on without assistance with no zippers, no buttons or clasps that were impossible. Being able to slip into slippers with no laces and that kind of thing. Twenty years on I still avoid certain clothes that I would not be able to fasten independently or put on without help.
>
> *(Jo, 47, embolic stroke as a result of endocarditis, 20 years post stroke)*

Sensory deficits

The somatosensory nervous system sustains sensation across different regions of the body acting as a pathway which links various sensory experiences and transmitting information from the body's periphery to the brain to interpret environmental stimuli (Raju and Tadi, 2022). This system is responsible for the perception of touch, pressure, pain, temperature, position, movement and vibration. It involves the perception and interpretation of tactile sensations received by the skin's receptors, enabling individuals to identify and distinguish various characteristics of objects or surfaces. Tactile discrimination is essential for performing tasks requiring manual dexterity, precision and sensory feedback, such as grasping objects, manipulating tools and recognising objects by touch. Tyson *et al.* (2008) explored the characteristics of sensory loss in stroke survivors and found that not only do somatosensory deficits often accompany motor impairments, but that the extent of weakness and stroke severity are significantly associated with sensory dysfunction. This dysfunction can present as absent, reduced, heightened or altered sensation when compared to usual (Lv *et al.*, 2022) and, as a result, stroke survivors experiencing somatosensory loss experience a decrease in participation in daily tasks such as washing and dressing (Carey *et al.*, 2018). This may increase the risk of injury during washing and dressing or lead to challenges in selecting appropriate items of clothing due to alteration in perception of temperature and texture.

> The constant feeling of having pins and needles, that's all I ever felt, like a numbness. I couldn't hold the shower head in my left hand. My partner would come in to help and he'd say, 'it's red hot, what are you doing?' My skin would go really red, and he'd touch the water and it would be really hot, but I couldn't feel it.
>
> *(Jacqueline, 42, ischaemic stroke whilst pregnant, 12 years post stroke)*

Additionally, changes in somatosensory association can further affect the washing and dressing process. For instance, individuals may need to see parts of their body or articles of clothing to identify and distinguish between them, whereas previously, this was done through spatial awareness and touch. Using a mirror or changing body position might become necessary to aid visualisation, which could increase the risk of accidents, such as falls.

> Even now I can't find the left-hand sleeve of a coat. If I can't see it and have to feel for it, I can't find it. Trying to find things in my pocket – I can't feel the difference between the pocket, and the things inside it.
>
> *(Jo, 47, embolic stroke as a result of endocarditis, 20 years post stroke)*

Spatial awareness and perceptual deficits

Body schema can be described as the internal representation of the body's spatial dimensions and the relative position of body parts in relation to each other, helping to coordinate movements and interact with the environment (Cardinali *et al.*, 2009). Both central and peripheral systems are involved in the development of body schema, which is learnt through movement and experience. Spatial awareness and perceptual deficits can occur due to damage in specific areas of the brain, particularly the parietal lobe and associated neural pathways. These are responsible for processing sensory information and developing perception of an individual's body and surroundings. These neural networks can be altered leading to difficulties in accurately interpreting sensory input, such as touch, proprioception and visual cues, which are critical in making continuous adjustments during movement (Barrett and Muzaffar, 2014). This can lead to difficulties in accurately judging distances, locating body parts and understanding the spatial relationships between objects and the body, leading to errors in judgement and coordination during washing and dressing activities. Tasks such as reaching for and grasping objects, coordinating movements to manipulate clothing and washing items, and self-orientation can become challenging and frustrating. Reduced awareness of the stroke-affected side causes further functional disability which can lead to un-recognised neglect of one side during self-care activities (Barratt, 2021).

> I never used to know where my arm was which is bizarre, so when getting dressed and stuff, I thought my arm was in front of me but actually it was behind me.
>
> I remember sitting down once and I could feel something touching my leg. I jumped up – 'what's that, what's that?', and it was my arm.
>
> *(Jacqueline, 42, ischaemic stroke whilst pregnant, 12 years post stroke)*

Rehabilitation interventions focusing on improving spatial awareness, proprioception and visual perception can be crucial in addressing these challenges (Barrett and Muzaffar, 2014), promoting independence in washing and dressing tasks for stroke survivors. Planning tasks in advance, adapting techniques, providing environmental modifications and offering appropriate assistive devices can support stroke survivors in regaining confidence and functionality in their daily routines.

Cognitive impairments

> Planning what I was going to wear, checking what went together, then the action of putting the clothes on was exhausting. The process was hard as I had lost the opportunity to do things that I once found simple, automatically – something that I took for granted before my stroke.
>
> *(Jo, 47, embolic stroke as a result of endocarditis, 20 years post stroke)*

EbyE Jo explains the cognitive impact of stroke and how it can lead to challenges when it comes to washing and dressing decision-making. Damage to the brain resulting from stroke can lead to cognitive deficits, including attention, memory and executive function impairments. Persson *et al.* (2017) found that cognitive changes such as impaired memory, changes in executive function, mental fatigue and reduced attention can remain present for many years post stroke, thus impacting the ability to plan, sequence and undertake the steps required to wash and dress independently. For example, people who have had a stroke may find it difficult to maintain focus while performing tasks such as bathing and their ability to remember the steps involved in washing and dressing activities can be compromised, resulting in confusion or frustration during the process. As the stroke may have affected the brain's ability to coordinate actions, the organisation of thoughts needed to complete these personal care tasks can become challenging. An inability to initiate and sequence tasks is often related to a reduction in executive function and this can impact the planning and decision-making capacity vital for undertaking washing and dressing activities. It is recognised that the addition of cognitive difficulties post stroke can impose a significant burden on stroke survivors and their caregivers and that clinicians must understand that sometimes, unseen aspects of stroke call for ongoing support following hospital discharge (Tang *et al.*, 2020).

> Having to think about it constantly – that is exhausting. Look at the jumper, put my left arm in first, then put it over my head. Having to consciously think about everything before I did it, every single stage.
>
> *(Jacqueline, 42, ischaemic stroke whilst pregnant, 12 years post stroke)*

Stroke may lead to anosognosia, a condition in which individuals are unaware of their own abilities, impairments and surroundings. This lack of insight can further complicate activities of daily living and people living with anosognosia are often unable to undertake the steps required to wash and dress both with assistance and independently (Grattan *et al.*, 2018). This is because they may not be fully aware of the extent of their cognitive deficits or recognise the need for support and might perceive themselves as functioning normally. Declining help and lack of engagement with rehabilitation activities aimed at improving cognitive functioning can negatively impact recovery and the potential for becoming independent with washing and dressing. Addressing anosognosia through education, therapy and support from healthcare professionals is crucial for maximising rehabilitation outcomes and promoting a better quality of life for stroke survivors (De-Rosende-Celeiro *et al.*, 2021).

Emotional and psychological factors

Al-Khindi *et al.* (2010) found that stroke survivors commonly experienced deficits in memory and executive function which were further compounded by depression, anxiety, fatigue and sleep disturbances. Depression, anxiety and frustration are prevalent in the subacute and chronic stages following stroke (Schottke and Giabbiconi, 2015). These mood problems can impact the level of participation and engagement in self-care activities such as washing and dressing (Andrenelli *et al.*, 2015). Clothing choices and preferences can be influenced by changes in body image, altered self-esteem and functionality, and grief over the loss of independence and changes in life circumstances can further affect the psychological and emotional experiences of stroke survivors. Depression, for example, can reduce motivation and energy, making it difficult to undertake personal care activities and anxiety symptoms can exacerbate cognitive difficulties and become overwhelming, leading to the avoidance of tasks that require concentration and focus.

> My outfits changed – loose t-shirts and leggings or loose sleeveless dresses and cardigans because it is easier to get dressed and I don't wear jeans because of the button.
>
> *(Jacqueline, 42, ischaemic stroke whilst pregnant, 12 years post stroke)*

> My clothes choices are based on fastenings, whether they are easy take on and off, and also on comfort, rather than self-image or fashion. I haven't worn heels for years due to fear of falling over and also as I live with daily pain. It is important not to make it worse by being in uncomfortable clothes or footwear.

> It's hard to know what to wear on special occasions or nights out – as I never feel as dressed up or feminine as others. It used to really upset me in my thirties

as I felt that flat footwear and a walking stick would take the shine out of an outfit. As time went on, I started buying different types of walking sticks with different colours and patterns to try and complement my outfit.

(Jo, 47, embolic stroke as a result of endocarditis, 20 years post stroke)

Addressing the emotional and psychological impact of stroke is crucial for supporting recovery and improving quality of life. Providing a supportive environment and involving social networks and caregivers in the rehabilitation process can contribute to a more positive experience and greater success in regaining independence in all aspects of washing and dressing.

Maintaining a washing and dressing routine including having a shower rather than a bedside wash where possible, even when in hospital, provides structure and consistency and can have a profound impact on physical and mental health.

I really feel that getting up and maintaining normality in personal care like getting dressed was really important and also good at the other end of the day getting undressed and getting into nightwear and under the covers. A normal routine at both ends of the day is important so that you don't become institutionalised, and it really helped my mental health and wellbeing.

(Jo, 47, embolic stroke as a result of endocarditis, 20 years post stroke)

- How can the physical environment be adapted to promote emotional wellbeing during washing and dressing routines?
- What communication strategies can be implemented to ensure individuals feel respected and involved in their personal care?
- Are there any specific activities that can be incorporated into the routine to enhance emotional wellbeing?
- How can caregivers support individuals in maintaining a sense of normality and autonomy during personal care?

Assessment

Imagine you are assessing the washing and dressing needs of a patient who has had a stroke.

- What questions would you ask?
- What observations would you make?
- Where else might you gather information from to support your assessment?

Assessing the personal care needs of stroke survivors is essential for developing rehabilitation plans which meet individual requirements. The National Institute for Health and Care Excellence (NICE) (2023a) recommend referral to an occupational therapist who has expertise in neurological disability. A comprehensive assessment should involve evaluating an individual's abilities and limitations when undertaking activities of daily living including washing and dressing. Standardised holistic assessment tools, observation and discussions with both the stroke survivor and those supporting their care can be used to obtain relevant information to support decision-making and care planning.

As part of a holistic assessment, consideration of an individual's motor, sensory, spatial and perceptual awareness and cognitive abilities should be used to gain a detailed understanding of the individual's functional status. Physical assessments focus on motor function, range of motion, strength and coordination, to gain an understanding of the impact that motor impairments are having on washing and dressing activities. Sensory assessments evaluate sensory perception and touch discrimination, identifying deficits that may affect the individual's awareness and safety during daily activities (Mak-Yuen *et al.*, 2023), while cognitive assessments explore memory, attention, executive function and problem-solving abilities, as cognitive deficits can impact the ability to sequence tasks and follow instructions. This is important when considering the potential dangers related to the accurate judgement of water temperature and the use of heated devices such as hairdryers, straighteners and curlers. In addition to physical and cognitive assessments, it is vital that emotional and psychological evaluations are undertaken when identifying the personal care needs of stroke survivors. The emotional factors resulting from stroke can impact engagement in rehabilitation and overall wellbeing (Andrenelli *et al.*, 2015). Assessing emotional and psychological needs enables healthcare professionals to identify and address mental health challenges that may impact an individual's ability to participate in washing and dressing and adherence to rehabilitation plans. The assessment should also consider environmental factors to determine the level of support and modifications needed to promote independence and safety.

The ISWP (2023) make recommendations in relation to the assessment of washing and dressing:

- People with stroke should be formally assessed for their safety and independence in all relevant personal activities of daily living by a clinician with the appropriate expertise, and the findings should be recorded using a standardised assessment tool.
- People with limitations of personal activities of daily living after stroke should:
  - be referred to an occupational therapist with knowledge and skills in neurological rehabilitation. Assessment should include consideration

of the impact of hidden deficits affecting function including neglect, executive dysfunction and visual impairments
- be assessed by an occupational therapist within 24 hours of admission to a stroke unit
- be offered treatment for identified problems (e.g. feeding, work) by the occupational therapist, in discussion with other members of the specialist multidisciplinary team.

When assessing the washing and dressing function of an individual, consider the points in Table 7.1.

- Identify a washing or dressing activity such as washing your hands, washing your hair or putting on an item of clothing
- How much effort does the activity take and does the activity usually require the use of both hands? What are the most important features of the activity?
- Break down the activity into the individual steps required to complete it successfully and in the correct sequence.

This activity helps you to develop a deeper understanding of the cognitive and physical aspects involved in activities of washing or dressing, enabling you to better assess individuals' functional abilities and tailor individual washing and dressing support strategies.

Person-centred care and empowerment in washing and dressing

> There is nothing that prepares you for the first time you have to endure a bed bath, the complete vulnerability that you feel in the hands of someone else, the emotions you feel at finding yourself in the position where you need one in the first place and despite being extremely weak and ill when I had my first experience of this my mind still flooded me with unhelpful body embarrassment, uncomfortable feelings and ridiculous thoughts.
>
> *(Jo, 47, embolic stroke as a result of endocarditis, 20 years post stroke)*

Person-centred care is essential when assisting an individual with washing and dressing after a stroke, to prioritise their dignity, while recognising their unique needs and preferences (Stevens *et al.*, 2022). This partnership approach requires actively involving the stroke survivor in their care decisions, respecting their autonomy, wishes and values, and tailoring support to their specific abilities and limitations (Martin-Sanz *et al.*, 2022). It is important that caregivers recognise and maintain an individual's established personal routines and preferences for

TABLE 7.1 Considerations when assessing the washing and dressing function of an individual

Point to consider	Rationale
How does the individual initially engage with the activity?	This can determine whether they are confident, hesitant, or unsure, which can impact positive outcomes (Horne *et al.,* 2014).
Does the individual demonstrate prior knowledge or experience with the activity?	This can indicate their level of cognitive function and memory, which can impact dressing ability (Walker *et al.,* 2003).
How does the individual address any challenges or unfamiliar aspects of the activity?	This assesses their cognitive flexibility and problem-solving skills, elements of executive function essential in stroke rehabilitation (Poulin *et al.,* 2012).
How does the individual start the activity? Do they require prompting or can they initiate it independently?	This can indicate their executive function and motor planning abilities (Rowland *et al,* 2008).
Does the individual maintain attention on the activity throughout its completion, or are they easily distracted?	This reflects their cognitive control and concentration, which affect functional recovery (Loetscher *et al,* 2019)..
Did the individual successfully finish the activity, and if so, how efficiently?	This evaluates their ability to follow through and complete actions to achieve a goal, and enables identification of individualised adaptations to promote independence (ISWP, 2023).
Can the individual modify their responses? This involves an individual's ability to adapt their actions based on feedback, changes in the environment, or unexpected circumstances during the washing and dressing activity.	This demonstrates executive functioning including their level of flexibility in problem-solving, their ability to adjust strategies as needed, and to correct errors. Executive functioning assessment is essential in post-stroke assessments (Poulin *et al.,* 2012).
Was the activity physically demanding for the individual? Did they appear to struggle or exert significant effort while completing it?	This helps to assess the individual's physical abilities and the presence of fatigue (ISWP, 2023).
Did the individual demonstrate good balance control while sitting or standing during the activity?	This indicates ability to maintain stability and control over their body position, which is essential for performing washing and dressing activities (Fujita *et al.,* 2015).
Was the individual able to position their body correctly and comfortably for the activity?	Proper body positioning reduces the risk of injury or strain while performing washing and dressing activity (National Advisory Committee for Stroke (NACS), 2022).

(*Continued*)

TABLE 7.1 (Continued)

Point to consider	Rationale
Did the individual use both sides of their body equally or as needed during the activity?	Washing and dressing often requires the use of both limbs or sides of the body simultaneously or sequentially. Observing bilateral task performance enables activity planning and support to be implemented (NICE, 2023b).
Can the individual concentrate on the purposeful actions required to complete the activity?	This assesses their ability to identify and focus on the most important aspects of an activity, organising actions to achieve a goal (ISWP, 2023).
Can the individual break the activity down into smaller steps, demonstrating a systematic approach and organisation of tasks?	This reflects higher intellectual functions of analysis, planning and conceptual ability (ISWP, 2023).

washing and dressing to ensure that care is comfortable and promotes a sense of normality and wellbeing. Person-centred care ensures that an individual's choices and values are respected, and their voice is heard within a collaborative and supportive environment. It is essential to focus on their strengths and to promote independence and control where possible. This respectful and compassionate approach enhances the effectiveness of care and contributes to the individual's overall emotional and psychological wellbeing and rehabilitation. Elvén *et al.* (2023) found that when stroke survivors feel unheard and insufficiently involved in their care during encounters with healthcare professionals, it can lead to a sense of exclusion, limiting their ability to understand and influence decisions. Jo explains the impact that those giving support in washing and dressing had on her while she was in hospital. She describes two approaches to the provision of assistance with personal care.; both of which were efficient and effective in keeping her clean and comfortable.

Approach 1: *That was important to me. I wasn't seen as an empty vessel, or someone who didn't understand what was going on just because I couldn't speak back to them.*

Approach 2: *It was like I was a dead weight that they were doing a task on, and it made me feel dehumanised and added to my distress and upset at having to be given personal care at that time.*
(Jo, 47, embolic stroke as a result of endocarditis, 20 years post stroke)

The first approach focussed on involving her in her own care, even when she was unable to communicate and represents person-centred care. The second approach showed a lack of recognition of Jo as an individual and failed to demonstrate person-centred care. This approach lacked inclusion and interaction, leaving Jo feeling disempowered.

Reflect on Jo's experiences during her time in hospital.
How did the different approaches to giving support in washing and dressing impact Jo's emotional wellbeing and sense of dignity?
How can healthcare professionals ensure that stroke survivors like Jo are included and empowered in decision-making regarding their personal care, even when communication barriers exist?
Jo expressed feeling dehumanised and distressed by the second approach to personal care. How can a culture of empathy and person-centred care be fostered?
Reflect on your own experiences or observations in healthcare settings. Have you encountered situations where individuals were treated similarly to either of Jo's scenarios? How do you think such experiences could be improved or prevented in the future?

In combination with a person-centred approach to care and support, empowerment is an essential process that promotes independence, fosters choice and decision-making and active participation in rehabilitation activities, enhancing the overall health and wellbeing of stroke survivors (Bravo *et al.*, 2015). Health empowerment helps to develop an individual's self-belief, enabling them to autonomously manage their own needs and exert influence over decisions and situations that affect them and their rehabilitation (Sit *et al.*, 2016). Disempowerment can lead to dependence in activities of daily living such as washing and dressing, feelings of helplessness and reduced self-esteem, and an exacerbation of the social consequences brought about by a loss of independence post stroke (Hörnsten *et al.*, 2016). Steph talks about the care that her Mum received in hospital following her stroke. Opportunities to empower and promote independence were missed and Steph explains how that made her Mum feel. Steph goes on to talk about the lack of collaboration and person- centred care that her Mum experienced whilst in hospital leading to feelings of disempowerment and further loss of independence.

She would say, 'I don't like being a burden and I don't like people helping me.' Washing and dressing, they did it for her. If they had given her a flannel in her right hand, she would have done it.

(Steph, daughter and carer)

It was really difficult when she was told to do something, and she was never asked to do anything. She had got all her faculties about her, but they always told her what they were doing, not asking her first. She had the capability to do a lot of things, but they never asked her, they told her.

(Steph, daughter of stroke survivor)

Consider these terms and what they mean to you:

| Promoting choice | Self-advocacy | Concordance |
| Active participation | Collaboration | Self-management |

- How do they relate to person-centred approaches and empowerment?
- How could you ensure that you apply these when supporting stroke survivors with washing and dressing activities?

Transfer of care from hospital to home

Imagine you are a stroke survivor preparing to leave the hospital.

- Write a journal entry describing your feelings, fears and hopes about returning home.
- Reflect on how your daily life might change and what adjustments you anticipate needing to make particularly in relation to washing and dressing.
- Consider the physical, emotional and social aspects of your transition.

While stroke is an acute medical event, it can lead to long-term health and social needs which may require nursing care and rehabilitation after the initial inpatient period. However, there are challenges associated with the transfer of individuals from hospital to community which often impact continuity and effective integration of services (Sit *et al.*, 2016). The most common transfer of care for stroke survivors is from the hospital to the home environment (ISWP, 2023). Adverse health outcomes and an increase in hospital readmissions result from fragmented transitions (Markle-Reid *et al.*, 2020) and, therefore, this is a critical phase which requires careful planning.

As individuals move from the structured environment of the hospital to the familiarity of their own homes, they often face challenges in maintaining washing and dressing routines. A key consideration is the need for continuity of care and support during this transition period. Health and care professionals must ensure that stroke survivors receive appropriate guidance and resources to continue their rehabilitation safely and effectively (ISWP, 2023). This may involve providing education and training to both the stroke survivor and their caregivers on safe and

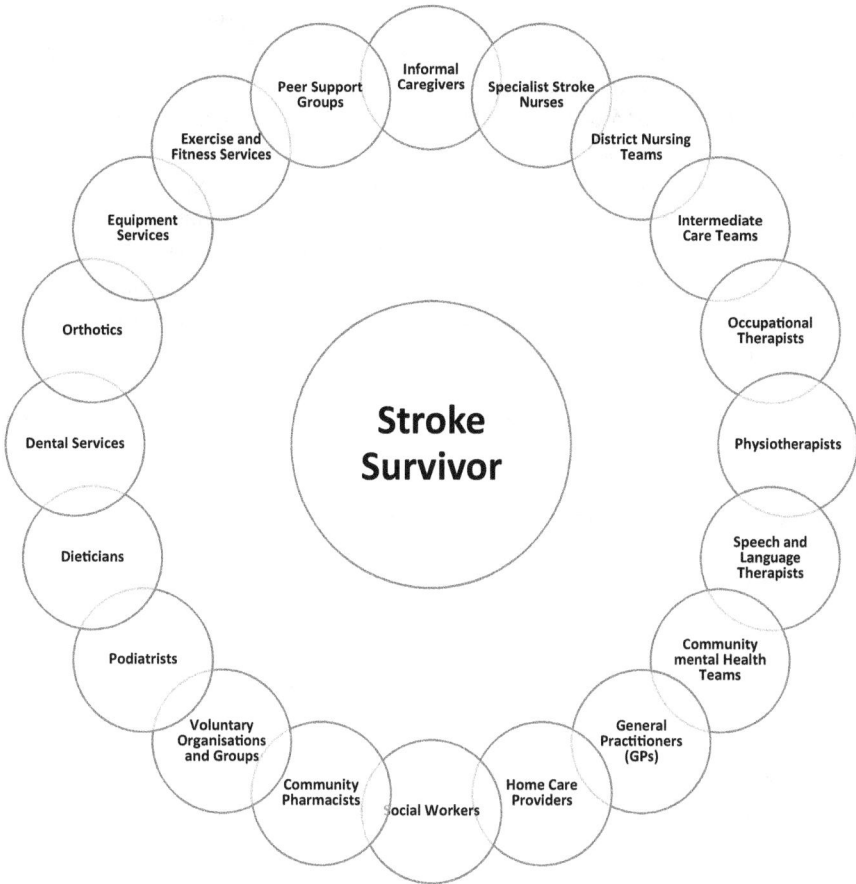

FIGURE 7.1 Professionals and groups involved in supportive discharge and ongoing rehabilitation.

effective strategies for washing and dressing, as well as the provision of assistive devices or adaptive equipment and guidance on their use. An interprofessional and interagency approach is important during the transfer of care from hospital to home and 'Early Supported Discharges' have long been shown to positively impact levels of independence with activities of daily living in stroke survivors (Fearon and Langhorne, 2012). Care and support at home will be provided by a number of different health and social care professionals, agencies and groups. The role of informal caregivers in the transfer of stroke survivors from hospital to home can support this collaborative approach, helping to ensure a smooth transition and to support an individual's recovery process, providing both practical assistance and emotional care, and is vital in achieving positive outcomes (Clarke and Forster, 2015).

When conducting an assessment within the home it is important to identify any barriers or hazards that may impact an individual's ability to wash and dress safely and independently. O'Callaghan *et al.* (2024) advocate for an individualised and comprehensive approach to stroke care that offers continual assessment of the needs of stroke survivors and their environments as they adjust to the transition between hospital and home. The assessment may identify any adjustments or modifications to the home that are needed, such as the installation of grab rails in the bathroom or the rearrangement of furniture to reduce the risk of falling. Healthcare professionals should give reassurance and encouragement during this transition time from hospital to home. Fostering a supportive environment that promotes the individual's confidence in washing and dressing is vitally important. Shared decision-making enhances stroke survivors' dignity and increases their sense of empowerment while respecting individual preferences. A holistic approach that addresses physical, environmental and emotional needs is required and health services should undertake needs assessments at regular intervals including at transition from hospital to home and 6 months post transition to meet the changing needs of stroke survivors (O'Callaghan *et al.*, 2024).

The ISWP (2023) make recommendations in relation to the transfer of stroke survivors from hospital to home:

- Before the transfer home of a person with stroke who is dependent in any activities, the person's home environment should be assessed by a visit with an occupational therapist. If a home visit is not considered appropriate, they should be offered an access visit or an interview about the home environment including viewing photographs or videos taken by family/carers.
- People with stroke who are dependent in personal activities (e.g. dressing, toileting) should be offered a transition package before being transferred home that includes:
  - visits or leave at home prior to the final transfer of care
  - training and education for their carers specific to their needs
  - telephone advice and support for 3 months

In the hospital, I saw a couple of physiotherapists and they had me on a walking stick going up and down the stairs. I got to the stage where I could do it holding onto the railing, and so then they were satisfied that I'd be okay at home, from that.

During the first week at home some physiotherapists came. They gave me some stretch bands and some exercises to do and then they left me to get on with it. I had a few visits just to check, 'oh you can walk round the block, you can do this', and then that was it. They were comfortable that I could do things, but in my head I thought 'well I can, but it's not how I used to be', I was struggling. I wouldn't go out, I had to have friends with me, and it was my friends who got me doing things.

Getting in and out of the bath to have a shower, I slipped because I was on my wet bathroom floor, a tiled floor, and obviously I couldn't feel my foot and I slipped. My bathroom didn't have any railings or any of that.

(Alan, 50, ischaemic stroke, 4 years post stroke)

Reading Alan's experiences of transitioning to home from hospital highlights the importance of undertaking a thorough assessment of the home environment to identify risks and barriers.

Imagine you are a healthcare professional visiting a stroke survivor's home:

- Create a checklist of safety measures you would recommend ensuring that their home is suitable for their personal care needs.
- Reflect on the role of support systems such as family, friends and professional caregivers in maintaining a safe home environment
- Research and create a list of community resources in your area that specialise in providing equipment, support and care services for stroke survivors
- How can stroke survivors access the services available to them?

Washing and dressing hints and tips from stroke survivors

Jo, 46, ischaemic stroke, 20 years post stroke and Jaqueline, 42, ischaemic stroke whilst pregnant, 12 years post stroke, discuss their hints and tips for washing and dressing post stroke.

I accessorise with patterned and colourful walking sticks.

I only wear leggings and pull over dresses as I avoid all clothing with any fastenings. Although this does limit my clothes options a lot, I try to show my personality in the bold and colourful prints I choose.

I wear oversized coats accompanied with large warm scarves in the winter to keep my front warm and to avoid having to fasten up coats, or I have coats with large buttons and will only fasten one of them, as I find zippers and smaller buttons to difficult.

I accessorise with trainers as I do not have many options in terms of footwear so I buy a range of trainers in different colours and styles so that I feel trendy. That allows me to be comfortable as they are practical and help to prevent trips and falls.

I have a whole wardrobe of clothes that have no fastenings at all so when on my own I have a variety of pull on joggers, flared skirts, tops and jumpers.

When clothes shopping I always go with someone that can help me in the changing room – as this is where you find out if an item can be out on or off without help, and there has been many time I have been able to get something on but not off independently. Any item I cannot use independently doesn't get bought unless for a special occasion when I know there will be someone around to help me.

I avoid buying any items with small buttons or fastening especially at the back. Or any items where they are very tight with no stretch about the arms. I do not wear tops that are fastened by bows I have to do as this can lead to embarrassing situations when the bows come undone.

It can be difficult getting your stroke side into clothes, so I have learnt that it is easier especially with my arm to put my left (affected side) in first. Coats can be particularly difficult, and I cannot feel to guide my arm in so never do this out of my line of sight. Where most people do by feeling for the arm hole, I look and place my hand into it. I also let friends and family help me by guiding my arm into the arm hole rather than struggle especially in the winter because this can become even harder when cold.

I wear jeans but not ones with only buttons as the they are too difficult and try to buy ones with some stretch in the denim as these always seem to be easier to get on and off than pure denim.

I choose coats with big zippers or easy fastenings and at first I hated people fastening my coats but now if I am cold or struggling or in a rush I just let someone do it for me, but I really test fastening out in the shop so to avoid where possible awkward zippers.

I wear snoods a lot as they are easy to get on and off over the head and keep my neck and top of my chest warm, as my pain and discomfort increases when I am cold and I seem to really feel the cold post stoke. Because of this in the winter I wear lots of layers: vest, t-shirt, long sleeve t-shirt then jumper or hoodie and have to make sure I buy sizes with room to layer.

Footwear = flat, comfortable and a lot of slip-ons like dolly shoes and pumps with decent size laces.

Cutting nails on my right hand using my left hand is very difficult so have learnt to ask for help from people I trust.

I cannot put necklaces or bracelets on unassisted so wear things that can just go over my head or bangles and often ask friends to assist me in changing jewellery then will wear a necklace for a while before changing it. I try to buy earrings with no backs, and simple hair clasps.

I limit my makeup to foundation, powder, eyebrows, eyeliner and mascara and this took a lot of practice and now is more about the containers than brand: simple tubes and things that can stand up. I buy pump bottle shampoo, conditioner and shower gels so I don't have to use two hands in the shower to get stuff out of bottle or have to squeeze things out of tubes, as all this is hard when you are wet, and containers are slippery. Some spray deodorants are impossible to use because I don't have the strength in my left fingers to spray on my right side, so I buy ones I now know are easy, or use roll on. Buying products and realising the container is impossible to use independently is a matter of trial and error. Now, with years of experience I know things I will find hard so just don't buy them.

Conclusion

Stroke can profoundly impact the ability to perform washing and dressing activities, presenting challenges due to physical, cognitive and emotional changes. Assessing these activities as part of a holistic, person-centred, collaborative recovery approach is essential, as it allows for a comprehensive understanding of an individual's needs and enables more effective rehabilitation. To mitigate the effects of stroke on washing and dressing, person-centred strategies must be tailored for both hospital and home settings. Focus on the transfer of individuals from hospital to home must include an interprofessional and collaborative approach which aims to empower stroke survivors and their care givers. Promotion of independence, self-management and maintenance of autonomy in washing and dressing activities can lead to improved physical, psychological and social wellbeing for stroke survivors.

References

Al-Khindi, T., Macdonald, R. L., and Schweizer, T. A. (2010) 'Cognitive and functional outcome after aneurysmal subarachnoid hemorrhage'. *Stroke*. 41(8): 519–536. Available at: https://pubmed.ncbi.nlm.nih.gov/20595669/

Andrenelli, E., Ippoliti, E., Coccia, M., Millevolte, M., Cicconi, B., Latini, L., Lagalla, G., Provinviali, L., Ceravolo, M. G., and Capecci, M. (2015) 'Features and predictors of activity limitations and participation restriction 2 years after intensive rehabilitation following first-ever stroke'. *European Journal of Physical and Medical Rehabilitation*. 51(5): 575–585. Available at: https://minervamedica.it/en/getfreepdf/UHNnTExJbHZa OUhCM01xMmZYeWp3Q01lMzBWRm5JTWtSbXZwcUk5cDhaODhZZkI0aGcya1Z VL29kRytQSldzTA%253D%253D/R33Y2015N05A0575.pdf

Barclay, T. (2023) The impacts of personal hygiene on your health. Available at: https://innerbody.com/impacts-of-personal-hygiene-on-your-health

Barratt, A. M. (2021) 'Spatial neglect and anosognosia after right brain stroke'. *Behavioral Neurology and Psychiatry*. 27(6): 1624–1645. Available at: https://ncbi.nlm.nih.gov/pmc/articles/PMC9421660/

Barrett, A. M., and Muzzaffar, T. (2014) 'Spatial cognitive rehabilitation and motor recovery after stroke'. *Current Opinion in Neurology*. 27(6): 653–658. Available at: https://ncbi.nlm.nih.gov/pmc/articles/PMC4455599/pdf/nihms634898.pdf

Belagaje, S. R. (2017). 'Stroke rehabilitation'. *Cerebrovascular Disease*. 23(1): 238–253. Available at: https://static1.squarespace.com/static/5bae3539ab1a622e64cb406b/t/62c5a 1faffd54208682dce91/1657119227137/ContinuumStrokeRehab2017.pdf

Bravo, P., Edwards, A., Barr, P. J., Scholl, I., Elwyn, G., McAllister, M., and The Cochrane Healthcare Quality Research Group, Cardiff University. (2015) 'Conceptualising patient empowerment: a mixed methods study'. *BMC Health Services Research*. 15: 252. Available at: https://bmchealthservres.biomedcentral.com/articles/10.1186/s12913-015-0907-z#citeas

Cardinali, L., Brozzoli, C. and Farne, A (2009) Peripersonal space and body schema:two labels for the same concept?' *Brain Topography*. 21(3–4): 252–260. Available at: https://doi.org/10.1007/s10548-009-0092-7

Care Quality Commission (CQC). (2011) *Supporting Life after Stroke – A Review of Services for People Who Have Had a Stoke and Their Carers*. London: CQC. Available at: https://cqc.org.uk/sites/default/files/documents/supporting_life_after_stroke_nati onal_report.pdf

Carey, L. M., Matyas, T. A., and Baum, C. (2018) 'Effects of somatosensory impairment on participation after stroke'. *American Journal of Occupational Therapy*. 72(3). Available at: https://ncbi.nlm.nih.gov/pmc/articles/PMC5915232/

Carke, D. J., and Forster, A. (2015) 'Improving post-stroke recovery: the role of the multidisciplinary health care team'. *Journal of Multidisciplinary Healthcare*. 8: 433–442. Available at: doi:10.2147/JMDH.S68764

De-Rosende-Celeiro, I., Rey-Villamayor, A., Francisco-de-Miguel, I., and Ávila-Álvarez, A. (2021) 'Independence in daily activities after stroke among occupational therapy patients and its relationship with unilateral neglect'. *International Journal of Environmental Research and Public Health*. 18(14): 7537. Available at: https://doi.org/10.3390/ijerph1 8147537

Dressler, D., Bhidayasiri, R., Bohlega, S., Chana, P., Chien, H. F., Chung, T. M., *et al.* (2018) 'Defining spasticity: a new approach considering current movement disorders terminology and botulinum toxin therapy'. *Journal of Neurology*. 265: 856–862. Available at: https://researchgate.net/publication/323017738_Defining_spasticity_a_ new_approach_considering_current_movement_disorders_terminology_and_botulinu m_toxin_therapy/link/5a9921b145851535bce183f4/download

Elvén, M., Holmström, I. K., Carlestav, M., and Endelbring, S. (2023) 'A tension between surrendering and being involved: an interview study on person-centredness in clinical reasoning in the acute stroke setting'. *Patient Education and Counselling*. 112. Available at: https://sciencedirect.com/science/article/pii/S0738399123000988?via%3Dihub

Fearon, P., Langhorne, P. (2012) 'Services for reducing duration of hospital care for acute stroke patients'. *Cochrane Database of Systematic Reviews*. 2012(9): 1–97. Available at: https://core.ac.uk/reader/9650460?utm_source=linkout

Fujita, T., Seto, A., Yamamoto, Y., Yamane, K., Otsuki, K., Tsuchiya, K., and Tozato, F. (2015) 'Relationship between dressing and motor function in stroke patients: a study with partial correlation analysis'. *Journal of Physical Therapy Science*. 27(12): 3771–3774. Available at: https://doi.org/10.1589/jpts.27.3771

Global Burden of Disease (GBD) 2019 Stroke Collaborators. (2021) 'Global, regional, and national burden of stroke and its risk factors, 1990–2019: a systematic analysis for the global burden of disease study'. *The Lancet Neurology*. 20(10): 795–820. Available at: https://thelancet.com/article/S1474-4422(21)00252-0/fulltext

Grattan, E. S., Skidmore, E. R., and Woodbury, M. L. (2018) 'Examining anosognosia of neglect'. *Occupational Therapy Journal of Research.* 38(2): 113–120. Available at: https://ncbi.nlm.nih.gov/pmc/articles/PMC5930481/

Horne, J., Lincoln, N. B., Preston, J., and Logan, P. (2014) 'What does confidence mean to people who have had a stroke? – A qualitative interview study'. *Clinical Rehabilitation.* 28(11): 1125–1135. Available at: https://doi.org/10.1177/0269215514534086

Hörnsten, C., Lövheim, H., Nordström, P., and Gustafson, Y. (2016) 'The prevalence of stroke and depression and factors associated with depression in elderly people with and without stroke'. *BMC Geriatrics.* 16: 174. Available at: https://doi.org/10.1186/s12 877-016-0347-6

Intercollegiate Stroke Working Party (ISWP). (2023) *National Clinical Guideline for Stroke for the UK and Ireland.* London. ISWP. Available at: www.strokeguideline.org

Kristensen, H. K., Tistad, M., Koch, L., and Ytterberg C. (2016) 'The importance of individual involvement in stroke rehabilitation'. *PLoS One.* 11(6): e0157149. Available at: https:// researchgate.net/publication/303904563_The_Importance_of_Patient_Involvement_in_ Stroke_Rehabilitation

Loetscher, T., Potter, K. J., Wong, D., and das Nair, R. (2019) 'Cognitive rehabilitation for attention deficits following stroke'. *Cochrane Database of Systematic Reviews.* 11. Available at: https://doi.org/10.1002/14651858.cd002842.pub3

Lv, Q., Zhang, J., Pan, Y., Liu, X., Miao, L., Peng, J., Song, L., Zou, Y., and Chen, X. (2022) 'Somatosensory deficits after stroke: insights from MRI studies'. *Frontiers in Neurology.* 13: 891283. Available at: https://doi.org/10.3389/fneur.2022.891283

Mak-Yuen, Y. Y. K., Matyas, T. A., and Carey, L. M. (2023) 'Characterizing touch discrimination impairment from pooled stroke samples using the tactile discrimination test: updated criteria for interpretation and brief test version for use in clinical practice settings'. *Brain Sciences.* 13(4): 533. Available at: https://mdpi.com/2076-3425/ 13/4/533

Markle-Reid, M., Valaitis, R., Bartholomew, A., Fisher, K., Fleck, R., Ploeg, J., and Salerno, J. (2020). 'An integrated hospital-to-home transitional care intervention for older adults with stroke and multimorbidity: a feasibility study'. *Journal of Comorbidity.* 10: 1–21. Available at: https://ncbi.nlm.nih.gov/pmc/articles/PMC7177995/pdf/10.1177_22350 42X19900451.pdf

Martin-Sanz, M. B., Salazar-de-la-Guerra, R. M., Cuenca-Zaldivar, J. N., Salcedo-Perez-Juana, M., Garcia-Bravo, C., and Palacios-Ceña, D. (2022) 'Person-centred care in individuals with stroke: a qualitative study using in-depth interviews'. *Annals of Medicine.* 54(1): 2167–2180. Available at: https://doi.org/10.1080%2F07853890.2022.2105393

National Advisory Committee for Stroke (NACS) (2022) *A Progressive Stroke Pathway.* Scottish Government. Edinburgh. Available at: www.gov.scot/publications/progressive-stroke-pathway/

National Institute for Clinical and Care Excellence (NICE). (2023a) Scenario: management of long-term complications of stroke. Available at: https://cks.nice.org.uk/topics/stroke-tia/management/management-of-long-term-complications-of-stroke/

National Institute for Clinical and Care Excellence (NICE). (2023b) Stroke rehabilitation in adults. Available at: https://nice.org.uk/guidance/ng236

O'Callaghan, G., Fahy, M., O'Meara, S., Chawke, M., Waldron, E., Corry, M., Gallagher, S., Coyne, C., Lynch, J., Kennedy, E., Walsh, T., Cronin, H., Hannon, N., Fallon, C., Williams, D. J., Langhorne, P., Galvin, R., and Horgan, F. (2024) 'Transitioning to home and beyond following stroke: a prospective cohort study of outcomes and needs'. *BMC*

Health Services Research, 24: 449. Available at: https://bmchealthservres.biomedcentral. com/articles/10.1186/s12913-024-10820-8

Persson, H. C., Törnbom, K., Sunnerhagen, K. S., and Törnbom, M. (2017) 'Consequences and coping strategies six years after a subarachnoid hemorrhage – a qualitative study'. *PLoS One*, 12(8): e0181006. Available at: https://pubmed.ncbi.nlm.nih.gov/28854198/

Poulin, V., Korner-Bitensky, N., and Dawson, D.R. (2013) 'Stroke-specific executive function assessment: a literature review of performance-based tools'. *Australian Occupational Therapy Journal.* 60: 3–19. https://doi.org/10.1111/1440-1630.12024

Raju, H., and Tadi, P. (2022) 'Neuroanatomy, somatosensory cortex'. In *StatPearls.* Treasure Island, FL: StatePearls Publishing. Available at: https://ncbi.nlm.nih.gov/books/NBK555 915/#__NBK555915_ai__

Rowland, T. J., Cooke, D. M., and Gustafsson, L. A. (2008) 'Role of occupational therapy after stroke'. *Annals of Indian Academy of Neurology.* 11 (Suppl 1): S99–S107. Available at: https://pmc.ncbi.nlm.nih.gov/articles/PMC9204113/pdf/AIAN-11-99.pdf

Schottke, H., and Giabbiconi, C. M. (2015) 'Post-stroke depression and post-stroke anxiety: prevalence and predictors'. *International Psychogeriatrics.* 27(11): 1805–1812. Available at: https://doi.org/10.1017/s1041610215000988

Sit, J. W., Chair, S. Y., Choi, K. C., Chan, C. W., Lee, D. T., Chan, A. W., Cheung, J. L., Tang, S. W., Chan, P. S., and Taylor-Piliae, R. E. (2016) 'Do empowered stroke patients perform better at self-management and functional recovery after a stroke? A randomized controlled trial'. *Clinical Interventions in Aging.* 13(11): 1441–1450. Available at: https:// ncbi.nlm.nih.gov/pmc/articles/PMC5072569/#:~:text=Conclusion,functional%20recov ery%20of%20stroke%20survivors

Stevens, E., Clarke, S. G., Harrington, J., Manthorpe, J., Martin, F. C., Sackley, C., McKevitt, C., Marshall, I. J., Wyatt, D., and Wolfe, C. (2022). 'The provision of person-centred care for care home residents with stroke: an ethnographic study'. *Health & Social Care in the Community.* 30: e5186–e5195. Available at: https://doi.org/10.1111/hsc.13936

Sturgeon, D. (2018) *Introduction to Anatomy and Physiology for Healthcare Students.* Abingdon: Routledge.

Tang, E. Y. H., Price, C., Stephan, B. C. M., Robinson, L., and Exley, C. (2020) 'Impact of memory problems post-stroke on individuals and their family carers: a qualitative study'. *Frontiers in Medicine.* 7: 267. Available at: https://doi.org/10.3389/fmed.2020.00267

Tyson, S. F., Hanley, M., Chillala, J., Selley, A. B., and Tallis, R. C. (2008). 'Sensory loss in hospital-admitted people with stroke: characteristics, associated factors, and relationship with function'. *Neurorehabilitation and Neural Repair.* 22(2): 166–172. Available at: https://doi.org/10.1177/1545968307305523

van Dongen, L., Hafsteinsdóttir, T. B., Parker, E., Bjartmarz, I., Hjaltadóttir, I., and Jónsdóttir, H. (2021). ''Stroke survivors' experiences with rebuilding life in the community and exercising at home: a qualitative study'. *Nursing Open.* 8(5): 2567–2577. Available at: https://europepmc.org/article/MED/33690972#free-full-text

Walker, C. M., Walker, M. F., and Sunderland, A. (2003) 'Dressing after a stroke: a survey of current occupational therapy practice'. *British Journal of Occupational Therapy.* 66(6): 263–268. Available at: https://doi.org/10.1177/030802260306600605

8

SLEEP, WORK AND PLAY

Hilalnur Küçükakgün and Zeliha Tulek

Learning objectives

- To understand the physiology of sleep.
- To explore how sleep disorders can be a risk factor for stroke.
- To examine how sleep is disturbed post stroke and discuss strategies to minimise the impact of this.
- To consider the factors that prevent returning to working life after stroke such as fatigue, mobility and coordination problems, aphasia, cognitive decline, depression and apathy.
- To consider the needs of carers and families.

Background

Sleep-related problems can lead to cognitive dysfunction, emotional instability, weakening of the immune system, metabolic problems and an increased risk of cardiovascular disease. Sleep problems are also common in stroke and there is a bi-directional causal relationship between stroke and sleep. Sleep problems can be both a factor that increases the risk of stroke and a factor that negatively affects the post stroke recovery. This chapter considers the impact of stroke upon sleep and vice versa as well as focusing on work and recreational activities.

Sleep

Physiology of sleep

Sleep is a fundamental physiological need for humans. Good sleep is essential for individuals to be able to perform activities of daily living and it has neural,

DOI: 10.4324/9781003426196-9

electrophysiological and behavioural characteristics (Landis and Heitkemper, 2014; McNamara *et al.*, 2025). Control over the sleep–wake cycle is provided by multiple centres distributed widely throughout the brain. The sleep–wake cycle is based on the interaction of the systems that ensure wakefulness and sleep. Sleep occurs when the systems that ensure sleep inhibit the systems that ensure wakefulness, and wakefulness occurs when the systems that ensure wakefulness inhibit the systems that ensure sleep.

Sleep is controlled by cortical and subcortical regions of the brain. Complex networks in the forebrain and brainstem areas work together to regulate the sleep–wake cycle. Wakefulness occurs through the activity of neurochemical systems. Neurotransmitters glutamate, dopamine, serotonin, histamine, acetylcholine and noradrenaline play a role in keeping a person awake (Landis and Heitkemper, 2014, McNamara *et al.*, 2025). Some of these are utilised by the ascending reticular activating system (RAS) (Herrera *et al.*, 2016). Sleep occurs when neurones in the hypothalamus inhibit the RAS system. Sleep ends with the release of the hormone melatonin which is secreted by the pineal gland in the brain. The secretion of melatonin, one of the elements that regulate the circadian rhythm (the biological 24-hour rhythm in the brain), is a process that responds to sunlight. Melatonin secretion peaks in the dark and circulating melatonin contributes to controlling the sleep–wake cycle (Landis and Heitkemper, 2014; Borbély *et al.*, 2016; McNamara *et al.*, 2025). In addition, neurotransmitters (gamma-aminobutyric acid (GABA) and galanin) inhibit the wakefulness centres by activating sleep-promoting systems and initiating the sleep phase.

Phases of sleep

Sleep has a cyclical structure and consists of phases. The sleep process is characterised by the alternation of rapid eye movement (REM) and non-REM (NREM) phases. An adult's sleep cycle begins with the NREM phase and continues with the REM phase. The REM and NREM phases of sleep occur in four to six cycles and alternate throughout the night. A sleep cycle lasts about 90–110 minutes, with about 75% of total sleep time being NREM and 20–25% being REM sleep (Bear and Paradiso, 2016; Kryger *et al.*, 2017).

- *NREM phase:* Sleep in adults begins with the NREM phase. NREM is the deep and restorative part of sleep that makes up the majority of sleep. No REMs are observed, neuronal activity decreases, brain metabolism slows down, sympathetic activity decreases and parasympathetic activity increases; therefore heart rate, blood pressure and respiratory rate decrease, but muscle tone and reflexes are maintained in this phase. Body temperature and energy expenditure drop to their lowest levels.
- *REM phase:* During this phase, brain waves similar to those observed during wakefulness are observed on electroencephalogram (EEG). REM sleep is

usually accompanied by active dreaming, and it is difficult to wake the person during this phase (Landis and Heitkemper, 2014; McNamara *et al.*, 2025). In this phase, the sympathetic nervous system dominates, and sometimes the tone of skeletal muscles decreases to the point of paralysis (except the muscles that control eye). The oxygen consumption of the brain increases, heart rate, blood pressure and breathing become irregular, and the regulation of body temperature is disturbed (Arı Sevingil and Ozdemir, 2022).

Effects of sleep problems on the body

Sleep is a fundamental physiological requirement to maintain health. Quality of sleep is just as important as duration. This refers to both adequate sleep and adequate wakefulness. Quality sleep can vary depending on time, environment, and mental and physical activity. During quality sleep, a person's physical and mental functions are restored. Sleep is important for improving memory and learning ability and for removing unnecessary information and waste products from the brain. Quality of sleep can affect a person's ability to perform social, occupational and daily activities. Sleep disorders are characterised by fatigue, non-restorative sleep and excessive daytime sleepiness. They can lead to an increased frequency of accidents and reduced quality of life (Bear and Paradiso, 2016; Kryger *et al.*, 2017).

Impairment of sleep quality can cause changes in bodily functions. These include irritability, weakening of the immune system, decrease in tissue repair, increase in blood pressure and cardiac arrhythmias, depression and cognitive problems. In addition, the effects of sleep deprivation accumulate over time. It is known that the risks of stroke, obesity, gastroesophageal reflux, insulin resistance and type 2 diabetes increase in people who are sleep deprived (McDermott *et al.*, 2018).

Every week is a stressful nightmare of consciously planning to pace my activities, work and home knowing I am doing more than I should, knowing that I will suffer pain and fatigue consequences. It's a vicious circle and sleep doesn't recharge or refresh me like it did before stroke. So, I just have to carry on, and sometimes it's really hard to push through and carry on, but there are no other choices.

(Jacqueline, 42, ischaemic stroke whilst pregnant, 12 years post stroke)

Sleep disorders as a risk factor for stroke

A systematic review examining sleep problems in stroke showed that there is a reciprocal relationship between sleep and stroke. Sleep disorders are both a risk factor for stroke and a consequence of stroke (Arı Sevingil and Ozdemir, 2022). Studies have found that sleep problems such as short sleep (<5 hours), long sleep

(>9 hours), poor sleep quality, difficulty falling asleep or staying asleep, snoring and breathing problems during sleep were significantly associated with an increased risk of stroke (Li *et al.*, 2015; Qu *et al.*, 2018; McCarthy *et al.*, 2023). It is not only a risk factor for the first stroke, but also for recurrent stroke. Obstructive sleep apnoea (OSA) and restless leg syndrome (RLS) in particular may be a risk factor for stroke. Breathing-related sleep disorders are common in stroke patients. The most common of these is OSA. It affects around 5–10% of the population and prevalence increases with age. OSA is reported to be a risk factor for various conditions such as cardiovascular disease, hypertension, diabetes, attention deficits, cognitive dysfunction and also stroke (Bassetti *et al.*, 2020). OSA is treatable and can be managed with a continuous positive airway pressure (CPAP) device. If treated, the risk of stroke can be reduced, especially in patients who adhere to treatment plans. Therefore, it is important to recognise and treat the problem early (Arı Sevingil and Ozdemir, 2022).

RLS is defined by the significant urge to move the legs accompanied by unpleasant sensations, such as itching, tingling, pulling, aching, throbbing or pins and needles. These worsen at rest, in the evening or at night and are relieved by movement. Moderate to severe RLS is associated with greater sleep-related sympathetic autonomic activation and is considered a risk for hypertension and stroke.

Periodic leg movements during sleep (PLMS) have also been suggested as a risk factor for stroke. PLMS is characterised by involuntary periodic jerky movements of the legs or arms during sleep, such as flexing the toes or foot, and bending the ankle (Lin *et al.*, 2018; Katsanos *et al.*, 2018; Bassetti *et al.*, 2020).

Sleep problems following stroke

> Since my stroke, I always wake up tired. I have a nightly pain management routine that involves using a TENS machine for half an hour every night before going to sleep in addition to pain meds. Pain is the main cause of my sleep being disrupted and this routine helps to take the edge off my pain making it easier to get to sleep.
>
> *(Jacqueline, 42, ischaemic stroke whilst pregnant, 12 years post stroke)*

Sleep is crucial for recovery post stroke. Not only does the person need to be alert and energised to take part in rehabilitation activities, but neuroplasticity (the brain's ability to relearn things) occurs in part during rest and sleep periods (Baillieul *et al.*, 2023; Iwuozo *et al.*, 2023). Motor learning begins during rehabilitation exercises and is consolidated during sleep. However, sleep is often disturbed after a stroke (Baillieul *et al.*, 2023; Iwuozo *et al.*, 2023). Fragmented sleep, reduced sleep efficiency and shorter total sleep time are frequently reported.

Various sleep problems can be observed post stroke. They can significantly affect recovery. These include:

- Insomnia
- OSA
- Limb movement sleep disorders – PLMS and RLS.

Insomnia is defined as difficulty initiating or maintaining sleep or waking too early. Episodes that occur more than three times a week and last longer than 30 minutes should be considered as insomnia. Chronic insomnia occurs when symptoms persist for more than 3 months (Yaremchuk, 2018). Insomnia affects more than 20% of the general population and 28–57% of post stroke patients (Matas *et al.*, 2022) with over a third of stroke survivors struggling with insomnia for over 3 months (Baillieul *et al.*, 2023; Iwuozo *et al.*, 2023). Sleep disturbance during post stroke rehabilitation is associated with slower functional recovery and poorer motor outcomes. However, it is not yet clear whether this association exists because post stroke sleep disorder directly interferes with memory consolidation, or whether it is due to other factors such as depression or lack of motivation because of the indirect effect of insomnia (Weightman *et al.*, 2024).

Insomnia is considered an independent risk factor for cognitive impairment. Studies in stroke patients have shown that participants with insomnia have a significantly higher risk of cognitive impairment than those without insomnia (Liang *et al.*, 2024). Therefore, sleep disorder may be considered an important modifiable risk factor affecting cognitive function in individuals who have had a stroke (Nedergaard and Goldman, 2020; Suzuki, 2024).

The effect of sleep problems on cognitive function relates to the glymphatic system. The glymphatic system is a waste clearance pathway in the brain, operating mainly during NREM sleep (Suzuki, 2024). Sleep deprivation is thought to lead to impaired function of the glymphatic system, resulting in an accumulation of waste proteins, which may contribute to the risk of dementia. Sleeping less than 6 hours per night in middle age is associated with a higher risk of dementia compared to a normal sleep duration (7 hours) (Sabia *et al.*, 2021). A recent meta-analysis found that insomnia symptoms such as delay in falling asleep and excessive time in bed are associated with the risk of cognitive impairment (Xu *et al.*, 2020). Therefore, it is important to address sleep problems to prevent cognitive problems in stroke.

OSA affects 5–66% of stroke survivors, although there are differences in severity. As previously discussed, the more serious forms of sleep-disordered breathing can be linked with a higher risk of having a stroke and this risk remains post stroke. Symptoms include loud snoring, or choking/gasping for air during sleep (Baillieul *et al.*, 2023; Iwuozo *et al.*, 2023). It can also cause excessive daytime sleepiness affecting mood and rehabilitation capabilities. Whilst snoring is not a definite symptom of OSA, if an individual snores on a regular basis, it may be worth being reviewed by a healthcare professional.

People with limb movement sleep disorders can find it very difficult to fall asleep and then are woken throughout the night. The prevalence of RLS is 12% after a stroke (Arı Sevingil and Ozdemir, 2022). Again, this can result in daytime sleepiness and lack of motivation to engage with rehabilitation and social activities.

Promoting good sleep and 'sleep hygiene'

The term 'sleep hygiene' refers to a set of healthy habits that can improve a person's ability to fall and remain asleep to improve the quality of their sleep. Avoiding smoking, alcohol and the consumption of beverages high in caffeine (e.g. tea and coffee) as well as environmental arrangements and mild exercise are recommended for a good night's sleep (Karna *et al.*, 2023). Creating routine, both during the day and at bedtime, can help promote sleep hygiene. A sleep diary can help with establishing patterns and sharing fact sheets ensure that patients get the correct information (Centre for Clinical Interventions, 2020).

Consider your sleep practices.

- Do you have a pre-bed routine? What is it?
- Do you like a particular pillow or type of material for your bedclothes?
- Do you wear pyjamas or sleep naked?
- Consider your preferred sleeping environment – warm or cold, fresh air or windows closed, blackout blinds or no curtains at all?
- How would the depth, length and quality of your sleep experience be affected if your preferences were not available to you?

To advise on good sleep hygiene, a detailed medical history should be taken first. This should include the following:

- Usual duration of sleep
- Usual bedtime and times for sleeping and waking
- Sleep interruptions and the reasons for them (anxiety, getting up to urinate, or pain/discomfort because they cannot change position if hemiplegic)
- Do they feel rested after waking up?
- Do they feel sleepy during the day?
- What impact does this have on their activities?
- Medication use – identify those that can cause sleep disturbances (diuretics, antihypertensives, central nervous system stimulants, antiepileptic drugs)
- Pharmacological and non-pharmacological methods used to manage sleep

Interventions for good sleep hygiene are planned according to the severity, duration and underlying causes of the insomnia.

One of the most important factors for poor sleep hygiene is an unfavourable sleeping environment in the bedroom. Noise or light in the bedroom can cause sleep problems. In addition, a bed partner who makes PLMS or snores loudly can impair sleep. The longer time it takes to fall asleep can increase anxiety. Therefore, people should be informed about how to organise their sleeping environment so that they can relax, and they should be encouraged to reduce light and noise levels.

How to have a good night's sleep. Tips and information health professionals can share:

- Adults should sleep at least 7–8 hours.
- It is important to go to bed and wake up at the same time every day. This regulates biological rhythms. This routine should also be maintained at weekends and on public holidays.
- Use the bedroom only for sleep and intimacy. Activities such as watching TV or talking on the telephone should be avoided. If the bedroom is only used for sleeping, the room will be associated with sleep when it is entered, and it will be easier to fall asleep.
- The room should be quiet, dark and cool. Noises from appliances, sounds from outside and the sound of the alarm clock should be minimised. Thick curtains that do not let light through ensure more effective sleep. If necessary, earplugs and eye masks can be used.
- It is important that the bed is comfortable. The bed should be selected according to the patient's functional status and time spent in bed. For assistance, refer to a physiotherapist or occupational therapist.
- Only go to bed when sleepy. If you do not fall asleep within 20 minutes of going to bed, get out of bed. Engage in a quiet activity without exposing yourself to too much light.
- Keep a sleep diary. There are smartphone applications that can be used for this purpose.
- Light should only be used when necessary. If the individual is mobile and gets up at night to urinate, a night light should be used for safety reasons.
- It is important to be exposed to daylight when waking up in the morning.
- Eating, drinking and exercise should be avoided before going to bed.
- Caffeinated drinks such as coffee, tea and cola should also be avoided.
- Reduce fluid intake before bedtime.
- Monitor daytime napping to determine if it has an impact upon quality of sleep at night.
- Limit exposure to bright (blue) light in the evenings and leave devices such as smartphones, televisions and computers outside of the bedroom. Screen exposure should be stopped at least half an hour before bedtime (Riemann *et al.*, 2017).

Importance of exercise in good sleep hygiene

An optimal cortisol level is necessary for sleep. Under normal circumstances, cortisol levels are lower in the evening before going to bed and peak in the morning just before awakening. This suggests that cortisol plays an important role in initiating wakefulness and plays a role in the body's circadian rhythm. Physical activity can influence sleep by regulating a person's cortisol hormones. For this reason, the importance of regular exercise for a good night's sleep has been emphasised in recent years. It has been shown that light to moderate physical activity, whether aerobic or mind–body exercises, appears to be beneficial in modulating both stress and sleep. Therefore, adults can benefit from physical activity that is tailored to their individual preferences and needs. However, exercise should not be performed before bedtime and heavy exercise should be avoided (De Nys *et al.*, 2022; Karna *et al.*, 2023).

Non-pharmacological and pharmacological approaches

Non-pharmacological methods should be the first step in promoting sleep. Educating the patient about sleep and sleep hygiene and the use of cognitive behavioural therapy and relaxation techniques are important non-pharmacological approaches. Commonly used behavioural approaches to promote sleep include reading or other activities which relax the mind.

Cognitive–behavioural therapies comprise a range of psychological and behavioural techniques developed specifically for the treatment of insomnia. The cognitive part of this treatment includes stress management techniques or relaxation strategies. The behavioural part includes limiting the time they stay in bed, setting a specific time to get up in the morning, only going to bed when feeling sleepy and getting up when they cannot sleep. The specific approach varies depending on the patient's needs (Espie *et al.*, 2019; Gao *et al.*, 2022).

Herbal solutions such as valerian, St John's wort, lavender, lemon balm and chamomile tea may also be used in the management of sleep problems. The most commonly used plants are valerian and lavender. These plants have an anxiolytic effect. It is reported that they can improve sleep quality (Guadagna *et al.*, 2020). However, care should be taken as it is unclear whether this active ingredient poses a risk with long-term use due to possible interactions with other medications (Shinjyo *et al.*, 2020).

When treating OSA, it is advisable to elevate the head of the bed and, if the person is overweight, refer them to a dietitian to help them lose weight. For some people, a CPAP machine with a mask is used. If the patient is not receiving CPAP, they should be informed about it if there are indications that OSA might be a problem (Bassetti *et al.*, 2020; Karna *et al.*, 2023).

If a sleep disorder persists despite non-pharmacological approaches, appropriate pharmacological methods might be initiated. Most medications used for insomnia work by promoting the initiation or maintenance of sleep. When deciding which medication to administer for sleep problems (benzodiazepines, non-benzodiazepine hypnotics and melatonin receptor agonists), the nature of the sleep disorder is taken into account (Riemann *et al.*, 2017). These medications should be used under the supervision of a physician and only for short periods of time. These medications should be taken shortly before bedtime and should aim to promote an average of 8 hours of sleep. The stroke survivor should be informed about, and monitored for, the effects and side effects of the medication. Medications used to treat insomnia can cause drowsiness and interfere with driving and other activities that require alertness. The person should be aware that they may be at risk of harm even if they feel fully awake.

Work and play

> I miss being a nurse I do still think about it – it was hard losing the career I loved because of my stroke, I think about what I would have been, friends I worked with have moved up in their career, I had ambition to move up the ladder – its depressing I will never know what I would of achieved, it depressing not having the same ability to earn as I did before my stroke – sometimes it makes me angry.
>
> *(Jacqueline, 42, ischaemic stroke whilst pregnant, 12 years post stroke)*

Work is defined as the regular activity a person performs to earn money. It is a specific task, performed as part of a professional routine or for an agreed price. It includes various forms of employment, including paid work, vocational training, therapeutic or voluntary work and adult education (ISWP, 2023). Returning to work refers to returning to a previous job, returning to a different position or returning to paid employment with a new job (Coutts and Cooper, 2021).

It is generally recognised that work is beneficial both for the individual and for society. It plays an important role in the fulfilment of psychosocial needs and the financial security of life. For most people, their work is the most important determinant of their self-esteem, family respect, identity and position in society and life satisfaction (Gard *et al.*, 2019; Coutts and Cooper, 2021). An unemployed person may feel incomplete in terms of all these social statuses. Unemployment has many negative consequences for people with stroke. The inability to return to work might adversely affect physical and mental health.

> I want to be working but I don't want to be working if I just have more hassle. My brain can't deal with any type of stress and if I am tired on top of that …. If I'm stuck in front of a laptop, I can't do it. I need to find something that won't trigger seizures or make me too tired. Mentally I'm capable but its just adapting. I have voice recognition software but its s***. I try and say something and it comes out with something different and I get frustrated. I then need to think, no, calm down, calm down.
>
> *(Alan, 50, ischaemic stroke, 4 years post stroke)*

It is reported that returning to work after an illness 'improves recovery, self-esteem, self-confidence, social identity and overall quality of life' (Coutts and Cooper, 2021). Returning to work is an important component and indicator of returning to normal life following stroke. If stroke survivors cannot return to work, it is a major burden on national economies. A report from the UK estimates the economic cost of stroke at around £9bn. It is reported that in addition to the cost of healthcare services and medication, job loss and missed workdays are important factors in this economic burden (Coutts and Cooper, 2021). The share of job loss in the economic burden is greater than the budget for healthcare expenditure. Individuals who give up their employed work to become caregivers also represent an economic loss for their country.

One-third of stroke survivors are under 65 years of age, therefore, they are people of working age. As young people live with the consequences of stroke for many years, the burden of stroke may affect young people more significantly (Krishnamurthi *et al.*, 2015). However, given the importance of the concept of work in life, being unable to return to work is a major concern not only for young patients but also for all age groups. There are many studies on the rates of return to work after a stroke (Gard *et al.*, 2019). While this rate is 20% in some countries, it can reach 80% in others. The differences can be explained by the different levels of wealth in the countries, social policies and differences in the treatment, management and rehabilitation of stroke (Schnitzler *et al.*, 2019). When analysing studies conducted on stroke patients of working age, it is generally found that less than half of patients are able to return to work (Gard *et al.*, 2019). The main reason for this is the difficulty in walking and performing activities of daily living as outlined in Chapter 9. Studies show that stroke survivors walk significantly slower and have a higher metabolic cost of walking than healthy individuals of the same age (Jarvis *et al.*, 2019).

The difficulties that people have in returning to work after a stroke are not only influenced by decreased mobility, but also by speech, cognitive and fatigue problems. Additionally, psychiatric issues such as depression and anxiety (Coutts and Cooper, 2021) can arise. Although not as visible as physical disabilities, these issues are similarly common.

As discussed in the communication chapter, a stroke can result in aphasia (difficulty processing speech) and dysarthria (difficulty expressing speech). The ability to interact is crucial for participation in working life. Therefore, any communication disorder can be a significant barrier to returning to work. Return to work is reported to be lower for people with aphasia.

Other factors that are a major barrier to return to work are cognitive difficulties and fatigue which are discussed in detail in Chapter 9. Such problems, as well as physical and communication difficulties, can persist in the long term (Coutts and Cooper, 2021). In addition, some sufferers report that they experience symptoms similar to those of a stroke, such as numbness, tingling and headaches when stressed at work, leading to fears of suffering another stroke. They are unable to return to work due to these concerns (Nuccio *et al.*, 2023).

> [When I'm stressed] I start getting a fuzzy head and vertigo feeling. I know I've got to try and calm it down because if it stays at that level, I will have a seizure. As soon as I get stressed or a bit elevated, I get pins and needles in my hand.
>
> *(Alan, 50, ischaemic stroke, 4 years post stroke)*

In addition to individual barriers, issues such as architectural barriers, lack of suitable transport and stereotypes about disabled people are also important barriers to return to work, despite legislation to protect them. Issues include:

- decreased ability to use public transport
- difficulties walking from the car park into workplace
- problems moving around within a building or workplace
- physical barriers in the work environment (Jarvis *et al.*, 2019).

The nature of work and whether there is an alternative in the workplace (e.g. part-time work) have a significant influence on the return to previous employment. White-collar workers are three times more likely to return to work than blue-collar workers (Nuccio *et al.*, 2023).

Stroke not only has a significant impact on patients, but also on the lives of family caregivers in physical, social and psychological terms. It can impact the working opportunities of caregivers. Literature shows that one-third of caregivers leave their jobs to care for their patients and around half develop depressive symptoms. This can lead to serious economic and financial problems. Considering the loss of income and healthcare costs related to the stroke survivor, the financial problems are further deepened when a caregiver loses his/her job too.

Returning to work, vocational rehabilitation, benefits and finances

Returning to work has positive effects on pain, depression, quality of life and participation in normal life, and gives a sense of autonomy. Therefore, returning to work after a stroke is an important goal of rehabilitation. The United Nations (UN) Convention on the Rights of Persons with Disabilities (ISWP, 2023) discusses the importance of work, education and recreation in equal measure. Specifically, Article 27 identifies 'the right of persons with disabilities to work, on an equal basis with others'.

However, it is often a complex process that depends on several interacting factors and the involvement of many stakeholders. Barriers and facilitators include personal factors, workplace factors and factors related to rehabilitation services, social rights and national health policy. Given the complexity of returning to work after a stroke, counselling by trained personnel who are familiar with the relevant legislation on this subject is required. It is also important to ensure that the stroke survivor understands their rights as a disabled person and that reasonable adjustments can be made (Stroke Association, 2024a).

Healthcare teams should ask questions about the working lives of stroke survivors as early as possible to better understand their role in society and ways in which to help them to return to their previous status. There is evidence that return-to-work support such as counselling and information should be provided as soon as possible to minimise problems on return to work. This support should not only address the barriers to returning to work, but also provide information on different work options that are suitable for the person concerned. Such support can be provided by employers and institutions. The concept that encompasses all these services is vocational rehabilitation (VR). The aim of VR is to use a multidisciplinary approach to reintegrate people of working age who have functional problems back into working life and enable them to perform the demands of their jobs within the limits of their abilities. VR is summarised as 'a coordinated plan, supported by the employee and all relevant parties to optimise the employee's work capacity' (ISWP, 2023). VR includes counselling and coaching, emotional support, adaptation of the work environment and strategies to compensate for functional limitations (e.g. communication, cognition, mobility and arm function, fatigue management). In this process, a coordinator is needed to provide information and support in planning the return to work. To ensure a healthy return to work, the expectations of the stroke survivor, their colleagues and superiors should be considered. It is important to support the rehabilitation of people of working age and inform them about services and policies (Coutts and Cooper, 2021; ISWP, 2023; NICE, 2023).

> I've gone from having a really good job to being on benefits and I don't like being on benefits. I'm embarrassed to be on benefits.
>
> *(Alan, 50, ischaemic stroke, 4 years post stroke)*

The Stroke Association have a complete guide to work and stroke. This resource includes useful information, tips and guidance for anyone who has had a stroke and is thinking about returning to work (Stroke Association, 2024a) www.stroke.org.uk/complete_ guide_work and stroke.pdf.

Driving

Being able to drive is important for individuals because it can improve their quality of life. It influences self-esteem and mood and being able to drive, or not, may likely have an impact upon whether someone can return to work particularly if the role itself involved driving or a commute. Further details and guidance regarding driving post stroke can be found in Chapter 9.

Hobbies, sports and leisure activities

Recreation or leisure time refers to the activities that people carry out other than those necessary for existence such as sleeping, eating and work. Leisure activities offer the individual pleasure and relaxation. It is beneficial to support people to participate in leisure activities after a debilitating and life-changing illness such as a stroke (Vincent-Onabajo and Blasu, 2016). Most survivors are confronted with obstacles that result in their dependence on others for daily living activities and limited participation in social and leisure activities. However, over time, the stroke gradually becomes a normalised life situation (Norlander *et al.*, 2018). It has been reported that incorporating leisure activities into stroke rehabilitation can help to improve physical, cognitive and psychological outcomes and provide therapeutic benefits (Dorstyn *et al.*, 2014). Recreational activities increase quality of life, create a sense of belonging to a community, support the development of skills, increase self-esteem and self-confidence. They have benefits such as support opportunities, stress reduction, social interaction and they enable personal and spiritual development. Therefore, the integration of social participation into rehabilitation programmes is necessary for patients and caregivers.

It can be challenging to guide patients who have difficulty with everyday activities and have little energy to participate in recreational activities. For the patient to participate, it may be necessary to consider the physical environment and choose activities based on the patient's cognitive abilities. For example, taking part in sports or using a computer may become activities that need to be carefully planned for a person with apraxia. It has been reported that the number of leisure activities utilised by people after a stroke decrease by half compared to before the stroke (Im *et al.*, 2015). The most common barriers to participation in leisure activities are mobility and balance problems, transport problems and financial problems. In addition, mood, age, cognitive abilities, communication skills, social support and motivation influence participation in activities (Norlander *et al.*, 2018).

Rehabilitation of stroke patients should include plans for leisure activities (Schnitzler *et al.*, 2019). Occupational therapy practices and upper extremity training, combined with cognitive training aimed at improving social participation, enhance leisure and social participation outcomes after stroke. Leisure activities that stroke patients can do are generally in four areas: recreational, social, cognitive and productive/creative activities (Vincen-Onabajo and Blasu, 2016; Schnitzler *et al.*, 2019).

It is important for an assessment to include finding out what types of recreational activities the stroke patient used to undertake and what they would like to be able to return to. If returning to previous activities is not possible, encouraging new activities and adjustments may be needed. Targeted therapeutic interventions and individualised plans for participation should be based on collaborative goal setting. Technological equipment can be used to carry out some activities. Identifying someone who can be a source of support from the patient's social network is also helpful. Local opportunities should also be explored and can include stroke clubs, aphasia groups and disability groups. Signposting family and the patient to visit the local library or to contact their local council or leisure centre for group information may also provide opportunities for suitable recreational activities (Canadian Stroke, 2021; Heart & Stroke Foundation, 2023; Stroke Association, 2024b).

The Stroke Association have a directory of local support available which you can search by area (Stroke Association).

Experiences and needs of family members of stroke survivors

A stroke affects not only the patient but also the wider family, especially the person primarily responsible as caregiver. This is especially challenging following a severe stroke or when care tasks are unevenly distributed. Caregivers can be extremely overwhelmed and experience conflicting feelings. Caregivers may feel helpless and that their lives are being taken away from them. Studies show some admit that sometimes they have no choice and have to accept the changes in their lives, which is why they find it difficult to adapt (Nuccio *et al.*, 2023).

Some caregivers see work as a 'breathing space' and a source of strength. However, the patient's dependency requires the caregiver to restructure their working life. Some caregivers have to reduce their working hours, postpone their return to work or quit their jobs completely. This situation has serious economic and financial consequences. Caregivers report that it is difficult to balance their career, family and caring responsibilities (Nuccio *et al.*, 2023). If the caregiver's needs are not supported during this period, this leads to psychological and social problems for the person and prevents them from adequately fulfilling their responsibility to care. Return to work should be supported for the stroke survivor's family caregiver as well as the survivor themselves. For both parties, regaining a sense of independence and participating in daily life becomes a priority to help them build a 'new' self-identity after a stroke (Nuccio *et al.*, 2023). Therefore, their return to work and participation in recreational activities should be supported.

Support systems for patients and caregivers

Although the multidisciplinary team provides rehabilitation for functional improvement in the clinical setting, most people who have suffered a stroke face challenges after returning to their home environment. Most survivors experience depression, social isolation and a decline in their quality of life after returning home. For people who have suffered a stroke, the primary goal is usually to ensure optimal functional recovery and the patient's safety both in hospital and at home, so psychosocial problems can be overlooked. Caregivers also have psychosocial issues and difficulty accepting the changes in their role.

Social habits also change fundamentally after a stroke. Individuals may react much more sensitively to stimuli and have problems due to fatigue. Even a normal conversation may be extremely tiring and require a lot of energy. This constant effort may leave some people socially isolated. They may avoid joining friends because it is exhausting and be wary of crowded places. Quiet places that they know well and feel comfortable may be preferred as it is difficult to process stimuli in crowded places (Meijering *et al.*, 2016).

Conclusion

This chapter has explored how sleep problems can increase the risk of stroke and negatively affect the recovery process after a stroke. Therefore, it is important to develop good sleep habits to both reduce the risk of stroke and improve the quality of life after a stroke. Regular exercise, stress management, adaptation of the sleep environment and, if necessary, pharmacological or non-pharmacological treatments should be used to establish a sleep routine.

In the post stroke period, a comprehensive approach and professional support are required to enable patients to return to work, drive and return safely to leisure activities. In addition, addressing the needs of families will improve the quality of life for both the patient and their family.

References

Arı Sevingil, S., & Ozdemir, A.O. (2022). Serebrovasküler Hastalıklar ve Uyku, in: Benbir Şenel G., (Ed.). *Uyku Nörofizyolojisi ve Hastalıkları İçinde* (345–362). Ankara: Bayçınar Tıbbi Yayıncılık.

Baillieul, S., Denis, C., Barateau, L., Arquizan, C., Detante, O., Pépin, J. L., Dauvilliers, Y., & Tamisier, R. (2023). The multifaceted aspects of sleep and sleep-wake disorders following stroke. *Revue Neurologique (Paris)*. 179(7):782–792. doi: 10.1016/j.neurol.2023.08.004

Bassetti, C. L., Randerath, W., Vignatelli, L., Ferini-Strambi, L., Brill, A. K., Bonsignore, M. R., & Papavasileiou, V. (2020). EAN/ERS/ESO/ESRS statement on the impact of sleep disorders on risk and outcome of stroke. *European Respiratory Journal*, 55(4). https://doi.org/10.1183/13993003.01104-2019

Bear, M.F., & Paradiso, M.A. (2016). Brain rhythms and sleep. In: Bear, M.F., Connors, B.W., & Paradiso, M.A. (eds.). *Neuroscience Exploring the Brain* (4th ed., 645–683). China: Wolters Kluwer.

Borbély, A. A., Daan, S., Wirz-Justice, A., & Deboer, T. (2016). The two-process model of sleep regulation: a reappraisal. *Journal of Sleep Research*, 25(2), 131–143.

Centre for Clinical Interventions. (2020). Sleep hygiene: how can i get a good night's rest?. Available at: www.centerformentalhealth.in/sleep-hygiene-how-can-i-get-a-good-nights-rest/

Canadian Stroke. (2021). Recreation & leisure after stroke. Available at: https://canadianstroke.ca/sites/default/files/inline-files/Resources%20-%20Rec%20%20Leisure%20FINAL.pdf

Coutts, E., & Cooper, K. (2021). Interventions, barriers, and facilitators associated with return to work for adults following stroke: a scoping review protocol. *JBI Evidence Synthesis*, 19(12): 3332–3339. doi:10.11124/JBIES-20-00386

De Nys, L., Anderson, K., Ofosu, E. F., Ryde, G. C., Connelly, J., & Whittaker, A. C. (2022). The effects of physical activity on cortisol and sleep: a systematic review and meta-analysis. *Psychoneuroendocrinology*, 143, 105843.

Dorstyn, D., Roberts, R., Kneebone, I., Kennedy, P., & Lieu, C. (2014). Systematic review of leisure therapy and its effectiveness in managing functional outcomes in stroke rehabilitation. *Topics in Stroke Rehabilitation*, 21(1), 40–51.

Espie, C. A., Emsley, R., Kyle, S. D., Gordon, C., Drake, C. L., Siriwardena, A. N., Cape, J., Ong, J. C., Sheaves, B., Foster, R., Freeman, D., Costa-Font, J., Marsden, A., & Luik, A. I. (2019). Effect of digital cognitive behavioral therapy for insomnia on health, psychological well-being, and sleep-related quality of life: a randomized clinical trial. *JAMA Psychiatry*, 76(1), 21–30. https://doi.org/10.1001/jamapsychiatry.2018.2745

Gao, Y., Ge, L., Liu, M., Niu, M., Chen, Y., Sun, Y., Chen, J., Yao, L., Wang, Q., Li, Z., Xu, J., Li, M., Hou, L., Shi, J., Yang, K., Cai, Y., Li, L., Zhang, J., & Tian, J. (2022). Comparative efficacy and acceptability of cognitive behavioral therapy delivery formats for insomnia in adults: a systematic review and network meta-analysis. *Sleep Medicine Reviews*, 64, 101648. https://doi.org/10.1016/j.smrv.2022.101648

Gard, G., Pessah-Rasmussen, H., Brogårdh, C., Nilsson, Å., & Lindgren, I. (2019). Need for structured healthcare organization and support for return to work after stroke in Sweden: experiences of stroke survivors. *Journal of Rehabilitation Medicine (Stiftelsen Rehabiliteringsinformation)*, 51(10).

Guadagna, S., Barattini, D. F., Rosu, S., & Ferini-Strambi, L. (2020). Plant extracts for sleep disturbances: a systematic review. *Evidence-Based Complementary and Alternative Medicine*, 2020:3792390. doi: 10.1155/2020/3792390.

Heart & Stroke Foundation. (2023). Leisure and recreation after stroke. Available at: https://heartandstrokenb.ca/post/leisure-and-recreation-after-stroke

Herrera, C. G., Cadavieco, M. C., Jego, S., Ponomarenko, A., Korotkova, T., & Adamantidis, A. (2016). Hypothalamic feedforward inhibition of thalamocortical network controls arousal and consciousness. *Nature Neuroscience*, 19(2), 290–298.

Iwuozo, E. U., Enyikwola, J. O., Asor, P. M., Onyia, U. I., Nwazor, E. O., & Obiako, R. O. (2023). Sleep disturbances and associated factors amongst stroke survivors in North Central, Nigeria. *Nigerian Postgraduate Medical Journal*, 30(3), 193–199. doi: 10.4103/npmj.npmj_56_23

Im Yi, T., Han, J. S., Lee, K. E., & Ha, S. A. (2015). Participation in leisure activity and exercise of chronic stroke survivors using community-based rehabilitation services in Seongnam City. *Annals of Rehabilitation Medicine*, 39(2), 234.

Jarvis, H. L., Brown, S. J., Price, M., Butterworth, C., Groenevelt, R., Jackson, K., Walker, L., Rees N., Clayton, A., & Reeves, N. D. (2019). Return to employment after stroke in young adults: how important is the speed and energy cost of walking? *Stroke*, 50(11), 3198–3204. doi: 10.1161/STROKEAHA.119.025614

Katsanos, A. H., Kosmidou, M., Konitsiotis, S., Tsivgoulis, G., Fiolaki, A., Kyritsis, A. P., & Giannopoulos, S. (2018). Restless legs syndrome and cerebrovascular/cardiovascular events: systematic review and meta-analysis. *Acta Neurologica Scandinavica*, 137(1), 142–148.

Karna, B., Sankari, A., & Tatikonda, G. (2023). Sleep disorder. In *StatPearls*. StatPearls Publishing.

McNamara, S., Spurling, B. C., & Bollu, P. C. (2025). Chronic insomnia. In *StatPearls*. StatPearls Publishing. https://ncbi.nlm.nih.gov/books/NBK526136/

Krishnamurthi, R. V., Moran, A. E., Feigin, V. L., Barker-Collo, S., Norrving, B., Mensah, G. A., Taylor, S, Naghavi, M., Forouzanfar, M. H., Nguyen, G, Johnson, C. O., Vos, T, Murray, C. J. L., & Roth, G., GBD 2013 Stroke Panel Experts Group. (2015). Stroke prevalence, mortality and disability-adjusted life years in adults aged 20–64 years in 1990–2013: data from the Global Burden of Disease 2013 study. *Neuroepidemiology*, 45(3), 190–202. doi: 10.1159/000441098

Kryger, M., Roth, T., & Dement, W. C. (2017). Normal human sleep: an overview. In: Kryger, M., Roth, T., & Dement, W. C. (eds.). *Principles and Practice of Sleep Medicine*. China: Elsevier.

Landis, C. A., & Heitkemper, M. M. (2014). Sleep and sleep disorders. In: Lewis, S. L., Burcher, L., Dirksen, S. R., Heitkemper, M. M., & Harding, M. M., *Medical Surgical Nursing, Assessment and Management of Clinical Problems* (9 edn., 99–113). Canada: Elsevier.

Li, M., Li, K., Zhang, X. W., Hou, W. S., & Tang, Z. Y. (2015). Habitual snoring and risk of stroke: a meta-analysis of prospective studies. *International Journal of Cardiology*, 185, 46–49.

Liang, W., Wu, D., Chuang, Y. H., Fan, Y. C., & Chiu, H. Y. (2024). Insomnia complaints correlated with higher risk of cognitive impairment in older adults following stroke: a National Representative Comparison Study. *Sleep and Biological Rhythms*, 22(1), 41–47.

Lin, T. C., Zeng, B. Y., Chen, Y. W., Wu, M. N., Chen, T. Y., Lin, P. Y., & Hsu, C. Y. (2018). Cerebrovascular accident risk in a population with periodic limb movements of sleep: a preliminary meta-analysis. *Cerebrovascular Diseases*, 46(1–2), 1–9.

Matas, A., Amaral, L., & Patto, A. V. (2022). Is post-ischemic stroke insomnia related to a negative functional and cognitive outcome? *Sleep Medicine*, 94, 1–7.

McCarthy, C. E., Yusuf, S., Judge, C., Alvarez-Iglesias, A., Hankey, G. J., Oveisgharan, S., … & Interstroke. (2023). Sleep patterns and the risk of acute stroke: results from the interstroke international case-control study. *Neurology*, 100(21), e2191–e2203.

McDermott, M., Brown, D. L., & Chervin, R. D. (2018). Sleep disorders and the risk of stroke. *Expert Review of Neurotherapeutics*, 18(7), 523–531. https://doi.org/10.1080/14737175.2018.1489239

Meijering, L., Nanninga, C. S., & Lettinga, A. T. (2016). Home-making after stroke. A qualitative study among Dutch stroke survivors. *Health & Place*, 37, 35–42.

Intercollegiate Stroke Working Party (2023) National Clinical Guideline for Stroke for the UK and Ireland. RCP:London. Available at: www.strokeguideline.org

Nedergaard, M., & Goldman, S. A. (2020). Glymphatic failure as a final common pathway to dementia. *Science*, 370(6512), 50–6. https://doi.org/10.1126/science.abb8739

NICE. (2023). Stroke rehabilitation in adults. Cinical guideline [NG236]. Published: 18 October 2023, returning to work. Available at: https://nice-org-uk.translate.goog/guidance/ng236/chapter/Recommendations?_x_tr_sl=en&_x_tr_tl=tr&_x_tr_hl=tr#returning-to-work

Norlander, A., Iwarsson, S., Jönsson, A. C., Lindgren, A., & Månsson Lexell, E. (2018). Living and ageing with stroke: an exploration of conditions influencing participation in social and leisure activities over 15 years. *Brain Injury*, 32(7), 858–866.

Nuccio, E., Petrosino, F., Simeone, S., Alvaro, R., Vellone, E., & Pucciarelli, G. (2023). The needs and difficulties during the return to work after a stroke: a systematic review and meta-synthesis of qualitative studies. *Disability and Rehabilitation*, 46(21), 4901–4914.

Qu, H., Guo, M., Zhang, Y., & Shi, D. Z. (2018). Obstructive sleep apnea increases the risk of cardiac events after percutaneous coronary intervention: a meta-analysis of prospective cohort studies. *Sleep and Breathing*, 22, 33–40.

Riemann, D., Baglioni, C., Bassetti, C., Bjorvatn, B., Dolenc Groselj, L., Ellis, J. G., Espie, C. A., Garcia-Borreguero, D., Gjerstad, M., Gonçalves, M., Hertenstein, E., Jansson-Fröjmark, M., Jennum, P. J., Leger, D., Nissen, C., Parrino, L., Paunio, T., Pevernagie, D., Verbraecken, J., Weeß, H. G., ... & Spiegelhalder, K. (2017). European guideline for the diagnosis and treatment of insomnia. *Journal of Sleep Research*, 26(6), 675–700. https://doi.org/10.1111/jsr.12594

Sabia, S., Fayosse, A., Dumurgier, J., van Hees, V. T., Paquet, C., Sommerlad, A., ... & Singh-Manoux, A. (2021). Association of sleep duration in middle and old age with incidence of dementia. *Nature Communications*, 12(1), 2289.

Schnitzler, A., Jourdan, C., Josseran, L., Azouvi, P., Jacob, L., & Genêt, F. (2019). Participation in work and leisure activities after stroke: a national study. *Annals of Physical and Rehabilitation Medicine*, 62(5), 351–355.

Shinjyo, N., Waddell, G., & Green, J. (2020). Valerian root in treating sleep problems and associated disorders – a systematic review and meta-analysis. *Journal of Evidence-Based Integrative Medicine*, 25. doi: 10.1177/2515690X20967323

Stroke Association (2024a). A complete guide to work and stroke. Accessed at: www.stroke.org.uk/complete_guide_work_and_stroke.pdf

Stroke Association. (2024b). Hobbies and leisure activities. Available at: https://stroke.org.uk/stroke/life-after/hobbies-and-leisure-activities

Suzuki, K. (2024). Link between insomnia, cognitive impairment and stroke. *Sleep and Biological Rhythms*, 22(1), 3–4.

Vincent-Onabajo, G., & Blasu, C. (2016). Participation in leisure activities after stroke: a survey of community-residing stroke survivors in Nigeria. *NeuroRehabilitation*, 38(1), 45–52.

Weightman, M., Robinson, B., Mitchell, M. P., Garratt, E., Teal, R., Rudgewick-Brown, A., ... & Johansen-Berg, H. (2024). Sleep and motor learning in stroke (SMiLES): a longitudinal study investigating sleep-dependent consolidation of motor sequence learning in the context of recovery after stroke. *BMJ Open*, 14(2), e077442.

Xu, W., Tan, C. C., Zou, J. J., Cao, X. P., & Tan, L. (2020). Sleep problems and risk of all-cause cognitive decline or dementia: an updated systematic review and meta-analysis. *Journal of Neurology, Neurosurgery & Psychiatry*, 91(3), 236–244.

Yaremchuk, K. (2018). Sleep disorders in the elderly. *Clinics in Geriatric Medicine*, 34, 205–216.

9

MOBILISING AND FUNCTIONAL MOBILITY

Lyndsey Shawe and Fiona Chalk

Learning objectives

- To understand what mobility is and what its importance.
- To recognise that mobility priorities vary for each person.
- To gain insight into the challenges that stroke survivors can experience with mobility.
- To explore stroke guidelines relating to mobility and enhance insight into rehabilitation of mobility.

Background

Mobility is defined as the ability to move freely (Cambridge Dictionary, no date). The NHS (2022b) states that mobility is not just the ability to walk or get around, it is also about receiving the right support to promote independence (Rantanen, 2013). Mobility primarily refers to walking, but this chapter will also consider transferring and other ways of moving around, for example driving.

Mobility is important for:

- Accessing services and facilities:
  - Hospital, medical, dentist appointments
  - Shopping
  - Library

- Allowing participation in social, cultural, faith-related and physical activities:
  - Attending a place of worship
  - Time with friends and family

DOI: 10.4324/9781003426196-10

- Social activities such as yoga, dancing, sports, meals out, cinema
- Maintaining independence
- Access to employment
- Psychological health – inclusion, social and emotional wellbeing
- Quality of life
- Promoting healthy living
  (Rantanen, 2013; NHS National Institute on Ageing, 2020)

As well as being an important contributing factor for lifestyle and quality of life, being active and mobile has health benefits. Benefits of mobility and the potential hazards of impaired mobility are outlined in Table 9.1.

Approximately half of people with stroke are unable or limited in their ability to walk (Intercollegiate Stroke Working Party (ISWP), 2023). Although most people post-stroke regain some mobility, few fully regain previous levels (ISWP, 2023).

Why is mobility and being able to get around important? Surely it is for everybody, don't you think?

(Olive, 82, TIA and ischaemic stroke, 8 years post stroke)

Reflect upon how much do you rely on your ability to mobilise day to day? How different would your life look if your mobility changed?

TABLE 9.1 Benefits of mobility and hazards related to immobility

Benefits of mobility	Hazards of immobility
Supports bone density, muscle bulk and joint movement	Loss of bone density, muscle wasting and joint stiffness
Supports circulation and prevention of deep vein thrombosis	Impaired circulation and potential predisposition to deep vein thrombosis
Supports respiratory function and prevention of respiratory infection	Impaired respiratory function and predisposition to chest infections
Prevents constipation, increasing intestinal transit rate	Constipation
Supports activities of living	Risk of pressure damage
Improves psychological wellbeing	Potential loss of psychological wellbeing, e.g. depression and anxiety
Supports social interaction	Potential for isolation and boredom
Maintains independence	Potential for dependence

Source: Adapted from Donnelly (2013).

Stroke guidelines around mobility and early mobilisation

Walking is not just about getting from place to place; it enables increased independence in daily functional tasks, participation in work and leisure activities, and access to the community. Therefore, it is unsurprising to find that walking-related goals are often a priority for patients (Moore *et al.*, 2022).

NICE Guidelines for Stroke Rehabilitation (NICE, 2023) and the (ISWP, 2023) National Clinical Guideline for Stroke both provide recommendations on rehabilitating mobility. NICE (2023) guidelines advise:

- Patients with movement difficulties post-stroke should receive assessment and management from suitably skilled physiotherapists. This input should continue until the patient can maintain or progress function independently or with assistance from others.
- Walking training should be offered to people who are able to walk with or without assistance, helping them build endurance and move more quickly.
- Treadmill training, one-to-one walking therapy and group training should be considered.
- Electromechanical gait training (EMGT), This involves the use of a robot-driven exoskeleton orthosis or an electromechanical device with two driven foot plates simulating the phases of gait. This reduces the physical dependence on therapists assisting with paretic limb movement. Most recently it has been identified there is moderate certainty evidence that EMGT alongside physiotherapy is more likely to achieve independent walking (Mehrholz *et al.*, 2025). Though this is not currently recommended in the NICE guidance (2023).

It is well documented that bed rest and immobility have detrimental effects on recovery. Early mobilisation (e.g. sitting out of bed, transferring, standing and walking) aims to minimise the risk of detrimental effects and improve functional recovery. The ISWP (2023) guidelines provide a long list of recommendations related to mobility, including advice on early mobilisation after stroke by appropriately trained staff:

- Patients with difficulty moving should be assessed as soon as possible within 24 hours of onset to determine the safest methods of transfer/mobilisation.
- Patients with difficulty moving, who are medically stable, should be offered frequent, short daily mobilisations (sitting out of bed, standing or walking).
- Mobilisation within 24 hours of onset should only be for patients who require little or no assistance to mobilise.

The ISWP (2023) also recommend that people with limited mobility after stroke should:

- Be assessed for, provided with and trained to use appropriate mobility aids, including wheelchairs.
- Be advised to participate in exercise to improve aerobic fitness and muscle strength, unless there are contraindications.
- Be offered repetitive task practice as the principal rehabilitation approach.
- Have access to equipment to enable intensive walking training such as treadmills or EMGT for those who wish to improve their mobility at any stage. To achieve this, training needs to be at 60–85% heart rate reserve for at least 40 minutes, three times a week, for 10 weeks.
- Be offered an ankle–foot orthosis or functional electrical stimulation (FES) to improve walking and balance, including referral to orthotics, for limited ankle–foot stability or limited dorsiflexion ('foot drop').
- Have access to specialist assessment, evaluation and follow-up for long-term FES use.
- Be assessed for real-world walking, such as road crossing, walking on uneven ground, including assessment of the impact of dual tasking, neglect, vision and confidence in busy environments.
- Have access to the voluntary sector and recreational fitness facilities such as gyms, leisure centres or outpatient departments to enable access to relevant fitness equipment.
- Not have risk assessment protocols used that limit training for fear of cardiovascular or other adverse events, given the good safety record of repetitive gait training.

The recommendations applicable to each patient will be different and implementation of the recommendations may be limited by resources and setting. The Sentinel Stroke National Audit Programme (SSNAP) (2024) identify that healthcare provision nationally does not currently meet recommendations.

Post-stroke mobility issues

Survivors can experience issues with function due to changes in sensation, proprioception, coordination, executive functioning, fatigue, vision, communication or muscle weakness (NHS, 2022a). This can affect one or both sides of the body. However, these symptoms rarely exist in isolation, commonly stroke survivors present with multiple interacting issues that have significant impact on functional ability. These issues can be further complicated by any pre-existing injuries or conditions.

> I was worried it [my mobility] would be like that for the rest of my life, that I wouldn't be able to go anywhere on my own, that there would always need to be someone to keep an eye of me. It took a lot of my confidence away.
>
> *(Olive, 82, transient ischaemic attack/ischaemic stroke,*
> *8 years post stroke)*

Safe mobilisation is important for confidence and independence (Stroke Association, 2023). A range of post-stroke symptoms that may affect mobility are outlined in Figure 9.1.

Stroke symptoms may cause a previously independent person to be bedbound, require assistance for sitting or transferring, or have an altered gait pattern. The most common disability following stroke is motor impairment of the contralateral limbs, affecting more than 80% of stroke survivors in the acute phase and 40% chronically (Khan *et al.*, 2022). However, hidden symptoms related to mobility including pain, fatigue and visual issues can be just as disabling.

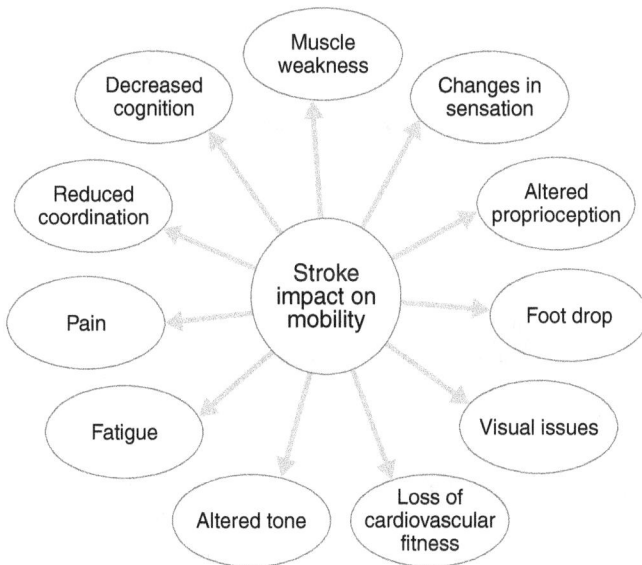

FIGURE 9.1   A range of post-stroke symptoms that may affect mobility.
Source: Adapted from Stroke Association (no date).

Post-stroke pain and mobility

Post-stroke pain is a common stroke-related issue, with varied prevalence (10%–45.8%) occurring in varying body parts and intensities (Atalan, Berzina and Sunnerhagan, 2021). This causes significant restriction of physical function. Stroke survivors who experience restricted mobility are more likely to experience pain 5 years post-stroke. Prevalence differs across post-stroke phases: acute, subacute and chronic. However, the highest prevalence is in the subacute phase with ongoing impact on rehabilitation potential (ISWP, 2023). Thus, professionals need to consider pain as a restrictor of mobility, but also consider prevention of post-stroke pain as part of their recovery programme (see Chapter 4 for further information about post-stroke pain).

Post-stroke fatigue and mobility

Post-stroke fatigue is characterised by a disproportionate sense of tiredness, need to rest greater than usual and lack of energy. For some, rest may not alleviate this fatigue. There are a range of definitions, without consensus, but there is agreement that post-stroke fatigue needs differentiation from apathy (ISWP, 2023). It is acknowledged that fatigue could significantly impact mobility and physical activity, return to work, mood, cognition and social activities (ISWP, 2023).

> I had a lot of fatigue so even a small activity like going for a walk would wipe me out.
>
> *(Jo, 47, embolic stroke as a result of endocarditis, 20 years post stroke)*

Stroke survivors should be assessed for fatigue early, to help plan ongoing rehabilitation. This should be repeated at the 6-month review (NICE, 2023) and include identification of factors that can precipitate or exacerbate fatigue. All healthcare professionals should explore issues relating to potential post-stroke fatigue and consider use of validated fatigue-related assessments.

Up to 92% of stroke survivors experience fatigue (ISWP, 2023), with some experiencing persistent fatigue for several years. Post-stroke fatigue seems to be multi-factorial, can fluctuate over the course of the day, and severity may vary. This can mean that mobility and, therefore, potential safety can vary depending on the level of fatigue.

- Consider the optimal time of day for rehabilitation to get the most out of each patient.
- Review the patient at the least optimal time of day to ensure all safety issues are considered.

Family and carers involved in supporting rehabilitation also need to understand post-stroke fatigue management strategies, as this may add to their burden of care (ISWP, 2023).

> Having to (visually) scan tired me out, as well constantly having to look … that along with trying to walk even a short distance, I was shattered.
>
> *(Alan, 50, ischaemic stroke, 4 years post stroke)*

Post-stroke vision issues and mobility

Visual problems after stroke are common, with some studies suggesting a prevalence of 58% (ISWP, 2023) whilst the Stroke Association (2022c) suggests prevalence of around two-thirds. They can present in a variety of ways including visual field deficits (loss of an area of vision), diplopia (double vision), nystagmus (involuntary, rhythmic and repetitive eye movements), blurred vision, light sensitivity, visual neglect (difficulties with visual processing) and dry eyes (RNIB, 2022).

Visual disturbances have a significant impact on mobility due to reduced confidence, balance, safety and independence (ISWP, 2023; Stroke Association, 2022c). Vision is important for mobility as it supports perception of the physical world. A range of assessments and behavioural observations are used to identify the impact of visual issues on function (NICE, 2023).

> I have got used to visual impairment; it's just I struggle in crowded places. Dim lighting and approaches from the left make me jump. I couldn't walk on the path properly, or next to a road because I lost all my sight to my left, so apart from not being able to feel my left side I didn't have any sight to my left.
>
> *(Alan, 50, ischaemic stroke, 4 years post stroke)*

Stroke survivors with visual field loss will need to compensate for the defect. Compensatory training will include visual scanning involving repetitive eye/head movements to each side, and visual search training which involves looking for specific objects on each side (ISWP, 2023).

> They walked me around the corridors and said 'you are going to have to scan now', … I have to turn my head constantly look where things are before I take any more steps, moving head for vision. I scan, scan, scan constantly.
>
> *(Alan, 50, ischaemic stroke, 4 years post stroke)*

Stroke survivors with visual changes who were previously driving should be advised of the relevant requirements and restrictions (ISWP, 2023).

Rehabilitating mobility

A key part of establishing an effective rehabilitation programme is thorough assessment.

Mobility-related subjective assessment should include information from the patient and family on:

- Pre-stroke mobility level
- Social situation (particularly home environment)
- Hobbies
- Pre-stroke exercise and fitness level.

Mobility-related objective assessment should include:

- Muscle strength
- Sensation
- Coordination
- Proprioception
- Current mobility level
- Balance (sitting/standing)
- Falls risk assessment.

Effective rehabilitation requires constant reassessment. This may be reassessment of the factors mentioned, or using mobility-related outcome measures, such as the 6-minute walk test, 10-metre walk test, the timed up and go test or the Berg Balance Scale (Dos Santos *et al.*, 2023).

Within the assessment process, it is also important to establish mobility-related patient-centred goals. What is important to the patient? They may say things such as "I just want to walk again", but it is important to clarify what this means. Do they want to be able to walk indoors, outdoors, across uneven terrain with their dog, run, play sport, cook, carry things while walking, participate in exercise or be able to manage steps/stairs?

Patients often have an opinion on their target gait quality:

- To get from A to B safely or quickly.
- To walk with minimal gait abnormalities
- To use a scooter at times to conserve energy or complete tasks more quickly, saving time/energy for activities contributing to quality of life.

When establishing goals and rehabilitation plans, considerations include the patient's ability to engage in therapy sessions, fatigue levels, information retention, available environment/equipment and the family/caregiver's engagement or availability. It is also important to remember that therapy is not just provided by therapists.

Within a day or week, a patient may see a therapist for a short period, spending the rest of the time with their family, carers, rehabilitation support workers and other health professionals supporting their recovery. Rehabilitation is a collaborative process between the patient and everyone who is involved in their day-to-day life.

Every functional activity or task is a rehabilitation opportunity

Once patient-centred goals are established, a step-by-step rehabilitation programme is developed. Depending on post-stroke abilities, limitations and goals, there are a wide variety of treatment options that may be used:

- Muscle strengthening
- Work to improve proprioception, coordination or sensation
- Pain and tone management
- Sitting balance work
- Gradual return to sitting out of bed in an appropriate chair
- Transfer practice with/without assistance and with/without a transfer aid – lying to sitting, sit to stand, or from bed to chair
- Mobility practice with/without assistance and with/without a mobility aid
- Use of an orthotic/FES
- Gait re-education
- Treadmill training
- Visual compensatory training.

Functional mobility-related goals are achieved through functional rehabilitation. For example, rehabilitation should include indoor walking, outdoor walking, walking whilst carrying items, dual tasking (e.g. walking and talking) and walking as part of completing a task/activity. This should include real-world walking as this is an important rehabilitation aspect which is a commonly identified goal (NICE, 2023; ISWP, 2023). If mobile, survivors should be assessed and rehabilitated for road crossing, walking on uneven ground, inclines, over distances or walking dogs. This should include assessment of the impact of dual tasking, neglect, vision and confidence in busy environments (ISWP, 2023).

So going down anything that is downhill or if the ground is wet because it has been raining, I was very tentative relying on the grip from walking boots, knowing that I had some grip.

(Alan, 50, ischaemic stroke, 4 years post stroke)

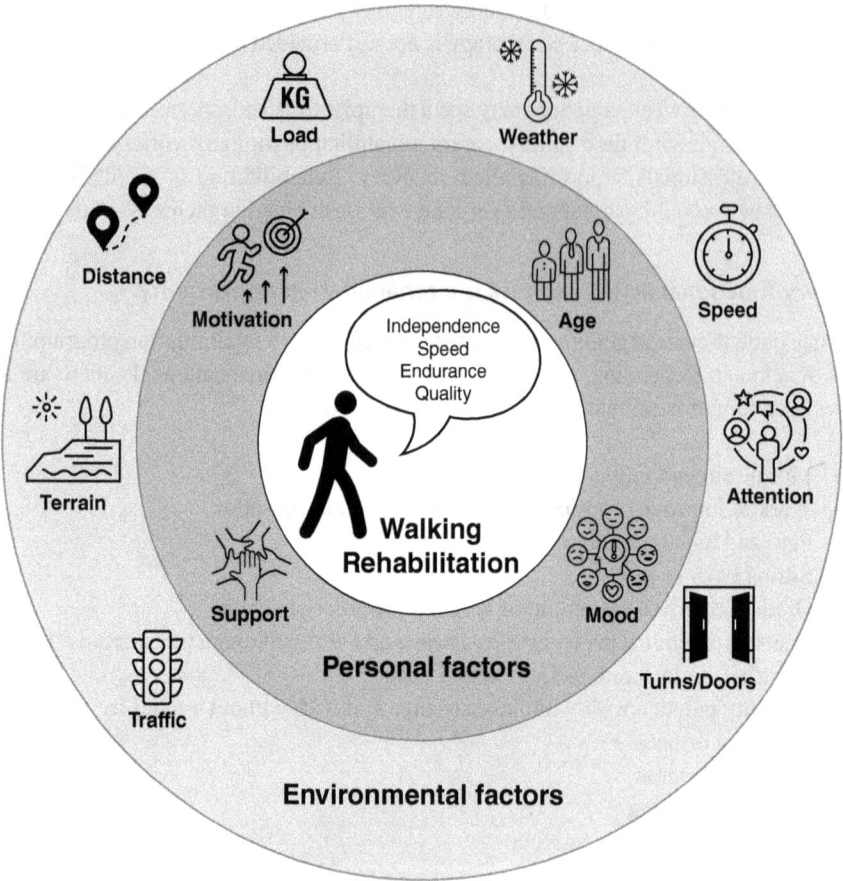

FIGURE 9.2 Walking recovery model for stroke.
Source: Adapted from Moore *et al.* (2022).

For real-world walking recovery, a range of complex and interlinking issues including environmental and personal factors need to be considered, as outlined in Figure 9.2.

Stairs

It is also important not to forget steps and stairs. A patient may need to be able to safely negotiate steps or stairs to access parts of their home, family/friend's houses, shops or other services. Rehabilitation may include practising steps, teaching an alternative method of ascending or descending (e.g. going up/down sideways with both hands on one rail or coming down backwards), providing additional handrails, stair lift or through floor lift.

I still think the most important to me is coming down the stairs backwards. Yeah, holding on to the rail.

(Olive, 82, TIA and ischaemic stroke, 8 years post stroke)

Return to hobbies/access to exercise

Physical deconditioning, with low cardiorespiratory fitness, muscle strength and muscle power, is common post stroke. Low physical fitness is associated with functional limitation and disability (ISWP, 2023), so regaining fitness and strength through regular activity and exercise is key to maintaining health. This includes healthy weight, blood pressure and cholesterol level. Exercise, mobility and fitness should be widely accessible and stroke survivors should understand that impairment or disabilities can be overcome (Donnelly, 2013). As well as returning to prior hobbies, sports and exercise for enjoyment, quality of life or social integration, it is important to consider access to exercise for secondary stroke prevention. There is ongoing research related to post-stroke rehabilitation intensity regarding cardiorespiratory fitness which may result in new guidelines in the future (Moncion *et al.*, 2024).

The ISWP (2023) provide many recommendations regarding physical activity and stroke secondary prevention. The most significant are:

- Stroke survivors should aim to be active every day and participate in physical activity for fitness unless contraindicated.
- Exercise prescription should be individualised, and all stroke survivors should be offered cardiorespiratory training.
- Stroke survivors at risk of falls should incorporate balance and coordination-based exercise at least twice per week.
- Stroke rehabilitation services should build links with community-based exercise facilities (such as support groups, gyms, leisure centres, Parkrun/Parkwalk or exercise referral schemes) to support stroke survivors with long-term access to exercise.

Professionals should support an increase in activity levels or access to hobbies, sports and exercise. This may require education on exercise importance, confidence building, graded return, adapted equipment and referrals to community-based facilities/groups.

Use of mobility aids

There are many types of mobility, including transferring or walking, with or without assistance, and with or without the use of aids.

TABLE 9.2 Overview of mobility related aids

Examples of walking aids
Walking/fischer stick
Quad/tri stick
Elbow crutches
Zimmer/rollator frame
3/4 wheeled walker

Examples of transfer aids
Stand aids, e.g. Rotastand, ReTurn, Molift, Sara Stedy, Quickmove.
Slide board
Stand aid hoist
Full body hoist

Other aids that may assist mobility
Wheelchair
Mobility scooter
Adapted car
Stairlift/through-floor-lift

Reflect upon how you mobilise? – walk, wheelchair, mobility scooter, drive? – with or without an aid, independently or with assistance? How would you feel if this changed?

Stroke survivors with mobility limitations should be assessed for, provided with and educated to use appropriate mobility aids, including wheelchairs, to enable safe and independent mobility (ISWP, 2023). There are a significant variety of mobility aids and equipment that can be provided by the NHS or purchased privately. This is dependent on the impact of the stroke and the stage of recovery. A selection of aids is shown in Table 9.2.

Mobility rehabilitation can be enhanced by aids/equipment to enable safety or to support walking earlier (ISWP, 2023). There are suggestions that the use of mobility aids improves the quality, stability and/or efficiency of walking and can also prevent falls in stroke survivors. However, other studies have identified the use of a mobility aid can be a prospective predictor of increased falls in stroke survivors, with a potential fivefold increase in falling (Kim and Kim, 2015). Using mobility aids requires attention and can compromise stability when a task is performed (Bertrand *et al.*, 2017). Therefore, these issues need to be considered as part of falls and other risk assessments.

Stroke survivor choices may contrast with evidence-based recommendations. Research suggests that mobility aid use has been significantly associated with long-term community ambulation (Durcan, Flavin and Horgan, 2016). Research has also explored perceptions of walking stick use in stroke survivors (Nascimento *et al.*, 2019). In this research, positive perceptions were outlined by individuals with more walking limitations, who overall identified that use of a walking stick could be helpful for safety, improving walking and supporting independence. Survivors with fewer walking limitations outlined more negative perceptions and may not have chosen to use aids for walking due to their perception of social stigma.

> To be honest I'm a bit proud and I don't want people to see I've got a walking stick.
> *(Alan, 50, ischaemic stroke, 4 years post stroke)*

> I would rather have the stick to feel safe, rather than go over.
> *(Olive, 82, TIA and ischaemic stroke, 8 years post stroke)*

Stroke survivors may require support and information about mobility aids and equipment. A range of support is available.

AbilityNet provides help with access and use of digital technology. https://ability net.org.uk

AGE UK factsheets cover the help you can get from the local authority to manage daily life at hope by the provision of equipment and adaptations https:// ageuk. org.uk/globalassets/age-uk/documents/factsheets/fs42_disability_equipment_ and_home_adaptations_fcs.pdf

Anything Left-Handed provides a range of equipment for people who use their left hand https://anythinglefthanded.co.uk

Red Cross offers a range of wheelchairs for hire https://redcross.org.uk/get-help/ hire-a-wheelchair/using-your-wheelchair

Gov.uk can be used to apply for equipment to support disabilities: https://www. gov.uk/apply-home-equipment-for-disabled in addition local councils can also be contacted for equipment and support

REMAP makes and adapts equipment to meet the unique needs of individuals https://remap.org.uk

Stroke Association advice and links for a range of aids: https://stroke.org.uk/stroke/life-after/equipment-independent-living

If you need to adapt your home because of a disability, you can apply to the council for equipment or help via https://gov.uk/apply-home-equipment-for-disabled

Use of orthotics to aid mobility

Foot drop is the limited ability to dorsiflex (pull the foot/ankle up towards the body) and has an incidence of 20–30% post stroke (Peishun *et al.*, 2021). This can cause mobility issues due to decreased floor clearance during the swing phase of gait (when the foot is off the floor), increased risk of trips/falls (due to the foot catching on the floor or altered balance) and causes gait pattern to alter.

Use of orthotics can address foot drop and include insoles, braces, splints, callipers and footwear. These help during the recovery phase or to manage long-term effects of stroke (NHS England, no date). Orthotics may also help with other lower limb issues affecting mobility, such as ankle or knee instability. The ISWP (2023) guidelines advise that people with foot drop should, in the first instance, be offered a lightweight, flexible ankle–foot orthosis to improve walking and balance.

The ISWP (2023) suggests use of FES as an alternative for foot drop management. FES is a rehabilitation treatment involving stimulation of the peripheral nerves supplying the paralysed muscle, using surface or implantable electrodes (NICE, 2009). Electrodes placed over the common peroneal nerve stimulate contraction of the dorsiflexor muscles. A footswitch is placed under the heel, triggering the stimulation to turn on and off at the correct time during the gait pattern, making walking safer, faster and less effortful. FES is used as an orthotic device, directly improving walking whilst in situ. However, for some users, FES may also have a therapeutic effect by improving walking/dorsiflexion even after the device has been removed.

Use of orthotics/FES should be evaluated and individually fitted. A referral to orthotics should be considered if required. The patient and their family/carers should be educated in applying, using and removing orthoses/FES as well as the risk of pressure damage, particularly if sensory loss is present (ISWP, 2023).

Stroke and falls

Healthcare professionals supporting patients at risk of falling should develop and maintain professional competence in falls assessment and prevention.

A fall is defined as an event that results in a person coming to rest inadvertently on the ground, floor or lower level (WHO, 2021). A 'simple fall' results from an impairment of vision, mobility or balance; these are distinguished from a 'collapse' caused by an acute medical problem, such as a vertigo, transient ischaemic attack or acute arrhythmia (NICE, 2019). It is important to be aware that a stroke survivor has a higher risk of simple falls or collapse due to stroke symptoms or stroke risk factors (ISWP, 2023). A Cochrane review of post-stroke falls highlights falls as one of the most common complications, with reported incidence between 7% in the first week and 73% in the first year (Denissen *et al.*, 2019). Around 40–60% of falls result in major lacerations, fractures or traumatic brain injuries. Falls can also increase risk of hip fracture (usually on the weaker side) for the stroke survivor (ISWP, 2023). Other significant effects are distress, loss of independence, loss of self-confidence, reduced quality of life, pain and mortality. Additionally, a cycle of fear of falls can be triggered, leading to social isolation, activity avoidance, depression, institutionalisation and functional decline (NICE, 2019). Non-serious falls are also a factor for predicting future falls (Denissen *et al.*, 2019).

> I blacked out due to my seizure about six months post stroke and woke up in hospital. I had pain on movement but used painkillers and carried on walking with soreness. It was only on a later scan that a fracture of my back was identified.
>
> *(Alan, 50, ischaemic stroke, 4 years post stroke)*

Research has found similar risk factors for stroke populations compared to general older populations (Persson and Hansson, 2021). The risk of falls is usually multi-factorial; however, specific risk factors are likely to play a greater role in stroke survivors. In addition, individuals with stroke are more likely to have other associated risk factors for falls (Table 9.3).

TABLE 9.3 Specific and associated risk factors for falls

Specific stroke-related risk factors for falls	*Associated stroke-related risk factors for falls*
• Unilateral weakness	• Diabetes
• Hemisensory or visual neglect	• Drugs which increase falls risk
• Impaired coordination	• Atrial fibrillation
• Visual field defects	• Other cardiovascular risk factors
• Perceptual difficulties	
• Cognitive issues	
• Balance/mobility problems	
• Requiring assistance from carers	
• Psychotropic or sedative medications	
• Depression	
• History of falls	

Source: Tan and Tan (2016), Xu *et al.* (2018), ISWP (2023)

> My left leg sometimes, as I'm walking, it just gives way. There's no warning it's gonna happen, and I've had lots of falls.
>
> *(Olive, 82, transient ischaemic attack/ischaemic stroke, 8 years post stroke)*

Balance problems are common as brain damage can result in weakness, poor coordination and balance issues. The Stroke Association (2022b) outlines common balance issues contributing to falls risk:

- Unilateral weakness/foot drop
- Sensation loss in a leg/foot
- Difficulty concentrating
- Vision problems or vertigo
- Medication side effects

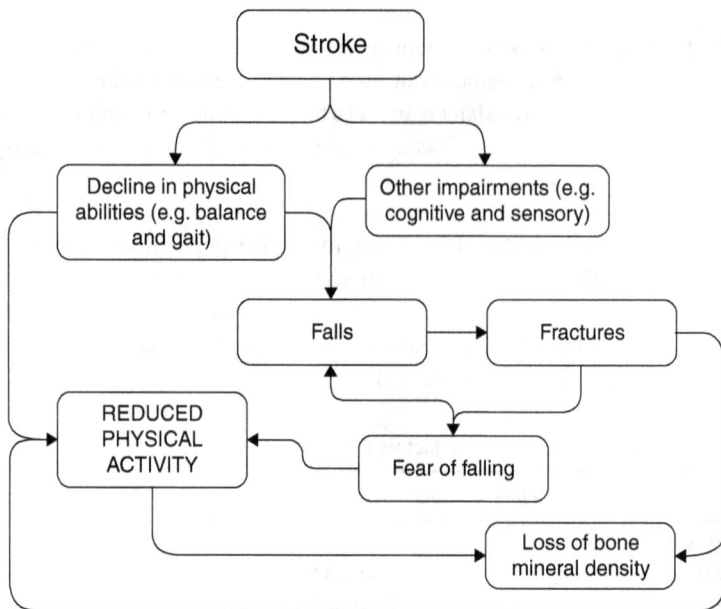

FIGURE 9.3 Interactions between risk factors, falls and consequences post stroke.
Source: Weerdesteyn *et al.* (2008, p. 1198).

In 2008, Weerdesteyn *et al.* provided an overview of the interactions post stroke between risk factors, fear of falling (FOF), falls and consequences (see Figure 9.3). This suggests a complex picture with multiple contributors.

Fear of falling (FoF)

Due to reduced mobility and balance, older survivors of stroke are more likely to experience a FOF, with 32–83% of stroke survivors identifying a FOF (Xie *et al.*, 2022). If there is a maladaptive response to FOF, this will cause a restriction of activity, recurrent falls and poor balance, causing a self-reinforcing cycle (Chen *et al.*, 2023; see Figure 9.4). In the stroke survivor, high levels of FOF and fall incidence can limit exercise, rehabilitation, independence, ability and mobility, thereby increasing mortality.

Post-stroke FOF higher risk predictors include:

- being female
- lower mobility levels
- impaired balance
- walking aid use
- falls history (Xie *et al.*, 2022).

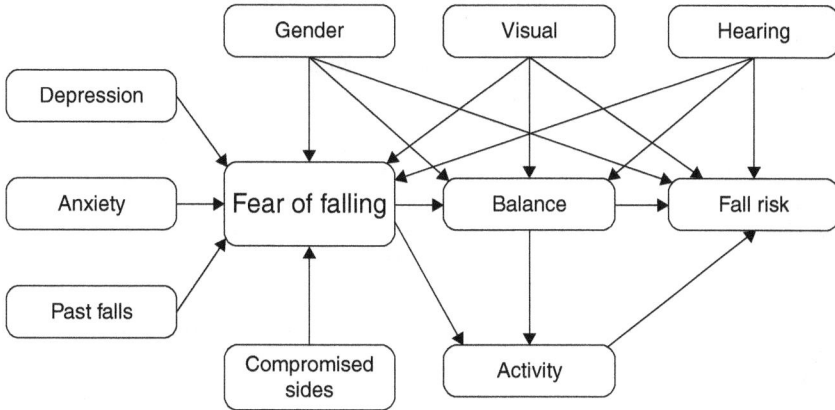

FIGURE 9.4 The hypothesised model with fear of falling.
Source: Chen *et al.* (2023, p. 4).

> I felt really very scared in the beginning about falling over and balance, and what more damage I could do if I fell over, and I felt quite vulnerable.
>
> *(Alan, 50, ischaemic stroke, 4 years post stroke)*

Reducing FOF

Support for the sensory, physical and psychological difficulties contributing to FOF should be available (ISWP, 2023), particularly during recovery (Chen *et al.*, 2023). Multifaceted interventions including psychological and physiological factors should be developed to address falls' prevention and FOF (Chen *et al.*, 2023). It is acknowledged that balance training, cognitive–behavioural therapy and physiotherapy are effective for reducing FOF post stroke (Liu *et al.*, 2018; ISWP, 2023).

> I think I took a lot longer (to go out) … because I was very scared of falling.
>
> *(Jo, 47, embolic stroke as a result of endocarditis, 20 years post stroke)*

Risk assessment and falls prevention

As risk of falling is multi-factorial, prevention is based on assessing multiple risk factors and should be completed by a skilled and experienced practitioner, usually in a falls' specialist service (NICE, 2013). This is no different post-stroke, with assessment addressing physical, sensory, psychological, pharmacological and environmental factors. Factors included in falls risk assessments are outlined in Table 9.4. The more risk factors someone has, the higher the falls risk (NICE, 2013).

TABLE 9.4 Falls risk, assessments and interventions

Risk and assessments	Interventions to minimise risks
Falls history – particularly in the last year Identifying balance/mobility issues – including premorbid issues Assessing gait/balance abnormalities Identification of muscle weakness	Advice on physical activity, incorporating balance and coordination at least twice weekly. Strength and balance training – particularly older people with recurrent falls and/or balance/gait deficits. Muscle-strengthening and balance programmes, individually prescribed and monitored.
General assessment to include identification of: • FOF • Low self-efficacy • Alcohol misuse • Potential changes someone is willing to make (including family/carers)	Education and falls prevention programmes should be accessible and address: • FOF • Low self-efficacy • Measures to prevent further falls • Staying motivated with falls prevention strategies • Psychological and physical benefits of falls risk modification • Encouraging negotiated activity change • Advice on seeking further support • How to cope if a fall occurs – summoning help and avoiding a 'long lie' • Group circuit training utilising peer support and education
Vision assessment	Referral for appropriate support
Cardiovascular examination, identifying postural/orthostatic hypotension	Management of cardiovascular issues
Cognitive state and mental health issues	• Address short-term confusion. • Support for long-term cognitive impairment. • Mental health support.
Medication review to identify potential issues	Modification of medicines to avoid polypharmacy and minimise unwanted side effects
Home hazard assessments	Address hazards – poor lighting, loose rugs, mats or fittings (handrails), uneven surfaces, wet surfaces and poor footwear
Identification of vitamin D deficiency, or at high risk and fragility fracture risk	Calcium and vitamin D supplements
Identification of ankle instability or foot drop	Consider orthotics referral

Source: NICE (2023), ISWP (2023).

Against a background of stroke diagnosis, management of recognised risks should be addressed with a falls prevention programme (NICE, 2023; ISWP, 2023). Multi-factorial intervention programmes utilising interdisciplinary approaches should be provided post stroke as shown in Table 9.4.

Unfortunately, some standard falls prevention measures cannot be implemented in stroke survivors. For example, drugs used to minimise further stroke risk in stroke survivors can increase falls risk. Anti-hypertensives may be linked to orthostatic hypotension; however, the benefit of effective blood pressure control for secondary stroke prevention outweighs potential falls risk. Anticoagulation is associated with increased risk of intracranial bleeding following a fall, but the risk of experiencing a further stroke outweighs risk of bleeding from a fall (Tan and Tan, 2016).

The individual needs to understand how they can ensure their own safety. The Royal College of Physicians (2016) have provided general guidance on what hospital patients can do to minimise falls. This guidance together with recommended educational information from NICE (2013) can be used to support stroke survivors in any setting (see Figure 9.5).

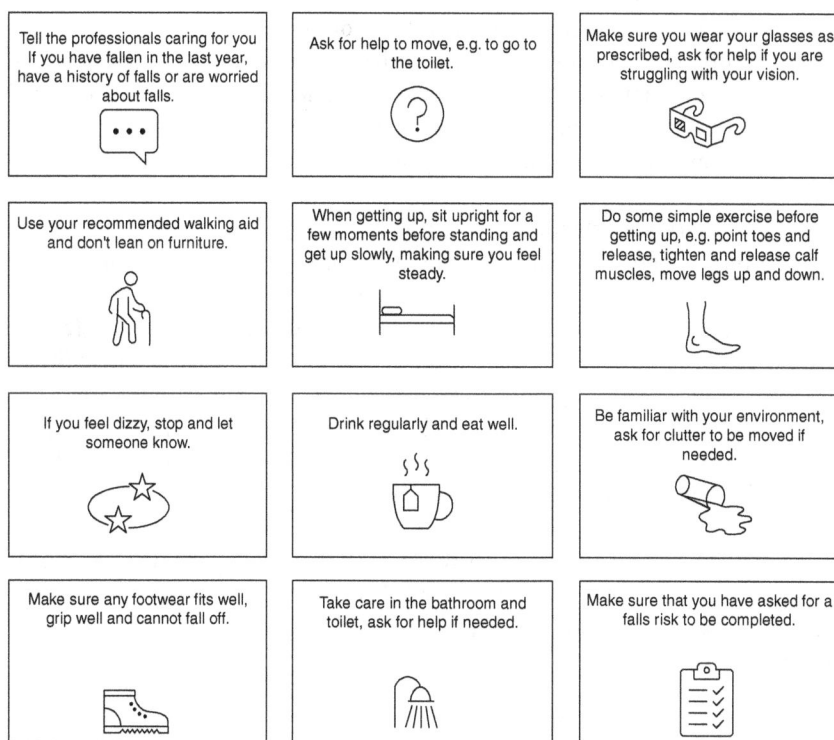

Tell the professionals caring for you If you have fallen in the last year, have a history of falls or are worried about falls.	Ask for help to move, e.g. to go to the toilet.	Make sure you wear your glasses as prescribed, ask for help if you are struggling with your vision.
Use your recommended walking aid and don't lean on furniture.	When getting up, sit upright for a few moments before standing and get up slowly, making sure you feel steady.	Do some simple exercise before getting up, e.g. point toes and release, tighten and release calf muscles, move legs up and down.
If you feel dizzy, stop and let someone know.	Drink regularly and eat well.	Be familiar with your environment, ask for clutter to be moved if needed.
Make sure any footwear fits well, grip well and cannot fall off.	Take care in the bathroom and toilet, ask for help if needed.	Make sure that you have asked for a falls risk to be completed.

FIGURE 9.5   What stroke survivors can do to minimise falls risk.

What is your role in falls prevention? What more could you do to promote falls prevention?

See also Chapter 2, which further explores falls as part of maintaining independence and safety post stroke.

Driving

Driving can be an important part of everyday life, socially and professionally. There are many reasons people want or need to drive: to commute, as part of their work role, for shopping, to support their children, or for social purposes. Driving gives independence and the opportunity to access a wider environment and social network. Therefore, returning to driving is frequently an identified goal (Driver and Vehicle Licensing Agency (DVLA), no date).

There are rules surrounding driving a car or motorbike in the UK post stroke. Currently, the DVLA (no date) states that a person must stop driving a car, motorbike or taxi for at least one month post stroke. If a full recovery has been made within 1 month, there is no obligation to inform the DVLA of the stroke. If any symptoms continue after one month, then the licence holder must inform the DVLA. Failure to inform the DVLA can incur a fine and, if involved in an accident, prosecution. There are different rules for professional drivers. Someone with a bus, coach or lorry licence must not drive the larger vehicle for at least one year post stroke, and require doctor's clearance before returning to professional driving. This could have a significant impact, both psychologically and financially.

- Stroke survivors should be asked about driving before they leave the hospital or outpatient clinic, be informed of the exclusion period and their responsibility to notify the DVLA if required (ISWP, 2023).
- Stroke survivors should be examined for absolute bars to driving (e.g. seizures, double vision, visual field deficits), be informed about eligibility for disabled concessions (e.g. Motability, Blue Badge scheme) and be offered an assessment of the impairments that may affect driving eligibility.
- People with persisting cognitive, language or motor disability should be referred for on-road screening and evaluation.

In relation to post-stroke epilepsy or seizure activity, the DVLA (2024) highlights that anyone with a medical condition likely to cause a sudden disabling event at the wheel, or who is unable to control their vehicle safely for any other reason, must not drive.

I cannot drive due to having two seizures and rely on my father to help me care for (child) and take him in the car to nursery.

(Nerys, 35, right frontal intracerebral haemorrhage from a ruptured arteriovenous malformation (AVM), 18 months post stroke)

Safe driving requires the involvement of many key elements from a range of skills (see Figure 9.6). Given these requirements, it follows that many body systems need to be functional for safe driving. A stroke may affect any of these abilities.

Driving a car is one of the most complex regular activities that we complete (DVLA, no date). It involves a complex and rapidly repeating cycle (see Figure 9.7) that requires a level of skill and the ability to interact simultaneously with both the vehicle and the external environment (DVLA, 2024).

Due to driving complexity, it can be difficult to assess whether a stroke survivor is safe to return to driving. Specific guidance is available from the DVLA (2024) for doctors and other healthcare professionals on the national guidelines to assist in advising patients about driving.

There are many standardised and non-standardised assessments that can assist healthcare professionals to understand the likelihood of fitness to drive post stroke (e.g. orthoptics/functional assessments). Clinicians can often struggle to predict driving safety due to its complex nature. A formal driving assessment is recommended if the stroke survivor has ongoing symptoms after 1 month.

Useful organisations and information sources for returning to driving

Current UK driving regulations: *https://gov.uk/guidance/general-information-assessing-fitness-to-drive*

DVLA: *Information on driving with medical conditions, Blue Badges and transport for people with disability: https://gov.uk/browse/driving/disability-health-condition*

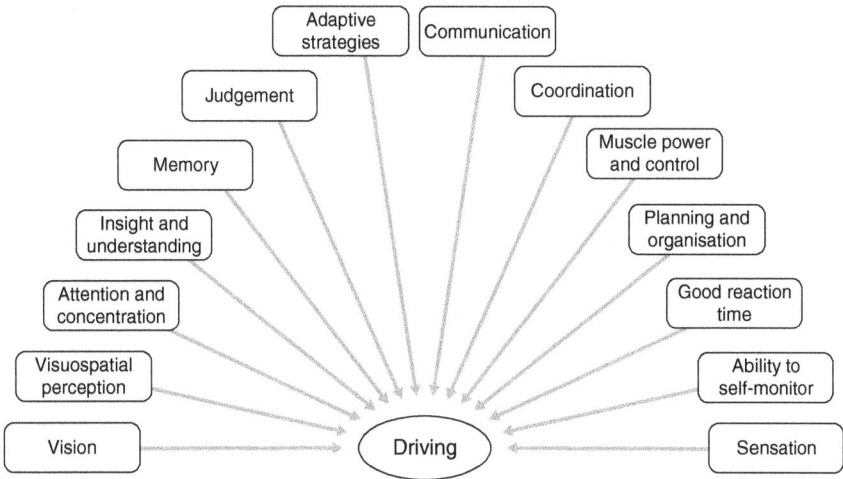

FIGURE 9.6   Key skills for safe driving.

Source: Adapted from DVLA (2024).

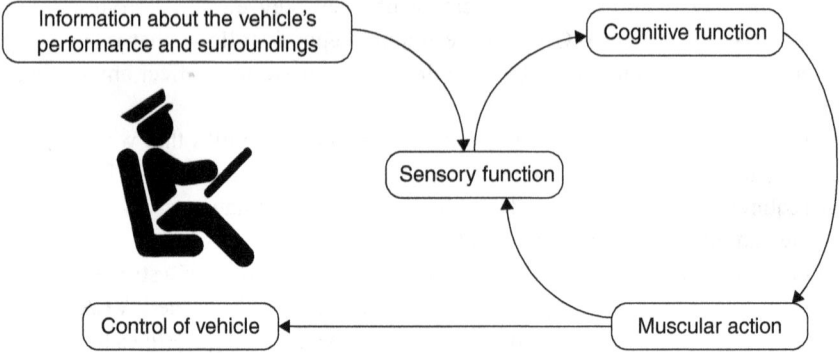

FIGURE 9.7 Diagram demonstrating driving complexity.

Blue Badge scheme: *Allows people with disabilities to park closer to their destination, either as passenger or driver: https://gov.uk/apply-blue-badge*

Motability: *If the individual is in receipt of the higher rate for the mobility part of Personal Independence Payment or Disability Living Allowance, they can join the Motability Scheme. The allowance can then be used for a car, wheelchair accessible vehicle, scooter or powered wheelchair: https://motability.co.uk/*

Driving mobility: *Help with driving accessibility and supported by the Department for Transport in England. This includes a driving safety assessment, identification of aids and potential vehicle modifications: https://drivingmobility.org.uk/*

Stroke Association information on driving: *https://stroke.org.uk/life-after-stroke/driving*

If someone is deemed safe to return to driving post-stroke, this does not necessarily mean they are confident. Driving can often be stressful, particularly if someone has not driven for a long time. Refresher driving lessons can be useful or having a trusted friend/relative accompany them until they feel more confident, starting with known routes.

> I feel much more confident when I am driving that someone is with me.
> *(Nerys, 35, right frontal intracerebral haemorrhage from a ruptured AVM, 18 months post stroke)*

Conclusion

Mobility is commonly an important goal in stroke rehabilitation, as it plays a central role in promoting independence and quality of life. There are well-established guidelines that provide direction for mobility management following a stroke.

However, a range of issues and symptoms may affect an individual's ability to regain mobility, requiring a tailored and flexible approach to rehabilitation. Various aids, orthotics, and treatment options are available to support mobility recovery and enhance safety. Falls and fear of falling remain key concerns that must be addressed through appropriate assessment and intervention. Stroke survivors who wish to return to driving should be provided with appropriate advice, support, and driving assessments to ensure both their safety and that of others..

References

Atalan, P., Bērziņa, G., Sunnerhagen, K.S. (2021) 'Influence of mobility restrictions on post-stroke pain', *Brain and Behavior*, 11(5), e02092. https://doi.org/10.1002/brb3.2092

Bertrand, K., Raymond, M.H., Miller, W.C., Ginis, K.A.M., Demers, L. (2017) 'Walking aids for enabling activity and participation: a systematic review', *American Journal of Physical Medicine & Rehabilitation*, 96(12), 894–903.

Cambridge Dictionary. (no date) *Independence*. Available at: https://dictionary.cambridge.org/dictionary/english/independence

Chen, Y., Du, H., Song, M., Liu, T., Ge, P., Xu, Y., Pi, H. (2023) 'Relationship between fear of falling and fall risk among older patients with stroke: a structural equation modeling', *BMC Geriatrics*, 23(647). https://doi.org/10.1186/s12877-023-04298-y

Denissen, S., Staring, W., Kunkel, D., Pickering, R.M., Lennon, S., Geurts, A.C.H., Weerdesteyn, V., Verheyden, G.S.A.F. (2019) 'Interventions for preventing falls in people after stroke', *Cochrane Database of Systematic Reviews*, 10, CD008728. Available at: https://doi.org/10.1002/14651858.cd008728.pub3

Donnelly, C. (2013) 'Mobility and immobility', in Brooker C., Waugh A. (eds.) *Foundations of Nursing Practice: Fundamentals of Holistic Care*. Missouri, USA: Mosby Elsevier. pp. 431–456.

Dos Santos, R.B., Fiedler, A., Badwal, A., Legasto-Mulvale, J.M., Sibley, K.M., Olaleye, O.A., Diermayr, G., Salbach, N.M. (2023, Feb. 21) Standardized tools for assessing balance and mobility in stroke clinical practice guidelines worldwide: a scoping review. *Frontiers in Rehabilitation Science*, 4, 1084085. Available at: https://doi.org/10.3389/fresc.2023.1084085

Durcan, S., Flavin, E., Horgan, F. (2016) Factors associated with community ambulation in chronic stroke. *Disability and Rehabilitation*, 38(3), 245–249.

Driving and Vehicle Licensing Agency (DVLA) (no date) *Stroke (cerebrovascular accident) and driving*. Available at: https://gov.uk/stroke-and-driving

Driving and Vehicle Licensing Agency (DVLA) (2024) *Assessing fitness to drive – a guide for medical professionals*. Available at: https://assets.publishing.service.gov.uk/media/65cf7243e1bdec001a322268/assessing-fitness-to-drive-february-2024.pdf

Intercollegiate Stroke Working Party (ISWP) (2023) *National Clinical Guideline for Stroke for the United Kingdom and Northern Ireland*. 5th Edition. Available at: www.strokeguideline.org

Khan, F., Abusharha, S., Alfuraidy, A., Nimatallah, K., Almalki, R., Basaffar, R., Mirdad, M., Chevidikunnan, M.F., Basuodan, R. (2022) 'Prediction of factors affecting mobility in patients with stroke and finding the mediation effect of balance on mobility: a cross-sectional study', *International Journal of Environmental Research and Public Health,* 19(24), 16612. https://doi.org/10.3390/ijerph192416612

Kim, O., Kim, J. (2015) 'Falls and use of assistive devices in stroke patients with hemiparesis: association with balance ability and fall efficacy. *Rehabilitation Nursing Journal,* 40(4), 267–274.

Liu, T.W., Ng, G., Chung, R., Ng, S. (2018) 'Decreasing fear of falling in chronic stroke survivors through cognitive behavior therapy and task-oriented training', *Stroke,* 50(1). https://doi.org/10.1161/strokeaha.118.022406

Mehrholz, J., Kugler, J., Pohl, M., Elsner, B. (2020) 'Electromechanical-assisted training for walking after stroke', *Cochrane Database of Systematic Reviews,* 5, CD006185. https://doi.org/10.1002/14651858.CD006185.pub6

Moncion, K., Rodrigues, L., De Las Heras, B., Noguchi, K.S., Wiley, E. Janice J., MacKay-Lyons, M., Sweet, S.N., Thiel, A., Fung, J., Stratford, P., Richardson, J.A., MacDonald, M.J., Roig, M., Tang, A. (2024) 'Cardiorespiratory fitness benefits of high-intensity interval training after stroke: a randomized controlled trial', *Stroke,* 55(9), 2202–2211. https://doi.org/10.1161/STROKEAHA.124.046564

Moore, S.A., Boyne, P., Fulk, G., Verheyden, G., Fini, N.A. (2022) 'Walk the talk: current evidence for walking recovery after stroke, future pathways and a mission for research and clinical practice', *Stroke.* 53(11), 3494–3505. https://doi.org/10.1161/STROKE AHA.122.038956

Nascimento, L.R., Ada, L., Rocha, G,M., Teixera-Salmela, L.F. (2019) 'Perceptions of individuals with stroke regarding the use of a cane for walking: a qualitative study', *Journal of Bodywork and Movement Therapies,* 23(1), 166–170.

NIH National Institute on Aging (2020) *Maintaining mobility and preventing disability are key to living independently as we age.* Available at: https://nia.nih.gov/news/maintaining-mobility-and-preventing-disability-are-key-living-independently-we-age

NHS (2022a) *Recovery – stroke.* Available at: https://nhs.uk/conditions/stroke/recovery/#:~:text=The%20injury%20to%20the%20brain,the%20symptoms%20and%20their%20severity.

NHS (2022b) *Walking aids, wheelchairs and mobility scooters.* Available at: https://nhs.uk/conditions/social-care-and-support-guide/care-services-equipment-and-care-homes/walking-aids-wheelchairs-and-mobility-scooters/

NHS England (no date) *Orthotic services.* Available at: https://england.nhs.uk/commissioning/orthotic-services/.

NICE (2009) *Functional electrical stimulation for drop foot of central neurological origin.* Available at: https://nice.org.uk/guidance/ipg278/documents/functional-electrical-stimulation-for-drop-foot-of-central-neurological-origin-interventional-procedures-consultation

NICE (2013) *Falls in older people: assessing risk and prevention.* Available at: https://nice.org.uk/guidance/cg161

NICE (2019) *Falls risk assessment.* Available at: https://cks.nice.org.uk/topics/falls-risk-assessment/

NICE (2023) *Stroke rehabilitation in adults.* Available at: https://nice.org.uk/guidance/ng236

Peishun, C., Haiwang, Z., Taotao, L., Hongli, G., Yu, M., Wanrong, Z. (2021) 'Changes in gait characteristics of stroke patients with foot drop after the combination treatment of foot drop stimulator and moving treadmill training', *Neural Plasticity,* 9480957. https://doi.org/10.1155/2021/9480957

Persson, C., Hansson, P. (2021) 'Determinants of falls after stroke based on data on 5065 patients from the Swedish Väststroke and Riksstroke Registers', *Scientific Reports*, 11(24035). https://doi.org/10.1038/s41598-021-03375-9

Rantanen, T. (2013) 'Promoting Mobility in older people', *Journal of Preventive Medicine & Public Health*, 46, S50–S54.

RNIB (2022) *Stroke-related eye conditions*. Available at: https://rnib.org.uk/your-eyes/eye-conditions-az/stroke-related-eye-conditions/?gad_source=1&gclid=CjwKCAjwnqK1BhBvEiwAi7o0X9PA7BV-xp67T3zcTRxPY1aOx-QiaPjKjBlEgUgE96AV5zsBI6bARRoCBgIQAvD_BwE#what-are-some-of-the-common-visual-symptoms-of-stroke (Accessed 26 July 2024).

Royal College of Physicians (2016) *Falls prevention in hospital: a guide for patients, their families and carers*. Available at: https://rcplondon.ac.uk/projects/outputs/falls-prevention-hospital-guide-patients-their-families-and-carers

Sentinel Stroke National Audit Programme (SSNAP) (2024) *National results – clinical*. Available at: https://strokeaudit.org/Results2/Clinical-audit/National-Results.aspx

Stroke Association (no date) *Physical effects of stroke*. https://stroke.org.uk/stroke/effects/physical

Stroke Association (2022b) *Preventing falls after a stroke*. Available at: https://stroke.org.uk/blog/preventing-falls-after-stroke

Stroke Association (2022c) *Vision problems after stroke*. https://stroke.org.uk/vision_problems_after_stroke_guide.pdf

Stroke Association (2023) *Staying safe at home*. www.stroke.org.uk/stroke/support/materials/stroke-news/staying-safe-home stroke

Tan, K.M., Tan, M.P. (2016) 'Stroke and falls – clash of the two Titans in geriatrics', *Geriatrics*, 1(4), 31. https://doi.org/10.3390/geriatrics1040031

WHO (2021) *Falls*. Available at: www.who.int/news-room/fact-sheets/detail/falls

Xie, Q., Pei, J., Gou, L., Zhang, Y., Zhong, J., Su, Y., Wang, X., Ma, L., Dou, X. (2022) 'Risk factors for fear of falling in stroke patients: a systematic review and meta-analysis', *BMJ Open* 12, e056340. https://bmjopen.bmj.com/content/12/6/e056340

Xu, T., Clemson, L., O'Loughlin, K., Lannin, N.A., Dean, C., Koh, G. (2018) 'Risk factors for falls in community stroke survivors: a systematic review and meta-analysis', *Archives of Physical Medicine and Rehabilitation*, 99(3), 563–573.e5. https://doi.org/10.1016/j.apmr.2017.06.032

10

RELATIONSHIPS, INTIMACY AND SEXUALITY

Fiona Chalk, Ruth Trout and Julia Williams

Learning objectives

- To understand the changes that stroke survivors may experience in their life roles, including with partners and loved ones.
- To understand the physical, cognitive and emotional challenges of relationships, intimacy and sexuality following a stroke.
- To understand the interpersonal and therapeutic support that may be needed by the stroke survivor and loved ones as they adapt to the new ways of living.

Background

Relationships, intimacy and sexuality are all essential aspects of good quality of life, but they can become complex or challenging for stroke survivors and their loved ones. Relationships exist between two or more people and are the regard and behaviour that exist towards others. Intimacy signifies the emotional aspects of a relationship, such as feelings of warmth, closeness and feeling connected, while sexuality refers to the physical aspects of a relationship, such as sexual functioning and intercourse. These aspects can mean different things to different people; therefore, it is an important part of the rehabilitation process to clarify the meaning for each person.

Surviving a stroke brings about many changes and challenges to the individual, as they adapt and adjust to this profound life-changing event (NHS, 2024). The experience of living with the aftermath of a stroke is often associated with physical and psychological anxieties which affect all aspects of life (Intercollegiate Stroke Working Party (ISWP), 2023). Whilst these anxieties may be attributed to the

DOI: 10.4324/9781003426196-11

practicalities of living with a stroke, it is not uncommon for individuals to express feelings of loss, altered or reduced self-esteem and stigma which can disrupt emotions, attitudes and relationships (ISWP, 2023; Kniepmann and Kerr, 2018; McGrath *et al.*, 2019). These issues can also be linked to body image or self-image and the alterations that can occur following a stroke. This requires a gradual process of adaptation and adjustment, which is rarely linear, with emotions fluctuating as the stroke survivor adjusts to a potential change from life as it was prior to the stroke (ISWP, 2023). Therefore, independent care management in isolation is not sufficient to foster adaptation and adjustment for return to a full and active life, as illustrated by this stroke survivor:

> Everyone at the hospital has been amazing, supporting my recovery but honestly, I wouldn't be where I am today without family and friends encouraging me to get out and be as active as I can... it's been really tough to adapt to all this, but you know, your mind is just as important as your body. I truly believe an active mind brings positivity and that's really helped me recover!
>
> *(Kelly, 55, ischaemic stroke, 7 years post stroke)*

Impact on loved ones and communication

In the initial days and weeks after a stroke, families can be dealing with stressful situations, including the shock of the event and a significant change in status of a loved one with stroke creates a ripple effect.

> I'm a ripple in this sea of everybody else: friends, family – I'm just in the middle. It's not me who is the only person who had a stroke, they did.
>
> *(Kelly, 55, ischaemic stroke, 7 years post stroke)*

Relationships after stroke are important for both the stroke survivor and family caregivers. During the initial acute care in hospital, families of stroke survivors can experience modification of their roles to support the stroke survivors' rehabilitation – introducing new stressors affecting family functioning (Zhang *et al.*, 2024). With approximately 54% of families experiencing relationship problems after stroke and up to 38% of couples experiencing conflict (McCarthy *et al.*, 2020), this is clearly a challenging time for all involved.

Within the ISWP guidelines for stroke (2023), there is significant discussion throughout about engaging with and utilising support from the family carer or carers for the stroke survivor.

> (My family) navigated all of that grown up, adult stuff, that we all take for granted that we can do, and I dread to think what people would do if they didn't have a family member to fix all of this.
>
> *(Jo, 47, embolic stroke as a result of endocarditis, 20 years post stroke)*

However, this in turn can lead to pressure for families. The American Stroke Association (2025) uses the term 'emotional roller coaster' and outlines the potential grieving process family members can experience due to their own personal 'loss'. However, within the recommendations from the ISWP (2023), there is the potential for early supported discharge from hospital with treatment at home within 24 hours (2023). This could place a high level of expectation on the family to provide support, despite a potential lack of adjustment period for significant changes in their life.

Lack of support for the stroke survivor and loved ones can present challenges to the relationship, including disagreement about boundaries and feelings of isolation or pressure. Family caregivers portray emotions of their own, including anger and sadness, and might become less invested in the relationship and slowly grow apart, contributing to further stroke survivor stress. Relationships need good communication and understanding to survive (McCarthy *et al.*, 2020), and communication may be adversely affected by stroke.

There are clear overlaps with how a stroke impacts the stroke survivor and the way that loved ones are impacted following a stroke (Figure 10.1). It can affect

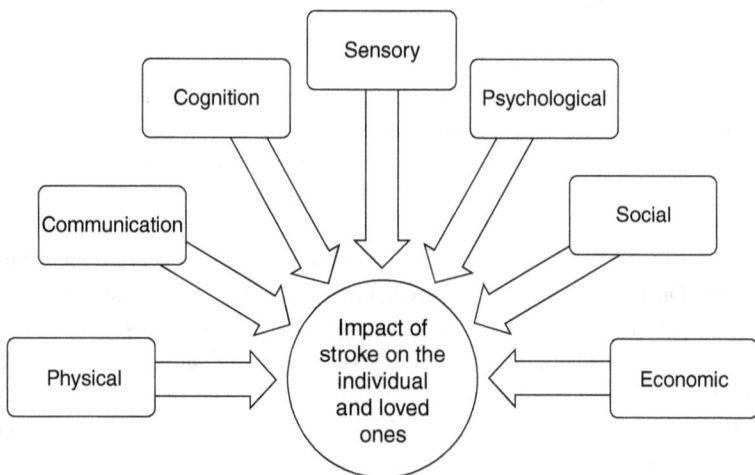

FIGURE 10.1 Impact domains in the stroke survivor and their loved ones.

Sources: Stroke Association (no date), American Stroke Association (2025), Suksatan *et al.* (2022), Tziaka *et al.* (2024).

body image, self-perception, mood, relationships, wellbeing, employment, social and leisure opportunities (ISWP, 2023).

All of these factors can potentially create tensions within the family unit as expectations may not change, despite the changes stroke survivors have experienced.

> Everybody expects you to function, (said by family members) are you not going down to dinner? There is the expectation that you will always do that.
>
> *(Jacqueline, 42, ischaemic stroke whilst pregnant, 12 years post stroke)*

> I feel like that there is expectation on myself and from other people that well you've been through shit before, you're hard, you're strong, you'll get through it and be fine.
>
> *(Jo, 47, embolic stroke as a result of endocarditis, 20 years post stroke)*

Relationship challenges can be related to the stroke survivors' behaviours and changes in personality, mood swings, frustration with their own ability, and the need for constant help and support in trivial tasks, such as doing up a button or tying a shoelace. Survivors can often become frustrated with their own limitations and the subsequent dependence on others and take such frustrations out on loved ones, leading to minor annoyances becoming big issues if left to fester (Fugl-Meyer *et al.*, 2019).

> He would talk about how 'I' was during that period (after stroke) and in my head I am thinking he never acknowledged to me that was happening, he never spoke to me about how I was losing it and I was in so much pain. But I've heard him telling other people that she is really tough she is, and she's dealt with loads.
>
> *(Jacqueline, 42, ischaemic stroke whilst pregnant, 12 years post stroke)*

> I said to a friend the other day ... can you just cheerlead me because I am doing my best ... just getting through the day ... and then I am exhausted.
>
> *(Jo, 47, embolic stroke as a result of endocarditis, 20 years post stroke)*

Any pre-existing relationship challenges before the stroke can sometimes be amplified afterwards, and it may not be possible to help families work through such historical challenges, as they are already embedded in the relationship and the 'norm' for that individual and their family. However, there are opportunities for families to take stock of the situation and re-evaluate what is important to them as a family, allowing them to work through past differences and grow together as a family (McGrath *et al.*, 2019).

…one day I had a little falling out with my son over something and nothing, and I realised I had a little breakdown… I had a mental health doctor to talk to me properly. Not only me, with the family, which gave us some kind of understanding why I am like that, because the behaviour wasn't me. That helped everybody, I think.

(Jacqueline, 42, ischaemic stroke whilst pregnant,
12 years post stroke)

Communication is an important part of any relationship, and aphasia following a stroke can impact existing relationships but also provide a challenge to the development of new relationships (Stroke Association, no date).

I'm missing the human interaction. I'm missing the social interaction massively… I'm quite happy being by myself and getting on with things. But I do need that interaction.

I've not been with anyone or seen anyone (romantically) for three years, ever since I had the stroke. I'm still a youngish guy and I still want to have some kind of relationship, and I don't have that, and I was a bit of, not a ladies man, but at a bar if I get the look from an attractive lady… I would saunter up and have a go… I can't do that any more.

(Alan, 50, ischemic stroke, 4 years post stroke)

I am a member of a group in the pub, every Wednesday with 8 or 9 people, an aphasia group, and it's fantastic and we have lunch and things and I am laughing, I really enjoy myself.

(Jeremy, 69, haemorrhagic stroke, 13 years post stroke)

Family as caregivers/carers

Figure 10.2 outlines the domains from the Burden Assessment Schedule used to estimate the impact on carers of young stroke survivors in the study from Aghoram *et al.* (2024). This study identified that it was interpersonal relationships in the 'Marital relationships' and 'Impact on relations with others' that were the most significant burden for carers.

The NHS (2024) acknowledges that caring for someone means that the carer will be a big part of a stroke survivor's recovery/life, whilst also stating that it can be frustrating, lonely and difficult, recommending to carers that they should access support.

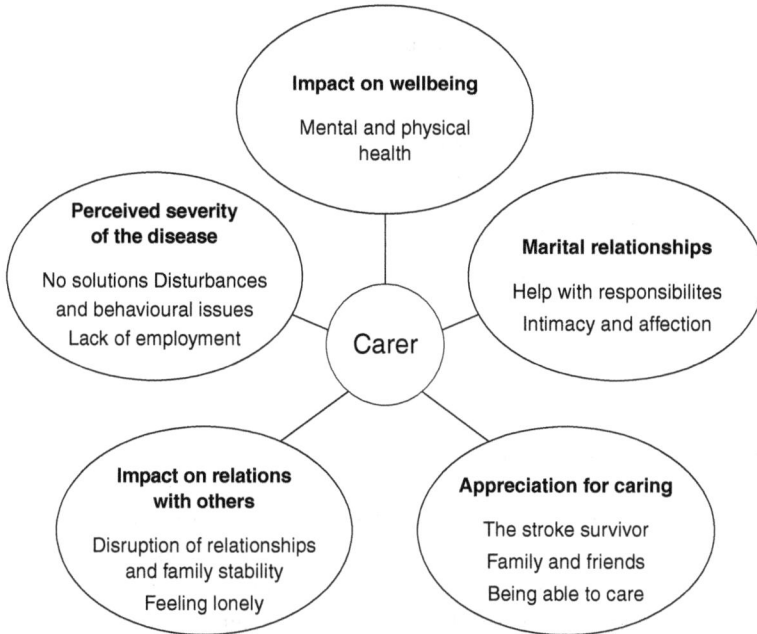

FIGURE 10.2   Carer impact domains from Burden Assessment Schedule.

I don't think I was thinking about myself at that point and how it was affecting me, I was just focused on Malcolm, just doing what I could to help him. Thinking back, I know I must have eaten, but I don't remember cooking anything for myself at all. I was literally on autopilot, because I was still trying to work as well.

(Gill, 71, partner to Malcolm, 80, bilateral thalamic infarct,
14 years post stroke)

Support from healthcare professional (HCPs) for loved ones who become a 'carer' is outlined in guidance (ISWP, 2023).

1. If agreed, HCPs should establish from the stroke survivor the extent of how a family member becomes involved in their care, and would act as a 'carer'
2. Family should be involved in significant decisions as an additional source of information about the person – clinically and socially
3. Educational programmes should be provided for the primary carer which:
   • provide clear information on stroke and dealing with post-stroke issues
   • teach them how to provide care and support, and provide opportunities to practise giving care
   • provide advice on secondary prevention

4. When transferred from hospital, the carer of the stroke survivor should be offered:
   - an assessment of their own needs
   - practical or emotional support
   - guidance on how to seek help
5. The stroke survivor's carer should be provided with the contact details of a named HCP who can provide further support
6. The carer should be reassessed whenever there is a significant change and be shown how to seek further help and support

Identity and self-image

For the stroke survivor and their loved ones, there are physical, emotional and social changes to adjust to, such as role responsibilities, isolation, and a loss of sense of closeness. Loss of role is notably affected in relation to employment abilities, managing finances and maintaining family and social networks. Fugl-Meyer *et al.* (2019) reported partners and loved ones of stroke survivors felt additional pressures to be the substitute parent – the main source of income whilst maintaining the stability of family life.

> When I had my stroke and I had to give up my full-time job, there was a lot of upset, it's a loss isn't it. When I started doing things, like expert by experience work, it felt like I am being able to use my skills from what I had as a professional and my (stroke) experience.
> *(Jo, 47, embolic stroke as a result of endocarditis, 20 years post stroke)*

> I feel everything has changed. I couldn't drive, I couldn't work, selling my house, I had a plan. I had a great job and the money was amazing, and you don't worry... I had a lovely family but some of my friends have left me.
> *(Kelly, 55, ischaemic stroke, 8 years post stroke)*

The effects of stroke can disrupt important strands of personal and social worlds that contribute to individual identity or 'self' of a stroke survivor. This can result in disruption across the key areas used by a stroke survivor to define who they are (Figure 10.3). They may need to face the loss of a previous sense of self and have to make adjustments through rebuilding a new or modified identity (Hall *et al.*, 2024). This in turn will impact the relationships with others in their life. The attempt to rebuild 'self' is also acknowledged as influencing the rehabilitation process (Da Costa Pato *et al.*, 2022); therefore, it is important for HCPs to understand how the individual has been impacted physically, emotionally and socially by their individual experience.

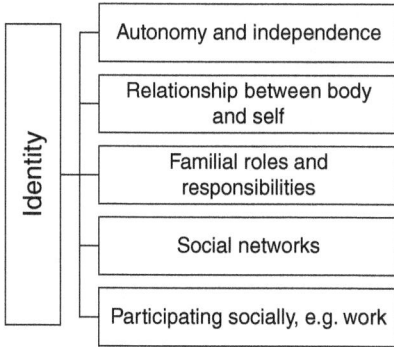

FIGURE 10.3 Elements of identity that may be disrupted by stroke.
Source: Hall *et al.* (2024).

As an example of this change in identity, a stroke survivor talks about what he wants in a potential partner:

> I want someone to be caring, more than I did previously, I liked the chase, and someone to give me a bit of hard time every now and again, but that's changed now, and I want someone a bit more caring.
>
> *(Alan, 50, ischaemic stroke, 4 years post stroke)*

Body image

Body image is also commonly impacted following a stroke (ISWP, 2023). This relates to how we see ourselves and how we feel we appear to others. The stroke survivor's disability can affect the 'self' with negative associations, which can result in anxiety and depression. As identity changes, this affects both the individual and their loved ones, this can generate a sense of 'threat' to the restoring of identity (Da Costa Pato *et al.*, 2022). If an attempt to restore identity fails, a mechanism adjustment is triggered, and a period of mourning for identity loss occurs with effort to rebuild a new 'self'. The attempt to rebuild 'self' can influence the rehabilitation process (Da Costa Pato *et al.*, 2022).

Therefore, it is important for HCPs to understand how an individual stroke survivor's body image may be individually impacted. The ISWP (2023) recommend that stroke survivors whose rehabilitation engagement and motivation appear reduced should be assessed for changes in identity and mood, self-efficacy or self-esteem. If there are significant changes in these characteristics, the stroke survivor should be offered support, advice and information, and be considered for psychological interventions, such as:

- increased social interaction.
- increased exercise.
- other psychosocial interventions, such as psychosocial education groups (ISWP, 2023)

Body image is multi-dimensional, with roots in identity, self-esteem and self-worth. On a basic level, if someone is happy with their physical appearance or body image, they are more likely to experience positive feelings of self-esteem. In contrast, a person who is unhappy with their physical appearance could have negative feelings regarding themselves. Self-esteem is related to the sense of personal value through acceptance and validation as a sexually desirable person. A stroke survivor can feel differently about their body image because of their altered physical function or emotions (Stott *et al.*, 2021).

There are many socio-cultural pressures relating to self-image and body image. These may be contributed to by a variety of sources, including family, friends and the media. Society could be seen to place significant value on physical appearance. It influences how a person is perceived by others and valued by them, and how people value themselves (Davidson, 2024). Stroke survivors may feel less valued than they did previously as a response to the physical and psychological changes experienced. This might include someone left with reduced mobility which now requires them to use a walking stick or wheelchair.

This stroke survivor echoes such feelings, which are felt by many,

> I can't see anybody wanting to be with a disabled person... the numbness on my right side means I've needed to adapt to how I live day to day... so, I totally understand if men don't find me physically – like, sexually attractive anymore, because I'm disabled and a burden.
>
> *(Anonymous female, 66, 2 years post stroke)*

A model was developed to help understand how body image might be perceived (Price, 1990). This model can also help to make sense of the altered body image being experienced by a stroke survivor. The model comprises three concepts (Figure 10.4): body ideal, body reality and body presentation, and can support the assessment of people with stroke to understand where they are in their journey towards recovery. This can offer focus on how they can continue to adapt and adjust to their new ways of living.

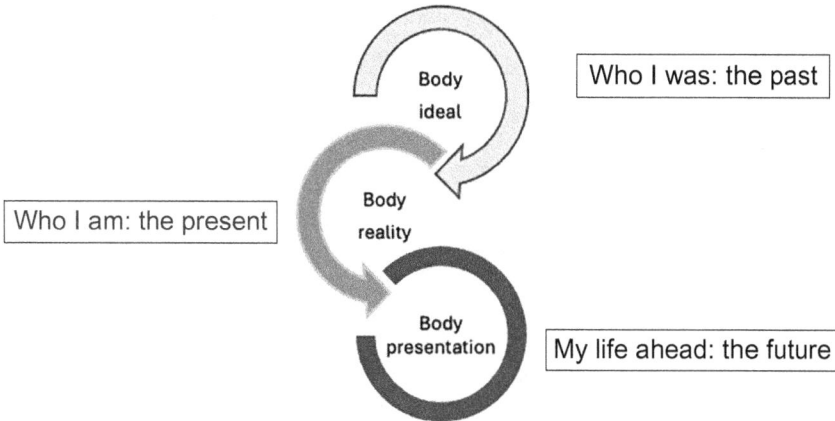

FIGURE 10.4 Body image illustrating the rehabilitative journey of the stroke survivor.
Source: Adapted from Price (1990).

The body ideal reflects how the individual would like their body to be and who they were in the past. For the stroke survivor, much of the research around lived experience refers to wishing to be as they once were, fully able and independent (Stott *et al.*, 2021), as described by this stroke survivor.

> I get very frustrated now I can't use my right hand or stand for long periods. I think back to my younger days and how active I was… if only… my wife and I share happy memories of those times as I try to come to terms with my 'new' way of living. It's tough. Just a constant feeling of loss with helplessness.
> *(Male, 70, 3 years post stroke)*

However, a specific definition for body image in stroke survivors has also been suggested (Davidson, 2024) (Figure 10.5). This acknowledges that there is variability in how stroke survivors will define their body image, identifying with some, though perhaps not all, of the outlined elements.

Body reality can relate to how the body is perceived by the individual; who am I or who have I become? For the stroke survivor, this will differ greatly depending on the area of the brain affected and its severity. In most cases, one side of the body is overtly affected. There may be complete paralysis (hemiplegia) or weakness (hemiparesis), which might involve the face, arms and/or legs, and might also affect abdominal and chest wall muscles. In severe cases, at rest, these problems are apparent through their effects, particularly on the face, where there may be lack of expression or drooling. In addition, a shoulder or limb might appear drooped or floppy, or the whole body might appear twisted or lopsided. These are all visible realities of a stroke; however, strokes may also cause changes to vision, perception, cognition, personality, mood and emotional expression which may not be immediately obvious to those who do not know the person.

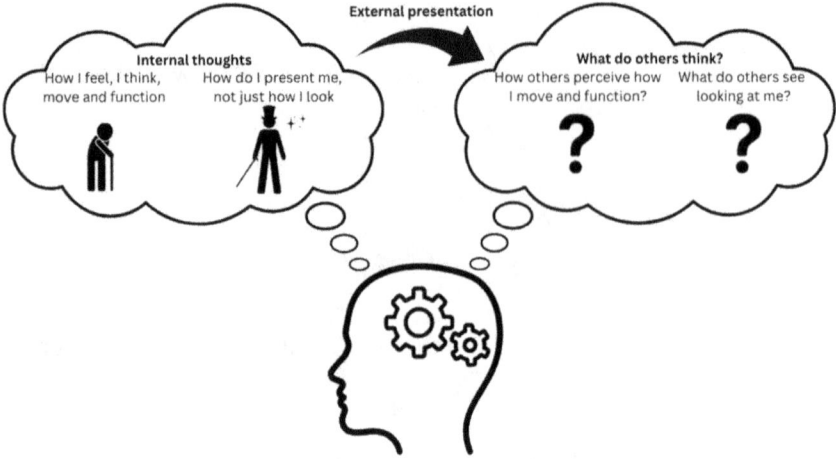

FIGURE 10.5 Stroke survivor specific definition for body image.

Source: Davidson (2024).

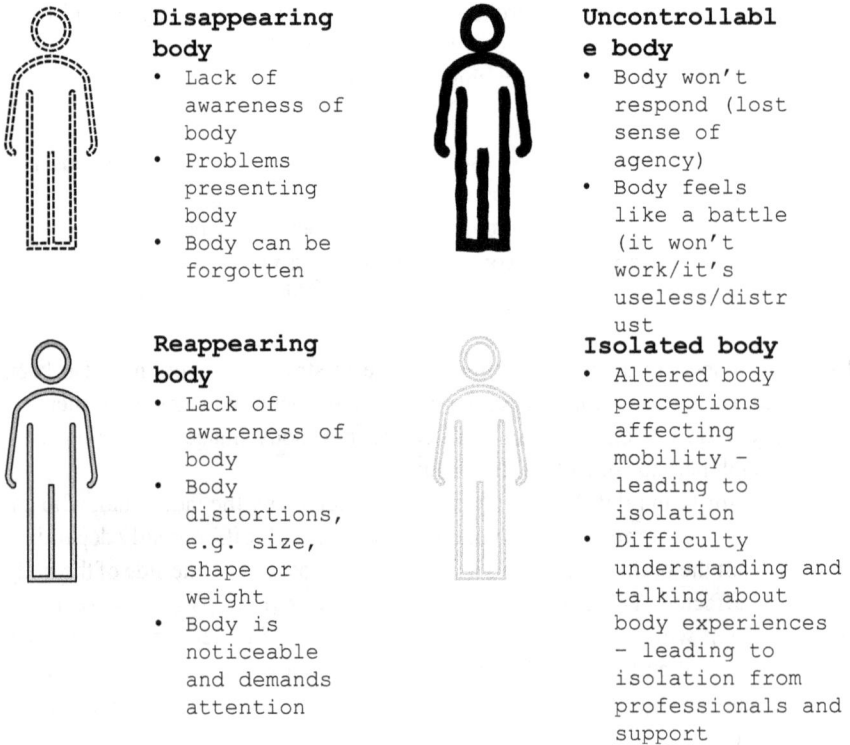

Disappearing body
- Lack of awareness of body
- Problems presenting body
- Body can be forgotten

Reappearing body
- Lack of awareness of body
- Body distortions, e.g. size, shape or weight
- Body is noticeable and demands attention

Uncontrollable body
- Body won't respond (lost sense of agency)
- Body feels like a battle (it won't work/it's useless/distrust

Isolated body
- Altered body perceptions affecting mobility – leading to isolation
- Difficulty understanding and talking about body experiences – leading to isolation from professionals and support

FIGURE 10.6 Stroke survivors' experiences of their 'body'.

Source: Stott *et al.* (2021).

Stott *et al.* (2021) outlined four themes which reflect shared body experiences (Figure 10.6). This research also identified that stroke survivors' body experiences were difficult to understand and communicate to healthcare staff.

Many stroke survivors are in a position of being unable to conceal their body reality. This can lead to a lack of healthy body confidence, which can result in a perception of their bodies being unfamiliar and unreliable, making the survivor feel fragile and vulnerable. This can have a profound impact on rehabilitation, as illustrated by this stroke survivor:

> I still feel like a freak. I just don't like going anywhere where I'm well known, and I feel now I'm not walking properly, and you know it's a funny feeling… It makes me wonder what others are thinking… which of course I don't know, but that's the thing, I just feel to myself and think, oh poor thing, and I don't like to feel that I'm like that. I mean, I still feel I want to be like I was before and I don't know whether I will. Not like I can cover it up, it's pretty obvious what's happened to me.
>
> *(Male, 65, 1 year post stroke)*

Some impacts of stroke can be concealed, e.g., whilst sitting by careful positioning, but as the person attempts to use or move the affected parts, the full extent of the problem becomes clear. It should be noted that brain damage can lead to a distorted sense of body representation, which can impact the planning, preparation and performance of movements. This might include standing up straight, maintaining balance, lifting the affected arm with the other or maybe pulling the affected leg in front of the other. Even if walking is manageable, muscles not normally required might be utilised to achieve a forward motion, which would contribute to an abnormal gait. There may be a lack of facial expressions, making communication difficult; there may be difficulties with smiling, swallowing or dribbling saliva.

Following a stroke, an individual enters a completely new world, experiencing fundamental psychological as well as physical challenges. The body becomes something foreign and separate from the self, essentially unfamiliar (Stott *et al.*, 2021). Some activities previously enjoyed no longer offer as much pleasure, and even when specific activities have been re-mastered by stroke survivors, the social meaning is lost. The realisation that no cure is available can come as a shock. It is perplexing when the body is no longer fully functioning, or if the individual does not understand why they have had a stroke. Once the stroke survivor returns home, they gradually build up a working relationship with their bodies; however, maintaining the status quo requires constant effort and concentration. The task of restoring the self-body split continues for most respondents in the face of the emotional, social and physical consequences of a changed body.

Download and read this article.

Stott *et al.* (2021) 'Somebody stuck me in a bag of sand': Lived experiences of the altered and uncomfortable body after stroke – PubMed Clinical Rehabilitation. 35(9), 1348–1359.

- What are the key points you can take away from the study's findings?
- How do the participants of this study resonate with the Price (1990) body image model (Figure 10.4)?
- Knowing this is how many stroke survivors feel about their new normality, how might you change your current practice?

Forster *et al.* (2014) identified that for stroke survivors who achieved meaningful recovery, adjustment and acceptance, the goal was not to return to their pre-stroke lives. Instead, recovery was about managing loss and creating a new, meaningful life. Conversely, those who experienced ongoing disruption tended to focus on trying to return to their pre-stroke bodies and lives. This finding challenges the traditional understanding in existing literature, which often links post-stroke recovery to the extent to which survivors can re-establish continuity with their previous selves and lives. This study suggests that stroke survivors develop varied understandings of what recovery entails, indicating a need for a more nuanced concept of recovery in the stroke literature and practice. Moreover, the findings indicate that meaningful recovery involves not just continuity with the past self, but also adapting to losses and creatively building new aspects of identity and life. For some, this process goes beyond merely reconnecting with their pre-stroke identity and existence.

Sexuality

The expression of human sexuality and body image are virtually inseparable within both health and illness (Das and Raman, 2019), with sexuality expressed throughout a life span. Sexuality encompasses much more than the physical act of intercourse, involving instead the totality of human being. Stroke has a profound impact on how sexuality is experienced by both the stoke survivor and partner due to changes in couples' interdependence and the relational ramifications (Abendschein *et al.*, 2021).

Each stroke survivor will have complex and individually experienced social circumstances, identity, coping strategies, sexuality and spiritual beliefs. All these factors are in addition to living with a stroke, involving adjustment and adaptation. The stroke survivor needs to come to terms with anxieties and concerns with body image, self-esteem, attractiveness, sexuality and fertility, and in some cases disclosure (Kniepmann and Kerr, 2018; McGrath *et al.*, 2019). The psychological and physical issues following a stroke can impact role identity and relationships with sexual partners, and sexual dysfunction can amplify these problems (ISWP, 2023).

Reports of sexual dysfunction following stroke are common. Among several surveys, declines in sexual activity have been reported (Stein *et al.*, 2013; Song *et al.*, 2011; Mountain *et al.*, 2020). Participants of one of the studies were given the support and opportunity to ask questions and were provided with tips to enhance sexual function. These individuals were ultimately more sexually active and experienced greater sexual satisfaction following stroke (Stein *et al.*, 2013).

Studies have demonstrated that as people age, their frequency of sexual activities declines. This has been identified as related to physical and psychosocial issues, including erectile dysfunction in men and lack of lubrication, inability to climax and reduced desire in women (Lindau *et al.*, 2007). However, the same study and others (Siegel *et al.*, 2021) demonstrated that some people continue to have intercourse, oral sex and masturbate into their eightieth and ninetieth years – so, ensuring stroke survivors are supported to re-engage with this activity, if desired, is important. Undiagnosed, or untreated sexual problems, can lead to depression or social withdrawal, as well as affecting relationships with intimate partners.

Following stroke, cranial nerve function can be affected. It has been demonstrated that olfactory nerve function, in particular, has a significant impact on sexual activity. The sense of smell plays an important role in sexual motivation and arousal. Decreased olfactory function has been associated with reduced sexual motivation and less emotional satisfaction with sex. However, this does not seem to decrease the frequency of sexual activity or the enjoyment of sex (Siegel *et al.*, 2021). Therefore, if a patient presents with concern regarding sexual motivation, an olfactory nerve assessment should be considered. Table 10.1 provides an overview of potential issues relating to physical intimacy for stroke survivors.

Sexuality and disability are still regarded as a taboo subject (McGrath *et al.*, 2019), with studies referring to stroke survivors being silenced or muted in such conversations even though they seek HCP support (Kniepmann and Kerr, 2018). Stroke survivors may also wish to discuss the changes to pre-stroke relationships,

TABLE 10.1 Stroke and sexual dysfunction

Male	*Female*
Increased erectile dysfunction	Reduced vaginal lubrication
Ejaculation difficulties	
Little or no orgasm	
Reduced arousal and satisfaction	
Decreased libido	
Reduced coital frequency	
Fear of another stroke during intercourse	
Depression	
Physical difficulties	
Decreased sense of smell	
Fatigue	
Avoidance, e.g., due to fear of increase in blood pressure	

Sources: Taman *et al.* (2008), Stein *et al.* (2013), Low *et al.* (2022).

changed relationship with the stroke survivor's own body and resuming sexual intimacy as they adapt to their loss (Kniepmann and Kerr, 2018).

Rehabilitation HCPs are not always comfortable or prepared to deal with sexuality and sexual function (Contrada *et al.*, 2023), with unmet psychological and sexuality-related care needs reported (Das and Raman, 2019). Despite the improvements across assessment, management and rehabilitation for stroke survivors, there are still unresolved clinical support issues related to sexuality that remain a concern for stroke survivors (Contrada *et al.*, 2023).

In their systematic review, McGrath *et al.* (2019) highlighted several initiatives and new evidence underscoring the critical role of sexual function restoration in rehabilitation, emphasising that it is as important to functional recovery as any other aspect.

> ...(I have) strong views on not allowing disability to prevent a good and healthy sex life and feels this has been positive factor in (how she views herself as) a disabled woman in her forties.
> *(Jacqueline, 42, ischaemic stroke whilst pregnant, 12 years post stroke)*

Bugnicourt *et al.* (2014) found that over one-third of younger patients reported difficulties with sexual activity 1 year after experiencing an ischaemic stroke. According to Low *et al.* (2022), the prevalence of sexual dysfunctions after a stroke ranges from 20% to 75%, largely due to the varying degrees of disability described by stroke survivors.

> My experience is that orgasm can lead to the weak side responding in a dramatic way i.e. heightening all effects of stroke, retract arm, slurred speech, so it can appear that a new stroke has taken place and this was scary at first and took time to get used to.
> *(Jo, 47, embolic stroke as a result of endocarditis, 20 years post stroke)*

As shown in Table 10.1, there are a variety of issues causing sexual dysfunction. After a stroke, reduced libido is particularly common, with reported rates of decreased sexual desire (Stein *et al.*, 2013). There is a notable decline in sexual activity, with only 28% of stroke survivors engaging in sexual activity 2–6 months post stroke (Nilsson *et al.*, 2017). Studies suggest the prevalence of erectile dysfunction among stroke patients is significantly higher than in the general population (Bugnicourt *et al.*, 2014; Contrada *et al.*, 2023). In addition, sociodemographic factors such as ageing, low income and high education levels can influence the development of sexual dysfunction in stroke patients. Gender does not appear to be a determining factor (Nilsson *et al.*, 2017).

Sexual dysfunction is commonly due to damage to the central nervous system areas controlling sexual behaviour, and the autonomic nervous system determining erectile dysfunction. For example, strokes in the right cerebellum might be associated with ejaculation disorders, while erectile dysfunction may be more frequent in patients with stroke in the middle cerebral artery territory, in the right hemisphere versus left hemisphere (Low *et al.*, 2022).

Post-stroke sexual dysfunction may also be influenced by psychological issues, such as anxiety or mood disorders, prior medical conditions such as hypertension or diabetes, or the use of particular medications to address these issues (McGrath *et al.*, 2019; Low *et al.*, 2022). Key factors include the use of angiotensin-converting enzyme (ACE) inhibitors and depression (Bugnicourt *et al.*, 2014; Nilsson *et al.*, 2017). Therefore, it is important that these aspects are considered during the rehabilitation phase, as there is a tendency to think that motor or cognitive problems are more significant. It is therefore important to consider the physical, psychological and behavioural changes that follow a stroke in terms of their potential to impair sexual function, during the acute and long-term rehabilitation phases (Contrada *et al.*, 2023). Low *et al.* (2022) recently identified that only 23% (*n* = 216 out of 958) of stroke rehabilitation professionals directly initiate conversations about sex with their patients. They demonstrated that sexuality education, religious affiliation, age of professionals and availability of programmes for sexuality rehabilitation predicted comfort in addressing this issue.

Information about sexual activity after a stroke is an area that rehabilitation facilities can undervalue. Prior *et al.* (2019) reported that over 30% of stroke survivors would have wanted to receive information about post-stroke sexual behaviour; however, only a small percentage of participants within the study (8.2%) received it. This study focused on creating new health education material that was authentic for the stroke survivors from immediately after the event through to the rehabilitation phase, with the emphasis on educating and reassuring the patient right from the start.

Studies have highlighted that whenever sex and disability are discussed during the counselling of a stroke patient, it is solely in terms of capacity, technique and fertility, and there is no reference to sexual feelings (Kautz and Van Horn, 2017; Prior *et al.*, 2019). Despite often being overlooked and underreported, it is essential to recognise the challenges that stroke patients encounter when seeking help for sexual difficulties. Patients frequently cite the predominance of neurological symptoms, the presence of family or friends during medical appointments, and the lack of inquiry from HCPs as the most common barriers to discussing sexual concerns (Stein *et al.*, 2013; McGrath *et al.*, 2019; Low *et al.*, 2022). This evidence is recognised by stroke survivors themselves, as illustrated by the following:

My wife asked the doctor before I was discharged for advice as to whether we could continue with intercourse, and we were told to speak to our GP; they were not interested in giving us advice in the hospital, By the time we saw the doctor we realised all was ok and continued with our life. But we wish we have had been reassured in the hospital. It is very important that this is discussed.

(Male, age 62, 3 years post stroke)

I think this subject is very important because I lost sexual drive after stroke which split my family up. My wife went somewhere else for sex, so she said that (she) doesn't need me anymore and kicked me out.

(Male, 54 years, 2 years post stroke)

Wider conversations are required, covering more than just the physical act of sexual intercourse and physical issues (Kautz and Van Horn, 2017; Nilsson *et al.*, 2017). This might include assessing other aspects of sexuality such as self-esteem, identity of sexual orientation, reproduction, intimacy, eroticism and sexual communication, inclusive of both physical and psychological aspects of sexual functioning (Song *et al.*, 2011). These conversations may require advanced communication skills and specialist training, which may not be easily accessible.

Read each of the expert by experience narratives within this chapter again and reflect upon what they are telling you as an HCP.

Consider

1. What are common themes amongst them?
2. What specific terms are used to describe recovery; it is positive or negative?
3. What can you learn from these experiences?
4. What are the key factors related to sexuality, intimacy and body image for the HCP to consider when supporting stroke survivors?

Although limited, some stroke survivors report positive changes in their sexuality, which they attribute to feelings of increased intimacy as a result of the changes in their relationships (Nilsson *et al.*, 2017).

It then takes a certain about of time to return to normal, so as you can imagine that requires great sensitivity from the person you are having sex with – but within the comfort of a good relationship and knowing its 'normal' it can also be a comical at times.

(Jo, 47, embolic stroke as a result of endocarditis, 20 years post stroke)

It is also acknowledged that regaining intimacy with a partner can positively impact self-esteem and quality of life and strengthen partner relationships (ISWP, 2023).

Strategies that can be suggested to improve partner intimacy following stroke can include:

- Managing unwanted negative changes, such as actively trying to adapt by planning time with a partner and decreasing pressure, anxiety and stress
- Open communication about emotions and sexuality with a partner
- Accessing a range of information to better understand how intimacy can be sustained and developed
- Encourage the exploration of alternative sexual positions to support physical adaptability and maintain intimacy
- Accessing counselling concerning intimacy and sexuality concerns (Nilsson *et al.*, 2017; Stroke Association, no date)

Support for sexuality

Clinicians supporting stroke survivors with sexual dysfunction should have a broad knowledge of neuroanatomy and physiology as well as the psychological and socio-relational issues involved in human sexuality and sexual function (Contrada *et al.*, 2023). Soon after discharge from hospital, at 6-month and annual reviews, stroke survivors should be asked if they have any concerns about sex, with partners also offered the opportunity to raise any concerns (ISWP, 2023). Understanding these issues as part of an assessment and rehabilitation process provides holistic, person-centred care (Contrada *et al.*, 2023). Specific considerations and areas of exploration for assessments should include:

- Sexual partnerships history: discuss the last 12 months, including frequency of sexual activity and participation in particular activities such as vaginal intercourse, oral sex and masturbation. If an individual has not had sex in the previous 3 months, explore why.
- Presence of sexual problems: explore interest, arousal, ability to orgasm, pain and satisfaction levels. If there are issues, how long have they been present? Are they purely 'post-stroke' issues? Explore the use of alternative sexual positions.
- Cranial nerve issues: particularly focussing on smell, taste and touch.
- Past medical history: including hypertension, diabetes, joint pain, arthritis.
- Drug history: is the individual taking any medications which could affect their sexual activity, e.g. blood pressure medications. Studies suggest that patients

may discontinue their tablets if they have side effects which detrimentally affect their sex lives (Lindau *et al.*, 2007).

• Consider a referral to a professional with expertise in psychosexual problems if sexual dysfunction persists (ISWP, 2023).

Partner perspective

McGrath *et al.* (2019) found that, for most couples, the functional impairments resulting from a stroke fundamentally altered the nature of their pre-existing relationship. These changes were driven by shifts in the dynamics between stroke survivors and their partners, as well as the survivors' altered relationship with their own bodies, some of which is illustrated by this stroke survivor:

> The feeling is that I miss my husband. I need a shoulder to lean on, someone to talk to, and someone who comforts me. I just don't have that ... maybe there are moments of loneliness.
>
> *(Anonymous, female spouse)*

A strong interpersonal relationship after stroke is important for the wellbeing of survivors and their family caregivers.

> The reality is over the years our co-dependence in different ways has caused issues, but it has also brought us closer together, and we couldn't be without each other.
>
> *(J, 75, stroke survivor and D, 78, partner, ischaemic stroke 15 years ago)*

A multidisciplinary approach to supporting the stroke survivor and their family is needed. Collaborative working requires nurses, physiotherapy, occupational therapy, social work medical support, psychology and counselling to come together with a goal to balance differing needs so that the relationship can remain strong and outcomes for both stroke survivor and partner can be enriched.

It is important for HCPs to provide encouragement and support for exploration of sexual function (ISWP, 2023). Kniepmann and Kerr (2018) suggest that embarrassment and awkwardness are commonly reported by stroke survivors and their partners as reasons to avoid sexual relations and closeness. Such feelings can make the partner feel uncomfortable, not wishing to cause further harm and feelings of neglect and a loveless relationship by the stroke survivor. This can result in a decrease in intimacy and sexuality, which can be associated with a reduced quality of life for both partners (Fugl-Meyer *et al.*, 2019).

If stroke survivors and their partners experience embarrassment about issues linked to intimacy and sexuality, they could be resistant to discussions with HCPs. Signposting to resources offering information about relationships, intimacy and sexuality could be offered instead.

Stroke Association website:
www.stroke.org.uk/stroke/life-after/sex-and-relationships

Different Strokes website:
https://differentstrokes.co.uk/stroke-information/sex-and-relationships/

American Stroke Association website:
www.stroke.org/en/about-stroke/effects-of-stroke/emotional-effects/intimacy-after-stroke

Australian Stroke Foundation website:
https://strokefoundation.org.au/what-we-do/for-survivors-and-carers/after-stroke-factsheets/sex-intimacy-and-relationships-after-stroke-fact-sheet

Canadian Guide for Stroke Recovery:
www.strokerecovery.guide/topics/getting-back-into-life/sex-and-intimacy/

Springrose website:
www.springrose.co/blogs/blog/sex-positions-for-stroke-survivors

Disability Horizons website:
https://disabilityhorizons.com/category/disabled-dating-relationships-and-sex/

Future research could specifically focus on understanding how rehabilitation services for stroke survivors and their families should be delivered to optimise post-stroke rehabilitation in relation to body image, sexuality and relationships.

Conclusion

This chapter has highlighted some of the relationship and intimacy challenges faced by stroke survivors and the importance of communication between all parties involved. Although issues connected to relationships, intimacy and sexuality may not be routinely considered as part of assessment, or supported effectively with stroke survivors, these issues continue to be important to the stroke survivor and their loved ones.

References

Abendschein, B., Basinger, E.D., and Wehrman, E.C. (2021) Struggling together: examining the narratives of interdependence and healing within romantic relationships after stroke. *Qualitative Health Research* 31(7), 1275–1289. https://doi.org/10.1177/1049732321 1004101

Aghoram, R., Priya, D.I., and Narayan, S.K. (2024) Burden of caregiving for young stroke survivors in the community: a cross-sectional study. *Journal of Stroke Medicine*, 7(1), 45–51.

American Stroke Association (2025) *Intimacy After Stroke.* Available at: www.stroke.org/en/about-stroke/effects-of-stroke/emotional-effects/intimacy-after-stroke

Bugnicourt, J.M., Hamy, O., Canaple, S., Lamy, C., and Legrand, C. (2014) Impaired sexual activity in young ischaemic stroke patients: an observational study. *European Journal of Neurology* 21(1), 140–146.

Contrada, M., Cerasa, A., Pucci, C., Ciancarelli, I., Pioggia, G., Tonin, P., and Salvatore Calabrò, R. (2023) Talking about sexuality in stroke individuals: the new era of sexual rehabilitation. *Journal of Clinical Medicine* 12, 3988. https://doi.org/10.3390/jcm1 2123988

Da Costa Pato, M.I.C., Ferreira, J.P., and Douglas, K. (2022) Body awareness, self-identity, and perception of exercise importance after stroke rehabilitation. *Advances in Orthopaedics and Sport Medicine* 2022(4), 1–7.

Das, K., and Raman, R. (2019) 'Mirror, mirror, on the wall… who is the fairest of them all?' – Body image and its role in sexual health. *Journal of Psychosexual Health* 1(3–4), 227–235. https://doi.org/10.1177/2631831819890778

Davidson, C. (2024) *Understanding and Defining People's Body Image Experiences After a Stroke.* DPhil Thesis. Available at: https://clok.uclan.ac.uk/49286/1/Catherine%20David son%2C%20G20751130%2C%20Minor%20Amendments%2C%2030.05.23.pdf

Forster, A., Mellish, K., Farrin, A., *et al.* (2014) Chapter 5 Project 4: adjustment after stroke study. *Development and Evaluation of Tools and an Intervention to Improve Patient and Carer Outcomes in Longer Term Stroke and Exploration of Adjustment Post Stroke: The LoTS Care Research Programme.* Southampton UK: NIHR Journals Library. Available at: www.ncbi.nlm.nih.gov/books/NBK269104/

Fugl-Meyer, K. S., Nilsson, M.I., Von Koch, L., and Ytterberg, C. (2019) Closeness and life satisfaction after six years for persons with stroke and spouses. *Journal of Rehabilitation Medicine* 51(7), 492–498.

Hall, J., van Wijck, F., Kroll, T., and Bassil-Morozow, H. (2024) Stroke and liminality: narratives of reconfiguring identity after stroke and their implications for person-centred stroke care. *Frontiers in Rehabilitation Sciences* 5, 1477414.

Intercollegiate Stroke Working Party (ISWP) (2023) *National Clinical Guideline for Stroke for the United Kingdom and Northern Ireland.* 5th Edition. Available at: www.strokegu ideline.org

Kautz, D.D., and Van Horn, E.R. (2017) Sex and intimacy after stroke. *Rehabilitation Nurse* 42, 333–340.

Kniepmann, K., and Kerr, S. (2018) Sexuality and intimacy following a stroke: perspectives of partners. *Sexuality and Disability* 36, 219–230. https://doi.org/10.1007/s11 195-018-9531-2

Lindau, S., Schumm, M., Laumann, E., Levinson, M., O'Muircheartaigh, C., and Waite, L. (2007) A study of sexuality and health among older adults in the United States. *New England Journal of Medicine* 357(8), 762–774.

Low, M.A., Power, E., and McGrath, M. (2022) Sexuality after stroke: exploring knowledge, attitudes, comfort and behaviours of rehabilitation professionals. *Annuals of Physical and Rehabilitation Medicine* 65(2), 101547. https://doi.org/10.1016/j.rehab.2021.101547

McCarthy, M.J., Lyons, K.S., Schellinger, J., Stapleton, K., and Bakas, T. (2020) Interpersonal relationship challenges among stroke survivors and family caregivers. *Social Work in Health Care* 59(2), 91–107. https://doi.org/10.1080/00981389.2020.1714827

McGrath, M., Lever, S., McCluskey, A., and Power, E. (2019) How is sexuality after stroke experienced by stroke survivors and partners of stroke survivors? A systematic review of qualitative studies. *Clinical Rehabilitation* 33(2), 293–303. https://doi.org/10.1177/ 0269215518793483

Mountain, A., Lindsay, M.P., Teasell, R., Salbach, N.M., *et al.* (2020) Canadian Stroke best practice recommendations: rehabilitation, recovery and community participation following stroke. Part 2 Transitions and community participant following stroke. *International Journal of Stroke* 15(7), 789–806. https://doi.org/10.1177/174749301 9897847

NHS (2024) *Recovering from a Stroke*. Available at: www.nhs.uk/conditions/stroke/ recovery/

Nilsson, M.I., Fugl-Meyer, K., von Kock, L., and Ytterberg, C. (2017) Experiences of sexuality six years after stroke: a qualitative study. *The Journal of Sexual Medicine* 14, 797–803. http://creativecommons.org/licenses/by-nc-nd/4.0/

Price, B. (1990) *Body Image – Nursing Concepts and Care*. London: Prentice Hall.

Prior, S., Reeves, N., Peterson, G., Jaffray, L., and Campbell, S. (2019) Addressing the gaps post-stroke sexual activity rehabilitation: patients' perspectives. *Healthcare* 7(25), 1–7. https://doi.org/10.3390/healthcare7010025

Siegel, J., Kung, S., Wroblewski, K., Kern, D., McClintock, M., and Pinto, J. (2021) Olfaction is associated with sexual motivation and satisfaction in older men and women. *Journal of Sexual Medicine* 18(2):295–302.

Song, H., Oh, H., Kim, H., *et al.* (2011) Effects of sexual rehabilitation intervention programme on stroke patients and their spouses. *Neuro-Rehabilitation* 28, 143–150.

Stein, J., Hillinger, M., Clancy, C., and Bishop, L. (2013) Sexuality after stroke: patient counselling preferences. *Disability Rehabilitation* 35, 1842–1847.

Stott, H., Cramp, M., McClean, S., and Turton, A. (2021) Somebody stuck me in a bag of sand: lived experience of the altered and uncomfortable body after stroke. *Clinical Rehabilitation* 35(9), 1348–1359.

Stroke Association (no date) *Effects of Stroke*. Available at: www.stroke.org.uk/stroke/ effects

Suksatan, W., Collins, C.J., Koontalay, A., and Posai, V. (2022) Burdens among familial caregivers of stroke survivors: a literature review. *Working with Older People* 26(1), 37–43.

Taman, Y., Taman, L., Akil, E., Yasan, A., and Taman, B. (2008) Post-stroke sexual functioning in first stroke patients. *European Journal of Neurology* 15(7), 660–666.

Tziaka, E., Tsiakiri, A., Vlotinou, P., Christidi, F., Tsiptsios, D., Aggelousis, N., Vadikolias, K., and Serdari, A. (2024) A holistic approach to expressing the burden of caregivers for stroke survivors: a systematic review. *Healthcare* 12(5), 565. https://doi.org/10.3390/healthcare12050565

Zhang, W., Gao, Y.J., Ye, M.M., and Zhou, L.S. (2024) Post-stroke family resilience is correlated with family functioning among stroke survivors: the mediating role of patient's coping and self-efficacy. *Nursing Open*, 11(7), e2230.

11

FACING MORTALITY AND LOSS

Catherine Hamilton and Hannah Mosley

Learning objectives

- To understand the potential impact of a stroke on an individual's perception of life and death.
- To consider the impact of a stroke on the person's feelings relating to their past, present and future.
- To explore the role of Advance Care Planning (ACP) and the legal context for end-of-life planning following a stroke.
- To gain an understanding of practical enhancements that might be used when caring for someone at the end of their life.
- To consider the potential impact of the death on family/loved ones and/or healthcare professionals (HCPs).

Facing the past

Stroke is a leading cause of disability (NICE, 2022). Stroke survivors may encounter abrupt and seismic changes to their physical abilities and cognitive functioning after a stroke. This can lead to feelings of grief and loss for their former self and past life, while trying to adjust to a new way of life and overcome the physical, cognitive and emotional obstacles that a stroke can cause.

Following a stroke, some people report a change in how they view themselves as a person. Not being able to complete or participate in daily activities in the same way as before is the main driving force for this change of identity. This can be from an individual perspective, or how they see themselves contributing to family and home life, their vocation or workplace and socialising (Kuluski

DOI: 10.4324/9781003426196-12

et al., 2014). This can then lead to feelings of disenfranchised grief and loss of former life (Hughes and Cummings, 2020). While there has been progress in survival and recovery following stroke, much of the care and interventions focus on physical deficits. People may feel that their feelings of loss for their former self, loss of relationships and loss of body autonomy are not recognised as being as important as their physical losses and changes (Hughes and Cummings, 2020).

A nurse and stroke survivor, explains, 'I do not think that a person who is not a stroke survivor has any idea of the magnitude of the loss' (Lanza, 2006):

...but that year was a terrible grief, that I didn't realise that I was grieving. I found the grief theory after a stroke and I just thought, that's it. That's how I feel. Everything has changed. I couldn't drive. I couldn't work.

(Kelly, 55, ischaemic stroke, 8 years post stroke)

For me, the grief never goes away. The disappointment never goes away and things trigger it.

(Jo, 47, embolic stroke as a result of endocarditis, 20 years post stroke)

Think about your personal perspective on life and death and reflect upon what factors or experiences influence your beliefs about life and death? Also consider, what roles or responsibilities are important in your life currently, and how would you feel if you could no longer fulfil these?

Facing the present

Shock, shocked and shocking. The most frequently reported emotion from people who have experienced a stroke is that of shock. Individuals are shocked by the event itself, as well as the treatments and subsequent loss of independence (Turgeman Goldschmidt, 2022). This feeling of shock not only affects the person with stroke, but it has been frequently documented and explored in the literature in relation to families and caregivers of stroke survivors. Shock has also been reported by family members and loved ones following the death of someone who had a stroke, as described by Rademeyer et al. (2020, p.12) there is 'shock in life and death'.

There is a sudden change to daily life, work and routines. People may have to change, adjust or give up employment entirely.

> I am in China and I am a project manager in turbine power stations and I have 2000 people reporting to me and it's fantastic... then I have a stroke. I have jumped out of bed and I have collapsed. And three weeks later I am in the hospital and it's... I have a coma...when you have your stroke and you get sick and your work life changes, there's a massive financial change.
>
> *(Jeremy, 69, haemorrhagic stroke, 13 years post stroke)*

Stroke is generally seen as a condition that affects the older adult, but evidence shows that stroke in people under 50 is increasing (Yahya *et al.*, 2020) with approximately 25% of strokes occurring in those under 65 (ISWP, 2023). The perception that it usually affects older adults can impact how younger people with stroke recognise and respond to the event – minimising, or rationalising symptoms based on other age-specific perceptions of health and illness (such as migraines or blood pressure related) which can lead to a delay in seeking medical treatment (Šaňáková *et al.*, 2024). This can lead to confusion and denial, from both the stroke survivor and their family/caregiver (Hughes and Cummings, 2020).

Confusion and denial of a stroke can continue even after a confirmed diagnosis, due to the way individuals viewed themselves prior to the stroke; that they were *too healthy* to have a stroke, or that they do not need to engage with all treatments and risk reduction measures because they see themselves as fit and healthy (Hughes and Cummings, 2020). In some cases, this perception can be replicated by HCPs who also dismiss signs and symptoms of a stroke, which can again delay diagnosis and timely, appropriate treatment (Kuluski *et al.*, 2014). Feelings of confusion have been reported by families due to mixed messages from HCPs regarding diagnosis and prognosis (Rademeyer *et al.*, 2020).

> After putting the phone down, I said to my husband 'her voice sounds like she has had a stroke, but they have sent her home from the hospital and said she is fine, so she can't have had a stroke, but it sounds like a stroke.'
>
> *(Catherine, relative of stroke patient)*

The person mentioned here was aged 26 at the time of her stroke. She was sent home by the Emergency Department (ED) staff. Twenty-four hours later, she returned and then was finally admitted. A few days later, she had a further, more serious stroke in hospital and remained an inpatient for several months.

This lack of responsieness is further described by Jacqueline who was heavily pregnant when she had a stroke two days before giving birth.

My first thought wasn't me; my first thought was my son. So, I phoned the maternity ward. The lady at the maternity ward said to me 'Oh, you can come in if you want'. And I said 'I've got pins and needles', and she said, 'well… maybe you have just slept on it funny'. And then she said, 'but you can come in if you want. But there is a really long wait. It's up to you. Why don't you give it an hour and then call me back?' So I put the phone down.

Phone her back an hour later. Said 'nothing's changed'.

At this point, my speech is really slurred. Even when I was talking to her on the phone, it was really difficult to understand what I was saying. And then I said 'I'm really worried about my baby. I'm coming in a taxi' so we jumped in a taxi, got to the hospital, went to the waiting room, sitting in the waiting room. Must have been about an hour at this point. But no one came to me. We went to the reception. My partner told them that, 'we think that she's had a stroke. Something's wrong with my Mrs. She can't feel the baby'. And that was that, sat down in the waiting room, was there for about an hour.

After that hour, my vision was really, really blurred and I couldn't see. And I started to lose consciousness again, and I was leaning up against the wall. And then I remember my partner jumping up and shouting, "So is anybody going to come and help? I think my Mrs had a stroke."

Somebody came out then when he shouted 'stroke' really loudly. All of a sudden some nurses came running through the doors into the waiting room. Nobody bought a wheelchair. So, my partner, grabbed hold of me and because I was really heavily pregnant, kind of managed to get me to a room where a triage nurse saw me. Within about two minutes of the triage nurse seeing me, she ran off. She ran away to get a doctor.

In the end, I wasn't responding very well to his questions. I was quite confused and…I didn't have the energy to get the words out of my mouth, and I was…I was trying to tell him what I need. So, my partner got really angry. And then he said to said to him, 'Can you stop? You know you're making her feel stressed out. You can see that you can't lift her arm. You can see that she can't lift the leg up'. And then he [the Doctor] said: 'I don't think you've had a stroke, but just to double check we're going to do CT scan'. I had had a stroke.

(Jacqueline, 42, ischaemic stroke whilst pregnant, 12 years post stroke)

These examples demonstrate how signs of a stroke can be dismissed or minimised by HCPs due to someone's age, or other healthcare needs.

Having a stroke is a highly significant experience, individuals report feeling frightened for their lives. While the clinical management of stroke is imperative, it is also important to consider the emotional impact of a stroke. This means assessing how someone is feeling and taking steps to acknowledge, explore and validate their emotions.

Reflect on the experience of Jacqueline and consider how having her signs and symptoms of a stroke dismissed by HCPs made her feel? What factors do you think influenced the lack of urgency from HCPs in this scenario and consider what steps You would take if you were in this situation as an HCP?

Facing the future

> There's many a time I've sat there and thought – I'm not going to kill myself, but I wouldn't be sad if I died.
>
> *(Jo, 47, embolic stroke as a result of endocarditis, 20 years post stroke)*

For individuals who have survived the acute phase of a stroke, the physical and cognitive sequalae that remain can severely impact their day-to-day life. They may experience feelings of prolonged suffering and may see death as a release from that – death would be easier. The risk of suicide and suicide attempt among stroke survivors is more than twice as high as that of people who have not experienced a stroke (Eriksson *et al.*, 2015). There are a variety of risk factors that can contribute to suicide attempts or ideation among stroke survivors which includes poor social support, low income or unemployment, living alone due to divorce or bereavement, having little interaction with others, and having a stroke at a younger age (Yokoi *et al.*, 2024). Post-stroke depression (PSD) is higher than following any other illness, but it may be difficult to assess and diagnose it due to the overlap between the symptoms of depression and those of neurological disease (Pompili *et al.*, 2015). As PSD is an important risk factor for suicide, the first step to avoid suicidal behaviour is to prevent PSD through screening measures and early treatment of depressive symptoms, which may significantly reduce suicide risk in stroke patients (Pompili *et al.*, 2015).

> I didn't realise I was depressed…I used to be frustrated because I couldn't say the word and I couldn't drive and I wasn't great for walking anyway. I didn't want to go anywhere in case anyone spoke to me. And I was isolated. I had lovely family, but friends had left… And I realised I had a little breakdown. I spoke to a doctor and I had a mental health doctor talk to me properly, not only me with the family. You know, which gave us some kind of understanding why I am like that, because the behaviour it wasn't me personally.
>
> *(Kelly, 55, ischaemic stroke, 8 years post stroke)*

Although many individuals report feelings that could be described as negative in the immediate aftermath of a stroke (shock, fear, frustration, anger), there are many who report a change in feeling over time, and although there is still an acknowledgement of a 'loss' of their former self, there are also positive feelings reported about sense of achievement or determination and some have described feeling 'like a hero' for overcoming the substantial challenges they face (Turgeman Goldschmidt, 2022). These changing emotions will ebb and flow throughout someone's life and may be influenced by a plethora of factors such as individual experiences, previous life experience, coping mechanisms and severity of stroke. The unknown and unpredictability of recovery can impact on how someone feels about their future and feelings of wanting to die may be present, even once the acute phase has passed and people know that they have survived:

I know that I'm going to get through this period now, but I still have moments, I still have days in the last couple of months where I've laid there or sat in the chair, and I've thought 'I just want it to be over'. So, for me, it's like encapsulating moments in time, rather than periods of time.

(Jo, 47, embolic stroke as a result of endocarditis, 20 years post stroke)

Young people with stroke are more likely to survive and, therefore, may live many years with physical and/or cognitive impairments (Kuluski *et al.*, 2014). The impact and experience of having a stroke, in addition to the long-standing effects caused by it, are linked to a higher prevalence of health anxiety – approximately 1/3 compared to 3.4% of general population (Diamond *et al.*, 2023). It is imperative that HCPs seek to understand these changing emotions and feel empowered to be able to have sensitive or difficult conversations about death and dying with stroke survivors.

Stroke can be described as a significant life event, and there is an adjustment period while an individual and their loved ones adjust to life after a stroke. There is an unpredictability to everyday life, both for the person who has had a stroke and their family and loved ones. Some report having to adjust to living with a different person, and there is the worry of another stroke (Gosman-Hedström and Dahlin-Ivanoff, 2012).

It's a double edged sword – I am able to work, I have tried to rebuild life differently, accept the reality of losing the ability to work full time and now I am deteriorating. I know I will have to constantly adapt as I deteriorate and change physically. It is very hard to be grateful for what you can do and not think about what you have lost.

(Jacqueline, 42, ischaemic stroke whilst pregnant, 12 years post stroke)

Reflect on your current perception of death and dying and if you have any clear wishes that you would want your family/loved ones to implement. Who are your current support networks and how you could clearly communicate these wishes.

Now consider your own professional practice. Do you encourage and enable patients and their relatives to begin these conversations?

Facing the future – practical considerations

Advance Care Planning

Advance Care Planning (ACP) may provide the person who has experienced a stroke with a sense of control and a forum to influence future decisions made about them. Expressing what matters most may enhance the current and future quality of life for the person and provide assurance to family and friends that they can uphold the wishes of the person they love. In March 2022, a collaborative initiative responded to the Care Quality Commission (CQC, 2021) report, *Protect, Connect, Respect: decisions about living and dying well,* to develop a national and consistent approach to ACP (Department of Health and Social Care (DHSC), 2022).

The shared aims are outlined in Table 11.1. To promote an individualised and holistic approach in ACP, six universal principles for best practice emerged (DHSC, 2022). All discussions with the person must engender a sense of ownership of the process and must respect and embrace the need for inclusivity of diverse cultures, spiritualities and ethnic groups.

TABLE 11.1 Universal principles for Advance Care Planning

1.	The person is central to developing and agreeing their advance care plan including deciding who else should be involved in the process
2.	The person has personalised conversations about their future care focused on what matters to them and their needs
3.	The person agrees the outcomes of their advance care planning conversation through a shared decision-making process in partnership with relevant professionals
4.	The person has a shareable advance care plan which records what matters to them, and their preferences and decisions about future care and treatment
5.	The person has the opportunity, and is encouraged, to review and revise their advance care plan
6.	Anyone involved in advance care planning can speak up if they feel that these universal principles are not being followed

ACP is best established through a series of conversations and should move at the pace expressed by the person. Gently and sensitively establishing the person's wishes and boundaries, while they have the mental capacity to engage in meaningful conversations, requires great emotional intelligence on the professional's part to sensitively navigate the breadth of emotions and accurately represent the person's wishes. This process may be complicated by the effects of stroke, specifically with cognitive functioning and the ability to receive and process information or express communication. Connolly *et al.* (2021) provide four specific suggestions on how communication should be approached to be cohesive. Firstly, it is necessary that HCPs are present and available; this is not just vital for when decisions are being made, but families appreciate HCPs being available to talk to and this builds positive communication relations. Acknowledging someone's current and future physical health status is the second recommendation. This 'sets the stage' for future conversations and is linked to a decrease in uncertainty for family members. Thirdly, setting expectations through stating facts. Families and loved ones of someone who has had an acute stroke should be involved in the decision-making process but may have to make decisions in a relatively quick time period and so need clear and factual information that isn't 'sugar coated' (p. 542). Finally, a coordinated and consistent message from all HCPs regarding an agreed treatment plan is required to reduce uncertainty about palliative care or end-of-life decision-making (Connolly *et al.*, 2021).

ACP may involve a number of ways to record the person's wishes (Department of Health and Social Care, 2022):

- An advance statement – of care wishes, preferences and priorities. It may include nomination of a named spokesperson such as a friend or family member or professional advocate. An advance statement is not legally binding, but it is useful to inform and guide decision-making in the future if the person subsequently loses their capacity to make decisions about their care.
- An Advance Decision to Refuse Treatment (ADRT) – Generally these are legally binding and are useful to inform and guide decision-making in the future if the person subsequently loses their capacity to make decisions about their care.
- Nomination of a Lasting Power of Attorney (LPA) for health and welfare identifies a person(s) who is legally empowered to make decisions up to, or including, life-sustaining treatment on behalf of the person if they do not have mental capacity at the time, depending on the level of authority granted by the person.
- Context-specific treatment recommendations, such as emergency care and treatment plans, treatment escalation plans, cardiopulmonary resuscitation decisions, etc.

- Seek and access your workplace's guidance, policies and procedures, and resources about ACP for patients.
- What support is in place for patients/clients, families/loved ones, or HCPs when making decisions about ACP?

Resources for patients and families/friends (Department of Health and Social Care, 2022):

For information about advance decisions/living wills and advance statements:
   Compassion in Dying: https://compassionindying.org.uk/
Do not attempt cardiopulmonary decisions: Do not attempt cardiopulmonary resuscitation (DNACPR) decisions – **NHS**
Lasting Power of Attorney for health and welfare decisions: www.gov.uk/power-of-attorney
Online support tool for ACP conversation: https://advancecareplanning.org.uk/planning-ahead
Why plan ahead? www.nhs.uk/conditions/end-of-life-care/why-plan-ahead

Resources for professionals

British Medical Association, Resuscitation Council UK and Royal College of Nursing. Decisions relating to cardiopulmonary resuscitation, 2016: https://www.bma.org.uk/advice-and-support/ethics/end-of-life/decisions-relating-to-cpr-cardiopulmonary-resuscitation

General Medical Council:

- Decision-making and Consent guidance 2020: https://www.gmc-uk.org/professional-standards/the-professional-standards/decision-making-and-consent

Decision-making and consent – professional standards – GMC
- Mental capacity tool
- Mental capacity – ethical topic – GMC Treatment and care towards the end of life: good practice in decision-making 2010. www.gmc-uk.org/guidance/ethical_guidance/6858.asp

Health Education England:

- E-learning programme for End-of-Life Care: www.elfh.org.uk/programmes/end-of-life-care/
- E-learning programme for Mental Capacity Act: www.elfh.org.uk/programmes/mental-capacity-act/

Mental Capacity Act 2005. www.legislation.gov.uk/ukpga/2005/9/contents
Mental Capacity Act Code of Practice: www.gov.uk/government/publications/
mental-capacity-act-code-of-practice#

National Guardian's Office:

- Implementing effective speaking up arrangements: www.nationalguardian.
  org.uk
- Confidential advice on speaking up process: https://speakup.direct/

National Institute for Health and Care Excellence (NICE).

- End-of-life care for adults: service delivery –www.nice.org.uk/guidance/ng142
- End-of-life care for infants, children and young people with life limiting
  conditions: planning and management –www.nice.org.uk/guidance/ng61
- Shared decision-making: www.nice.org.uk/guidance/ng197

**Resuscitation Council UK. Recommended Summary Plan for Emergency
Care and Treatment (ReSPECT) process:** www.resus.org.uk/respect
End of Life Care Think Tank (2025):: www.whatmattersconversations.org/

**Royal College of General Practitioners and Marie Curie Daffodil Standards
for General Practice:** Core standards for advanced serious illness and end-of-life
care: www.rcgp.org.uk/daffodilstandards

**Royal College of Physicians. Talking about dying. How to begin honest
conversations about what lies ahead, 2021. Talking about dying 2021:** How to
begin honest conversations about what lies ahead | RCP London

Royal College of Physicians, National Council for Palliative Care, British Society
of Rehabilitation Medicine, British Geriatrics Society, Alzheimer's Society, Royal
College of Nursing, Royal College of Psychiatrists, Help the Aged, Royal College
of General Practitioners. Advance care planning. Concise Guidance to Good
Practice series, No 12. London: RCP, 2009. ACP final

**Social Care Institute for Excellence & National Institute for Health and Care
Excellence. Advance care planning:** A quick guide for registered managers of
care homes and home care services, 2019. Advance care planning | Quick guides to
social care topics | Social care | NICE Communities | About | NICE

**UK Government Office of the Public Guardian: Information on Lasting
Powers of Attorney (2021) Make, register or end a lasting power of
attorney:** Overview – GOV.UK

Helping to support someone at the end of life – feelings and emotions

At the end of life, families and carers speak of the importance of fulfilling all their loved one's physical needs. This includes relieving pain, nausea, agitation and distress, breathlessness and respiratory symptoms (Young *et al.*, 2009). The essential role of maintaining physical comfort is frequently referred to in guidance and policy, with recommendations on how to meet these needs through prescribed medication and treatment available from the NICE guidelines – Care of dying adults in the last days of life (2015).

However, the importance of fulfilling the holistic needs of all involved cannot be underestimated. Considering aspects of care that fulfil any spiritual and sensory needs can provide a rounded, person-centred and individualised approach and engage the family/loved ones in assuring a good end of life and death.

A wide-ranging list of elements may need to be considered. These might include utilising the taking of comfort from food and taste; scent and evocative smells; music, sounds, images, videos and pictures. The benefits of touch and human contact; pets and animals, should all be considered when engaged in fulfilling the needs and wishes of the dying person.

Consider how you could gain knowledge and facilitate the following potential wishes and needs:

- Spiritual
- Food and taste
- Music and sounds
- Imagery
- Physical touch
- Pets and animals

Spiritual

It is important to acknowledge small differences in terminologies associated with spirituality which may sometimes be used interchangeably by patients, relatives or staff. The Department of Health (2011) describes them as follows – religion is participation in particular beliefs, rituals or activities of an organised religious group, spirituality is a subjective experience of an individual in the way they understand their life in context of core experiences, and wellbeing is the subjective emotional experience that relates to the way in which a person perceives themselves to be and to feel within any given situation. Spirituality is often used as a broad term, but it can incorporate any/all of the above elements. Higher spirituality is linked to better outcomes for stroke survivors (Li *et al.*, 2024).

Marie Curie (2025) suggests that spirituality may lead the person to seek or express the need:

- for meaning, purpose and value in life
- for love

- to feel a sense of belonging
- to feel hope, peace and gratitude.

Spiritual needs may also change with the person's prognosis. There may be a need to resolve a relationship conflict or link with estranged loves. They may wish to re-engage with formalised worship or religion or to reprioritise plans and wishes, perhaps form a 'bucket list' (Marie Curie, 2025).

It is important to take steps to assess someone's spiritual needs and to look for signs of spiritual distress. Tools such as the Queen's University HOPE (H – Sources of Hope: O – Organised religion; P – Personal spirituality and practices, and E – Effects on medical care and end-of-life decisions) and FICA (Faith or beliefs; Importance and influence; Community; Address) can aid in your assessment (Marie Curie, 2025). All HCPs can be involved in helping patients meet their spiritual needs. This can include talking with patients about their spirituality, practically helping them to engage with any religious activities, or referring to other professionals such as chaplain or spiritual coordinator.

Food and taste

As the end of life becomes near, food and nutrition can often take on a different role. Taste for pleasure and the emotive role of memories associated with different foods, drinks and textures become important. The focus is not on achieving nutrition but on engendering pleasure and wellbeing (Perkins, 2024).

Supporting someone to drink to promote hydration should be done, if the person is able to do so. But the ability to swallow may be altered in someone following a stroke, and so it is important to consider the role and necessity of artificial hydration and whether this is appropriate depending on the patient's status.

Focussing on promoting pleasure and comfort to enhance quality of life may be achieved through providing a taste through mouthcare with a flavour to meet the person's desire, such as tea, coffee, soft drinks, whisky or wine.

This experience may also provide comforting memories for the family and a sense of providing a positive shared experience and opportunity to reminisce and reflect together.

Feeding with acknowledged risk

Sometimes even though a patient has limited or unsafe swallow, the decision is made to allow 'feeding with acknowledged risk'. This refers to the decision to allow the stroke survivor to continue eating and drinking (in most cases drinking) despite the risks of coughing, choking and aspiration (ISWP, 2023). Guidelines state that rigid adherence to recommendations related to nutrition and hydration should be suspended in this situation if appropriate. This is because it may be that restrictions on nutrition and hydration (keeping an individual nil by mouth) are burdensome in this scenario and can exacerbate suffering (ISWP, 2023). One of the most commonly cited scenarios might be a person receiving end-of-life care, requesting a cup of tea.

The decision to allow a person to eat and drink with acknowledged risk should be individualised and made in collaboration with the multidisciplinary team, the stroke survivor and their family where possible. It may include a further swallowing assessment and strategies to minimise risk as much as is possible prior to allowing the individual to eat or drink (ISWP, 2023) as discussed in chapter 5. At the decision-making stage, a plan should be put in place about what actions should be implemented in the event of aspiration or a chest infection. Generally, these issues would not be considered problematical in this context, and a stroke survivor would not usually have their nil by mouth status resumed, but there should be clear guidance about the plan for interventions to manage complications if they occur, before they occur. This might include considering if chest physiotherapy or antibiotics might be initiated. The underlying concept is that there should not be a crisis situation if aspiration occurs. Everyone should have clearly documented instructions, which generally should not escalate treatment. The Royal College of Speech and Language Therapists (2021) has produced multidisciplinary guidance in their 'Eating and drinking with acknowledged risks: Multidisciplinary team guidance for the shared decision-making process (adults)' document, which sets out a best practice approach to feeding with acknowledged risk.

Scent and evocative smells

The link between scent and evocative smells is thought to transport the person to a memory and experience. The links between the psychological wellbeing of the person and positive memory triggered by scent have been recorded by Herz (2016) who emotes the power of scent in memory. Kreye *et al.* (2022) suggest there may also be physiological benefits to the use of aromatherapy; however, this is yet to be fully established (Gonçalves *et al.*, 2024).

The family can take a key role here in creating a positive and evocative environment using different and favourite scents, perfumes and foods. However, caution needs to be used, as one person's positive link can be another's negative trigger.

Music and sounds

Music and sound have the potential to produce a psychological and physical reaction – from ocean and rainforest sounds to choral singing and instrumentals, audio books and every genre of sound and music in between. There may be times for energising the environment or quiet contemplation and music and sound has the power to transport the soul and provide comfort on all levels.

Music has the potential to:

• reduce distress and anxiety
• promote emotional expression

- evoke memory and transport the mind to better times
- engender positive connections
- promote comfort and dignity
- link together friends and family.

Those moving towards the end of life should be encouraged to share their preferences and perhaps even develop a playlist for others to facilitate.

In collaboration with Marie Curie, Radio DJ and TV presenter Edith Bowman explores the impact of music as a source of comfort during life's final moments in conversation with three expert guests. Search music platforms such as Spotify and YouTube for Music for the End, a podcast hosted by Edith Bowman with Marie Curie.

Images, videos and pictures

There is little published literature about the use of images, videos and pictures at the end-of-life phase. However, from experience the authors feel there can be benefits to the person and those accompanying them of sharing in the reminders of enjoyable and significant times through the use of images and videos.

Austen *et al.* (2018) considered the role of charting someone's life pictorially and found there were many benefits to the person, family and professionals. It can change perspectives of HCPs, which is also felt by patients, that they are viewed as a unique individual. Using familiar pictures can also help staff, patients and loved ones feel more comfortable in an environment that feels more personal and homely.

Touch and human contact

Respecting the person's wishes regarding touch and human contact is key when considering this enhancement at the person's end of life. There may be significant benefits to the person's sense of wellbeing and symptoms (Freeman *et al.*, 2025). However, it is important to consider who, how, where and when this is to be used (Candy *et al.*, 2020). The person may be able to express their wishes; however, if communication of these is not attainable, proceed with caution and encourage others around the person to take the same approach.

Pets and animals

A companion animal may provide the person receiving palliative, end-of-life care significant comfort and engender positive emotion. Many organisations and services promote the benefits of therapy animals; however, evidence as to the benefit is largely anecdotal (MacDonald and Barrett, 2016; Quintal and Reis-Pina, 2021).

If the person has a meaningful relationship with a particular animal, then continuing to promote this contact may fulfil the wish for touch and comfort. During the end-of-life phase many palliative care services will facilitate the person's access to a companion animal and where possible, this should be encouraged.

Bereavement support

> The reality is that you will grieve forever. You will not "get over" the loss of a loved one; you will learn to live with it. You will heal and you will rebuild yourself around the loss you have suffered. You will be whole again, but you will never be the same. Nor should you be the same, nor should you want to.
>
> *(Kübler-Ross, 2014)*

When someone dies, it can affect their family and loved ones, whether the death was unexpected, as in the case of an acute stroke, or expected and someone had been receiving palliative care or hospice care. Therefore, the family and friends of someone who has died as a result of a stroke may need support.

Grief can evoke strong emotions, and not everyone will feel the same way or experience the same emotions. Macmillan (2025) lists some common emotions people may experience:

- Shock and numbness – expecting the person who has died to 'walk through the door' at any moment.
- Anger – that the loss is unfair.
- Guilt – people may feel like they could have, or should have, done more to prevent the death.
- Relief – there may be relief that the person is no longer suffering.
- Loneliness – people can feel lonely even when surrounded by family and friends.
- Longing – having a strong desire to see, speak to, or hold the person who has died.
- Fear – of the future, how to cope and support others/their family.
- Sadness – sadness can be overwhelming and is often described as a physical pain in the chest.

Useful resources to support someone who is grieving

Hospice UK (2025a): www.hospiceuk.org/information-and-support/i-need-support-bereavement/coping-grief

Good Grief: https://goodgrief1.wpengine.com/resources/

Sue Ryder: www.sueryder.org/grief-support/online-bereavement-support/

To support someone who is grieving there are some practical things to consider, along with providing emotional support. There are many useful charities that provide a wealth of resources, including practical advice such as registering a death, seeing the person after death, getting a death certificate and planning funerals:

Good Life, Good Death, Good Grief (2025)– www.goodlifedeathgrief.org.uk/support-after/

Hospice UK (2025b) – www.hospiceuk.org/information-and-support/i-need-support-bereavement/what-do-when-someone-dies

Macmillan – www.macmillan.org.uk/cancer-information-and-support/supporting-someone/coping-with-bereavement/how-to-plan-a-funeral-for-someone

Reflect on your place of work and consider what support mechanisms are in place to support relatives following the death of a patient? Are there any specific stroke-related support mechanisms or advice that you could offer relatives following the death of a loved one from a stroke?

Impact of stroke on healthcare professionals

HCPs involved in caring for someone who has had a stroke can experience feelings of grief and loss. It can create demanding situations for nurses, which can lead to feelings of secondary traumatic stress (STS), which is mainly felt when caring for younger people who die as a result of stroke (Wilkinson *et al.*, 2022). It can also be challenging to balance the care needs for the individual, whilst also trying to support relatives through a very difficult and stressful situation which can make HCPs feel that they are not adequately fulfilling their job roles (Wilkinson *et al.*, 2022). This may lead to burnout and reduction in job satisfaction (NHS England, 2023). Therefore, it is important to consider the working environment, personnel and team dynamics and make use of restorative supervision if available. While it is imperative the care needs of patients and their families are met, the death of patient should also be recognised for the potential impact it can have on HCPs.

Reflect upon your current place of work and consider what support mechanisms are in place for staff following the death of a patient? Do you know how to access mental health and wellbeing support from your employer? Is there anything that your current clinical area/workplace/unit could implement following the death of a patient that might improve staff wellbeing?

Conclusion

Stroke can be linked to the past, present and future in relation to grief and loss for many different people. This can include the individual who has a stroke, their loved ones and family, and HCPs providing care for someone who is dying. While these experiences will be different, and vary on an individual basis, each is a valid experience that can be explored and affirmed. A stroke causes many people to have to adjust to loss and grief and to face mortality, whether that be their own, a loved one, or a patient. While survival rates following a stroke have improved, it remains a leading cause of mortality. A stroke can cause disenfranchised grief, and individuals may grieve for their former selves or previous life. The dismissal of signs and symptoms of a stroke (especially in younger people) by themselves or HCPs can delay treatment and exacerbate feelings of fear and death due to the unknown. Communication with people who have had a stroke regarding their wishes and preferences about palliative care and end-of-life care should be considered through ACP. Practical, emotional, psychological and spiritual support towards the end of life for someone who has had a stroke should be explored and steps taken to implement any specific desires or wishes wherever possible. HCPs should be mindful of the impact of the death of someone from a stroke can have on the individual's family or rather than/ loved ones and provide onward support and guidance for bereavement support. The death of someone from a stroke, particularly in the acute phase, can also impact HCPs and create challenging situations requiring high emotional intelligence and clinical competence to adequately care for those individuals while balancing communication and expectations of the family or loved ones.

References

Austen, E., Wheatland, S., Timms, S., and Partridge, M. (2018) *All about me: the patient as a person in palliative care (poster presentation)*. Available at: https://spcare.bmj.com/content/bmjspcare/8/Suppl_2/A55.3.full.pdf

Candy, B., Armstrong, M., Flemming, K., Kupeli, N., Stone, P., Vickerstaff, V., and Wilkinson, S. (2020) The effectiveness of aromatherapy, massage and reflexology in people with palliative care needs: a systematic review. *Palliative Medicine*, 34(2), 179–194.

Care Quality Commission (CQC) (2021). *Protect, connect, respect – decisions about living and dying well during covid-19*. Available at: www.cqc.org.uk/publications/themed-work/protect-respect-connect-decisions-about-living-dying-well-during-covid-19

Connolly, T., Coates, H., DeSanto, K., and Jones, J. (2021) The experience of uncertainty for patients, families and healthcare providers in post-stroke palliative and end-of-life care: a qualitative meta-synthesis. *Age and Ageing*, 50(2), 534–545. https://doi.org/10.1093/ageing/afaa229

Diamond, P. R., Dysch, L., and Daniels, J. (2023) Health anxiety in stroke survivors: a cross-sectional study on the prevalence of health anxiety in stroke survivors and its impact on quality of life. *Disability and Rehabilitation*, 45(1), 27–33. https://doi.org/10.1080/09638288.2021.2022778

Department of Health and Social Care (DHSC), (2011). Spiritual care at the end of life: a systematic review of the literature. Available at www.gov.uk/government/publications/spiritual-care-at-the-end-of-life-a-systematic-review-of-the-literature

Department of Health and Social Care (DHSC) (2022). *Universal Principles for Advance Care Planning (ACP) – co-produced by 28 national organisations*. Available at: www.england.nhs.uk/publication/universal-principles-for-advance-care-planning/

Eriksson, M., Glader, E.-L., Norrving, B., and Asplund, K. (2015) Post-stroke suicide attempts and completed suicides: a socioeconomic and nationwide perspective. *International Journal of Stroke*, 10, 33.

Freeman, J., Klingele, A., and Wolf, U. (2025) Effectiveness of music therapy, aromatherapy, and massage therapy on patients in palliative care with end-of-life needs: a systematic review. *Journal of Pain and Symptom Management*, 69(1), 102–113.

Gonçalves, S., Marques, P., and Matos, R. S. (2024) Exploring aromatherapy as a complementary approach in palliative care: a systematic review. *Journal of Palliative Medicine*, 27(9), 1247–1266. https://doi.org/10.1089/jpm.2024.0019

Good Life, Good Death, Good Grief (2025). *After a death*. Available at: www.goodlifedea thgrief.org.uk/support-after/

Gosman-Hedström, G., and Dahlin-Ivanoff. (2012). Mastering an unpredictable everyday life after stroke'– older women's experiences of caring and living with their partners. Scandinavian Journal of Caring Sciences, 26, 587–597. https://doi.org/10.1111/j.1471-6712.2012.00975.x

Herz R. S. (2016). The role of odor-evoked memory in psychological and physiological health. Brain Sciences, 6(3), 22. https://doi.org/10.3390/brainsci6030022

Hospice UK (2025a) *How to cope with grief. How to cope with grief.* Hospice UK.

Hospice UK (2025b) *What to do when someone dies. What to do when someone dies.* Hospice UK.

Hughes, A. K., and Cummings, C. E. (2020). Grief and loss associated with stroke recovery: a qualitative study of stroke survivors and their spousal caregivers. Journal of Patient Experience, 7(6), 1219–1226. https://doi.org/10.1177/2374373520967796

Intercollegiate Stroke Working Party (2023) *National Clinical Guideline for Stroke for the UK and Ireland*. London. Available at: www.strokeguideline.org.

Kreye, G., Wasl, M., Dietz, A., Klaffel, D., Groselji-Strele, A., Eberhard, K., and Glechner, A. (2022) Aromatherapy in palliative care: a single-institute retrospective analysis evaluating the effect of lemon oil pads against nausea and vomiting in advanced cancer patients. *Cancers*, 14, 2131. https://doi.org/10.3390/cancers14092131

Kübler-Ross, E. and Kessler, D. (2014) *On grief and grieving: finding the meaning of grief through the five stages of loss.* London: Simon & Schuster, Limited.

Kuluski, K., Dow, C., Locock, L., Lyons, R. F., and Lasserson, D. (2014) Life interrupted and life regained? Coping with stroke at a young age. *International Journal of Qualitative Studies on Health and Well-being*, 9(1). https://doi.org/10.3402/qhw.v9.22252

Lanza, M. (2006) Psychological impact of stroke: a recovering nurse's story. *Issues in Mental Health Nursing*, 27(7), 765–774. https://doi.org/10.1080/01612840600781154

Li, Z.-Y., Cao, X., Li, T.-J., Huang, T.-J., Liu, Y.-X., and Qin, L.-H. (2024) Spiritual needs and influencing factors among people with stroke in China: a cross-sectional study. *BMC Nursing*, 23, 507. https://doi.org/10.1186/s12912-024-02182-7

MacDonald, J. M., and Barrett, D. (2016) Companion animals and well-being in palliative care nursing: a literature review. *Journal of Clinical Nursing*, 25(3–4), 300–310. https://doi.org/10.1111/jocn.13022

Macmillan Cancer Support (2025). Support with grief. Available at: Grief support after someone dies | Macmillan Cancer Support

Marie Curie (2025) *Proving spiritual care*. Available at: www.mariecurie.org.uk/profession als/palliative-care-knowledge-zone/spiritual-care

National Institute for Health and Care Excellence (NICE) (2022) *Stroke and transient ischaemic attack in over 16s: diagnosis and initial management*. Available at: www.nice.org.uk/guidance/ng128

NHS England (2023) *Professional nurse advocate A-EQUIP model: a model of clinical supervision for nurses Version 2*. Available at: www.england.nhs.uk/publication/profe ssional-nurse-advocate-a-equip-model-a-model-of-clinical-supervision-for-nurses/

Perkins (2024) Nutrition and hydration: best practice towards the end of life. *Nursing Times [online]*, 120, 10.

Pompili, M., Venturini, P., Lamis, D. A., Giordano, G., Serafini, G., Belvederi Murri, M., Amore, M., and Girardi, P. (2015) Suicide in stroke survivors: epidemiology and prevention. *Drugs and Aging*, 32(1), 21–29. https://doi.org/10.1007/s40266-014-0233-x

Quintal, V., and Reis-Pina, P. (2021) Animal-assisted therapy in palliative care. *Acta Médica Portuguesa*, 34(10), 690–692. https://doi.org/10.20344/amp.13164

Rademeyer, M., Roy, D., and Gasquoine, S. (2020) A stroke of grief and devotion: a hermeneutic enquiry of a family's lived experience two years post-stroke. *Nursing Praxis in New Zealand Inc.*, 36(1), 8–19.

Royal College of Speech and Language Therapists (2021). Eating and drinking with acknowledged risks: multidisciplinary team guidance for the shared decision-making process (adults). Available at www.rcslt.org/members/clinical-guidance/eating-and-drinking-with-acknowledged-risks-risk-feeding/

Šaňáková, Š., Gurková, E., Štureková, L., Bartoníčková, D., Machálková, L., & Mazalová, L. (2024). How to return? Experiences of patients in working age after first Ischaemic stroke: an interpretative phenomenological analysis of patient's perspective at 12 – 24 months post-stroke. International Journal of Qualitative Studies on Health and Well-Being, 19(1). https://doi.org/10.1080/17482631.2024.2398249

Turgeman Goldschmidt, O. (2022) Narratives of stroke survivors: between trauma and redemption. *Journal of Loss and Trauma*, 27(8), 703–716. https://doi.org/10.1080/15325024.2022.2037889

Wilkinson, M., Cox, N., Witham, G., and Haigh, C. (2022) Hyperacute stroke and the specialist nursing impact: exploring the cause and context of feelings of secondary traumatic stress – a qualitative inquiry. *Journal of Research in Nursing*, 27(4), 343–354. https://doi.org/10.1177/17449871211018739

Yahya, T., Jilani, M. H., Khan, S. U., Mszar, R., Hassan, S. Z., Blaha, M. J., Blankstein, R., Virani, S. S., Johansen, M. C., Vahidy, F., Cainzos-Achirica, M., & Nasir, K. (2020). Stroke in young adults: current trends, opportunities for prevention and pathways forward. American Journal of Preventive Cardiology, 3, 100085. https://doi.org/10.1016/j.ajpc.2020.100085

Yokoi, T., Oguma, E., Inagaki, K., and Fukuda, T. (2024) Suicide in stroke survivors and social work. Health & Social Work, 49(4), 279–281. https://doi.org/10.1093/hsw/hlae029

Young, A. J., Rogers, A., Dent, L., and Addington-Hall, J. M. (2009) Experiences of hospital care reported by bereaved relatives of patients after a stroke: a retrospective survey using the VOICES questionnaire. *Journal of Advanced Nursing*, 65(10), 2161–2174.

INDEX

For Product Safety Concerns and Information please contact our EU
representative GPSR@taylorandfrancis.com
Taylor & Francis Verlag GmbH, Kaufingerstraße 24, 80331 München, Germany

www.ingramcontent.com/pod-product-compliance
Lightning Source LLC
Chambersburg PA
CBHW060239220326
41598CB00027B/3980